Transcutaneous Electrical Nerve Stimulation (TENS)

Research to support clinical practice

Mark I. Johnson

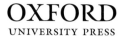

OXFORD
UNIVERSITY PRESS

OXFORD
UNIVERSITY PRESS

Great Clarendon Street, Oxford, OX2 6DP,
United Kingdom

Oxford University Press is a department of the University of Oxford.
It furthers the University's objective of excellence in research, scholarship,
and education by publishing worldwide. Oxford is a registered trade mark of
Oxford University Press in the UK and in certain other countries

Published in the United States of America by Oxford University Press
198 Madison Avenue, New York, NY 10016, United States of America

British Library Cataloguing in Publication Data
Data available

Library of Congress Control Number: 2013947886

ISBN 978-0-19-967327-8

Printed in Great Britian by
Clays Ltd, St Ives plc

Dedication

The book is dedicated to Professor John W. Thompson and Professor C. Heather Ashton who gave me the opportunity to undertake a career studying the science of transcutaneous electrical nerve stimulation (TENS), and to my long-suffering family: Neera, Nayan, Piyusha, Krishan, Mam, Dad, Craig, Smig, and Mark.

Preface

Electrical stimulation of the skin to reduce pain is an age-old technique. Nowadays, portable current generators are used to administer mild electrical currents across the intact surface of the skin to stimulate nerves in a technique called transcutaneous electrical nerve stimulation (TENS). TENS is used by practitioners throughout the world and is readily available to the general public. Thousands of research studies on TENS have been published, yet there is still uncertainty about effectiveness and the best way to administer TENS in clinical practice.

I have been investigating the factors that influence the analgesic effects and clinical efficacy of TENS since 1987, originally under the supervision of Professor John W. Thompson and Professor C. Heather Ashton at the University of Newcastle upon Tyne, UK. During this time there have been remarkably few textbooks devoted to TENS. The most recent textbook of note was written over 15 years ago by Professor Deirdre Walsh (*TENS: Clinical Applications and Related Theory*, Edinburgh: Churchill Livingstone), before the first systematic reviews of randomized controlled clinical trials on TENS or national guidelines on the cost-effectiveness and safe practice had been published. The last decade has seen a proliferation of investigations into the mechanism of action and optimal technique for TENS. Clearly, there is a need for a textbook that evaluates recent research on efficacy and TENS techniques to use in clinical practice.

The primary goal of this textbook is to synthesize research findings to inform safe and appropriate technique for TENS. The secondary goal of the textbook is to offer solutions to challenges associated with conducting research on TENS. Constructing the textbook has been challenging, with early drafts containing over 2000 references and the word count three times over the desired limit. Prioritizing what remained in the final text has proved extremely difficult. Hopefully, the balance between research evidence and clinical technique will satisfy practitioners and researchers alike. The book is aimed at healthcare professionals who are experienced in TENS or considering using TENS for the first time. This includes general practitioners, pain specialists, physiotherapists, nurses, sports therapists, acupuncturists, osteopaths, chiropractors, students and, hopefully, the occasional patient. The textbook should also appeal to experienced investigators and undergraduate and post-graduate students undertaking research on TENS.

As a scientist I am inspired by people and events that change the way I think. Therefore, feel free to challenge, comment, or correct any information contained within the book. I willingly accept responsibility for all omissions, errors, inaccuracies, and misinterpretations.

Professor Mark I. Johnson, PhD

Acknowledgements

I am grateful to the dedicated scholars who have contributed to the knowledge and wisdom on TENS, and to staff and student colleagues at Leeds Metropolitan University who have provided the infrastructure and personnel to conduct our research or have taken part in our research as participants. Special thanks go to Dr Ghazala Tabasam and Dr Osama Tashani, and to our PhD students, Dr Dimitrios Stasinopoulos, Dr Chih-Chung Chen, Dr Richard Francis, Dr Anabela Silva, Dr Matthew Mulvey, Dr Alex Benham, Dr Lesley Brown, Dr Oras Alabas, Dr Carole Paley, Dr Raga Elzahaf and Ms Helen Radford.

Contents

Abbreviations

AAN	American Academy of Neurology	MeSH	Medical Subject Header
AC	alternating current	MHRA	Medicines and Healthcare products Regulatory Agency
ACID	anode current into device		
APS	action potential simulation	NICE	National Institute of Health and Clinical Excellence
ATP	Adenosine triphosphate		
bps	bursts per second	NMES	neuromuscular electrical stimulation
CABG	coronary artery bypass graft	NSAIDs	non-steroidal anti-inflammatory drugs
CGRP	calcitonin-gene-related peptide		
CI	confidence interval	PAG	periaqueductal grey
CID	cathode current departs	PENS	percutaneous electrical nerve stimulation
CONSORT	Consolidated Standards of Reporting Trials		
		PONV	post-operative nausea and vomiting
Cox	cyclo-oxygenase		
CRPS	complex regional pain syndrome	pps	pulses per second
DC	direct current	PubMed	US National Library of Medicine National Institutes of Health
DNIC	diffuse noxious inhibitory controls		
		RCT	randomized controlled clinical trial
DVT	deep-vein thrombosis		
ECG	electrocardiogram	STRICTA	Standards for Reporting Interventions in Clinical Trials of Acupuncture
ECT	electroconvulsive therapy		
ES	electrical stimulation		
fMRI	functional magnetic resonance imaging	TEAS	transcutaneous electrical acupoint stimulation
		TENS	transcutaneous electrical nerve stimulation
FDA	Food and Drug Administration		
GABA	gamma-amino-butyric acid	tNMES	transcutaneous neuromuscular electrical stimulation
HVPC	high-voltage pulsed current		
Hz	hertz	TSE	transcutaneous spinal electroanalgesia
IASP	International Association of the Study of Pain		
		VIP	vasoactive intestinal polypeptide
ICD	implantable cardioverter defibrillator	VVI	a pacemaker mode that paces the right ventricle, senses the right ventricle and will be inhibited from firing if an intrinsic beat is sensed
IMMPACT	Initiative on Methods, Measurement, and Pain Assessment in Clinical Trials		
mA	milliamperes	WDR	wide dynamic range

Chapter 1

Introduction

Introduction

It is intuitive to stroke, massage, or rub painful parts of the body because this tends to relieve the pain. Local stimulation somehow affects the perception of pain. If a pain is severe it may be necessary to use stimulation that produces its own pain, before the original pain is reduced to any useful degree. Throughout history, many techniques have been used as a means of stimulating the skin for the relief of painful conditions, termed stimulation-induced analgesia. These include heat packs, ice, laser, massage, manipulation and mobilization, vibration, ultrasound and acupuncture.

Electrical currents are known to excite tissues of the body including nervous system tissue and therefore electricity can be used to produce local stimulation of the body for therapeutic purposes (electrotherapy) and the relief of pain (electroanalgesia). Stimulating nerves close to the surface of the body is relatively easy to achieve by delivering electrical currents across the intact surface of the skin (i.e. transcutaneous). The electrical currents can be generated by a battery-powered, portable, stimulating device and can be administered through the skin using conducting pads called electrodes (Figure 1.1). This technique is called transcutaneous electrical nerve stimulation (TENS) and it has become one of the most commonly used non-pharmacological techniques to relieve pain. The purpose of this chapter is to overview the use of TENS in health care by covering:

- ◆ TENS, what it is and why it is used
- ◆ A brief history of TENS
- ◆ Goal of the textbook
- ◆ TENS terminology

TENS, what it is, and why it is used

TENS is the delivery of electrical currents across the intact surface of the skin to stimulate nerves (Johnson 2008). TENS is used as a stand-alone treatment or as an adjunct to core treatment for symptomatic relief of any type of pain, including acute, chronic, malignant, musculoskeletal, nociceptive, or neuropathic. TENS has also been used to manage ailments not primarily associated with pain such as nausea, vomiting, ileus, constipation, incontinence, ischaemia, healing of wounds, nerve damage, and psychomotor disturbances.

TENS is popular with patients and practitioners because it is non-invasive, easy to administer, and has few side effects or drug interactions. Patients can administer TENS themselves at home and can titrate the dosage as required as there appears to be no

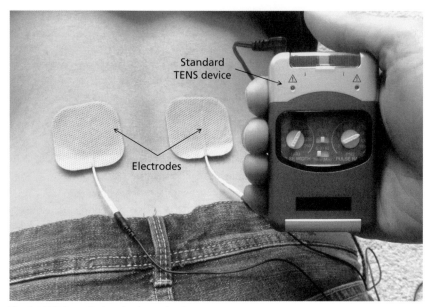

Fig. 1.1 TENS applied to the lower back.

potential for toxicity or overdose. The pain-relieving effects of TENS are immediate for most patients and some patients report prolonged effects after treatment. TENS treatment is relatively inexpensive when compared with long-term drug therapy, with a TENS device and accessories retailing between GB£15.00 and GB£100.00 with minimal running costs for batteries and electrodes.

TENS is used throughout the world. In most countries TENS devices can be purchased over the counter or via the internet without the need for a medical prescription. This makes TENS readily accessible to those who can afford it. However, it also means that individuals may not receive support from health-care professionals on whether TENS is appropriate for their condition and how to use TENS properly. As a consequence individuals may not achieve maximal benefit from TENS therapy. Individuals should be assessed by a health-care practitioner to make sure that TENS is an appropriate treatment. Individuals should also be given a supervised trial of TENS from a practitioner experienced in the principles and practice of TENS to ensure that they can administer safe and effective TENS technique. Clearly, the practitioner assessing the medical status of an individual should be a professionally qualified health-care specialist, although the person educating and training the individual about the principles of application of TENS does not necessarily need to be a health-care professional. For example, a health-care trainer or expert patients could undertake the role.

Despite widespread use, scepticism about the efficacy of TENS has persisted for decades. A vast amount of experimental and clinical research has accumulated trying to determine whether TENS effects are due to specific actions on the body or nonspecific 'placebo' effects. If TENS effects were predominantly a placebo response there would be no need to put batteries in the TENS device to get beneficial effects because the delivery of electrical currents were not contributing to outcome. There is inconsistency in clinical research findings on TENS and this is reflected in clinical guidelines. For example, the UK National Institute for Health and Clinical Excellence (NICE) recommends that TENS should be offered for short-term relief of musculoskeletal pain associated with osteoarthritis (National Institute for Health and Clinical Excellence, 2008) and rheumatoid arthritis (National Institute for Health and Clinical Excellence, 2009a), but not for persistent non-specific low back pain (National Institute for Health and Clinical Excellence, 2009b). In the USA, the North American Spine Society recommends that TENS should be offered for chronic low back pain (Poitras & Brosseau, 2008) whereas the American Academy of Neurology does not (Dubinsky & Miyasaki, 2010). You can be certain of uncertainty when evaluating the clinical effectiveness of TENS.

A brief history of TENS

Using electricity to relieve pain is an age-old technique that pre-dates the discovery of electricity (Table 1.1). Stone carvings which date from the Egyptian Fifth Dynasty (c2500 BC) suggest that electric catfish (Malapterurus electricus) and electric rays

Table 1.1 Historical milestones in the history of electrotherapy

Date	Source	Milestone
c.2500 BC	Egyptian Fifth Dynasty	Stone carvings of electric fish to treat ailments
c. 400 BC	Hippocrates	Electric fish used to treat headache and arthritis
c. AD 46	Scribonius Largus the Roman physician	First written report of the medical use of electric fish in the book Compositiones Medicae
c. 1745	Pieter van Musschenbroek of Leiden (Leyden) and Ewald Georg von Kleist of Germany	Invention of the Leyden Jar enabling static electrical energy to be stored and discharged as needed
1759	John Wesley	Wrote the book Electricity made plain and useful by a lover of mankind and of common sense which described using medical electricity to treat sciatica, headache, gout, and kidney stones
1965	Melzack & Wall (1965)	Publication of 'Pain mechanisms: a new theory' known colloquially as the gate control theory of pain
1967	Wall & Sweet (1967)	Reported using high-frequency (50–100 Hz) percutaneous electrical nerve stimulation to relieve chronic neuropathic pain
1967	Shealy et al., (1967)	Reported using dorsal column stimulation implants for pain relief
1969	Reynolds (1969)	Reported that stimulation of periaqueductal grey (PAG) in the midbrain of rat produces surgical anaesthesia

Table 1.1 (continued) Historical milestones in the history of electrotherapy

Date	Source	Milestone
1967–1973	Various	TENS used to predict response to dorsal column stimulation implants
1973	Long (1974)	Reported that TENS was successful as a stand-alone treatment for chronic pain, post-operative pain, cancer
1976	Sjölund & Eriksson (1976)	Reported that strong muscle contractions generated by low-frequency high-intensity TENS relieved pain and endogenous opioids were involved. The technique was termed acupuncture-like TENS (Chapter 3)
1977	Augustinsson et al., (1977)	Reported that labour pain was relieved using dual-channel TENS with an intensity 'boost' control when delivered to the thoracic and sacral areas of the back (Chapter 7)
1980s	Various	RCTs published with conflicting findings (Chapter 8)
1980s	Various (Chung et al., 1984b)	Evidence that electrical nerve stimulation reduced activity of spontaneous and noxiously evoked dorsal horn cells (Chapter 9)
1990s onwards	Various (Claydon et al., 2011)	Studies using experimentally induced pain suggested that pulse amplitude was critical for TENS effects but the role of other electrical characteristics remained unclear (Chapter 4)
1991	Johnson et al., (1991c)	An in-depth study of long-term users of TENS found no relationship between patient, stimulator, and outcome variables (Chapter 4)
1996	Carroll et al., (1996)	Publication of the first systematic reviews provided limited evidence that TENS relieved post-operative pain (Chapter 8)
1999 onwards	DeSantana et al., (2008c)	Studies using animal models of nociception suggested that TENS actions involved many neurochemicals including opioids, GABA, serotonin, and acetylcholine with differences between high- and low-frequency stimulation (Chapter 9)
2003	Chandran & Sluka (2003)	Evidence that repeated administration of TENS led to opioid tolerance (Chapter 9)
2003	Bjordal et al., (2003)	Publication of the first meta-analysis with assessment of optimal treatment parameters found TENS reduced postoperative analgesic consumption (Chapter 8)
2007	Johnson & Martinson (2007)	Largest meta-analysis to date found that TENS provided three times more pain relief than placebo (no current TENS) (Chapter 8)

Table 1.1 (continued) Historical milestones in the history of electrotherapy

Date	Source	Milestone
2003 onwards	(National Institute for Health and Clinical Excellence, 2003; National Institute for Health and Clinical Excellence, 2007; 2008; 2009a, b; 2011)	The UK National Institute for Health and Clinical Excellence recommended that TENS should be offered for multiple sclerosis, and rheumatoid and osteoarthritis but not for labour pain, early management of persistent non-specific low back pain, or stable angina (Chapter 8)
2008–2009	Nnoaham & Kumbang (2008) Robb et al., (2008) Walsh et al., (2009)	Cochrane reviews of TENS for chronic pain, acute pain, and cancer pain found inconclusive evidence (Chapter 8)
2011	Bennett et al., (2011)	Sources of implementation fidelity in RCTs were quantified and inadequate TENS technique was found to contribute to under dosing (Chapters 8 and 12)
2012	Jacques et al., (2012)	Medicaid in the USA recommended was found to that insurance coverage for TENS to manage chronic low back pain should expire in June 2015 unless methodologically robust RCTs demonstrating effectiveness became available

(Torpedo marmorata), which are capable of generating 300–400 V were used to treat a variety of painful ailments (Figure 1.2). Over 2000 years later, Hippocrates (400 BC) referred to the use of electric fish to treat headache and arthritis, although it was Scribonius Largus (AD 46), a Roman physician, who is often credited with the first written report of the medical use of electric fish in *Compositiones Medicae* (Gildenberg, 2006).

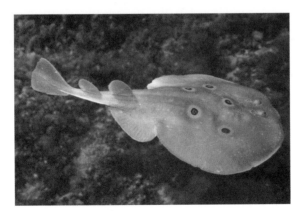

Fig. 1.2 Electric ray, *Torpedo marmorata*.

Reproduced from Joan Hester et al. (eds), *Interventional Pain Control in Cancer Pain Management*, Figure 11.1, p. 220, Copyright © 2012, by permission of Oxford University Press.

The use of medical electricity began in the 1700s with the invention of the Leyden Jar enabling static electrical energy to be stored and discharged as needed. The development of batteries coupled with experimental procedures on humans and animals by electrotherapy pioneers such as Giovanni Aldini, Alexandro Volta, Johann Krüger, and Christian Kratzenstein meant that medical electricity became popular with the masses. The Christian theologian and founder of the Methodist movement, the Reverend John Wesley, pioneered the use of electricity to treat illness in his book *The desideratum: or, Electricity made plain and useful* which was published in 1759. The use of electrotherapy continued until the late 1800s when popularity declined because of variable clinical results and an increasing reliance on pharmacological treatments.

Electrotherapy practice remained dormant until the beginning of the 1900s when a range of battery-powered transcutaneous electrical stimulators were developed in the USA, including Electrotreat® in 1919. Electrotreat® remained popular until 1941 when the Food and Drug Administration (FDA) banned advertisements that claimed that Electrotreat® relieved pain. Nevertheless, investigators in Russia remained enthusiastic about the effects of transcutaneous electrical stimulation on the body for a range of medical conditions including pain, depression, and anxiety. Serious interest in the use of transcutaneous electrical stimulation for pain relief was rekindled in Europe and the USA by the publication of *Pain mechanisms: a new theory* (Melzack & Wall, 1965). The 'new theory' became known as the gate control theory of pain providing a physiological explanation of how stimulating the skin using electricity could relieve pain.

Melzack and Wall proposed that the transmission of noxious (pain-related) information by small-diameter nerve fibres in the nervous system could be reduced if there was simultaneous activity in larger-diameter nerve fibres that normally transmit non-painful touch-related information. They used a metaphor of a 'pain gate' being open when pain was present, or closed when pain was absent. They suggested that the gate was open when high-threshold peripheral afferents that conduct pain-related information were active resulting in pain sensation. The pain gate could be closed by rubbing skin which activated low-threshold nerve fibres that transmit non-painful touch-related information (Figure 1.3). They suggested that electricity could artificially stimulate low-threshold nerve fibres that transmit non-painful touch-related information to close the pain gate and reduce pain. In 1967 Wall and Sweet stimulated large peripheral nerve fibres using needles inserted through the skin to deliver high-frequency (50–100 pps), non-painful electrical currents percutaneously, and found that patients reported relief from their chronic neurogenic pain (Wall & Sweet 1967).

Melzack and Wall also suggested that the pain gate could be closed by activity in central nervous system pathways that transmit information from the brain to the spinal cord (Figure 1.3). These descending pain-inhibitory pathways become active when motivational or distraction techniques are used to reduce pain—for example, when a person sustains an injury during a competitive sporting event but he or she does not feel pain until he or she returns to the locker room. In 1967 Shealy and colleagues implanted electrodes into spinal cord and administered electrical currents to stimulate nerves in the dorsal columns and found that this relieved chronic pain, providing the forerunner of modern day spinal cord stimulation (Shealy et al., 1967). The dorsal columns form the central transmission pathways for low-threshold peripheral nerve fibres.

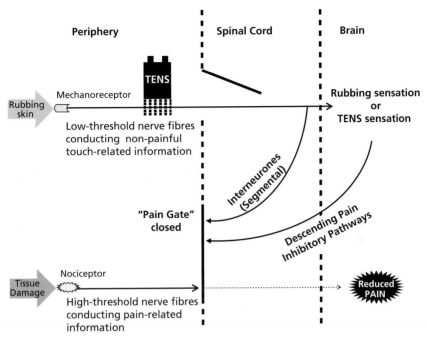

Fig. 1.3 The pain gate. Rubbing the skin or using TENS activates low-threshold afferents that conduct non-painful touch-related information to the brain and also close the 'pain gate', preventing pain-related information reaching the brain.

In 1969, Reynolds demonstrated that surgical anaesthesia could be achieved in rats by electrically stimulating the periaqueductal grey (PAG) region of the midbrain which acts as a relay station on the descending pain inhibitory pathways (Reynolds, 1969). This led to the development of deep brain stimulation techniques to relieve pain in humans (Richardson & Akil, 1977).

In the early 1970s TENS was being used to predict whether individuals would respond to dorsal column stimulation implants until it was realized that TENS could be used successfully on its own for various types of pain, including neuropathic pain, postoperative pain, and cancer pain (Long, 1974). Low-intensity, high-frequency pulsed electrical currents were delivered through the skin via electrodes attached to the intact surface of the body to stimulate nerve fibres with low thresholds of activation, and patients experienced a non-painful TENS sensation (i.e. electrical paraesthesiae). Nowadays this technique is termed 'conventional TENS'.

At the same time interest in the use of acupuncture in Europe and the USA had occurred following the visit of President Nixon to China. Observations that acupuncture needles were manually twirled at low frequencies (e.g. 2 Hz) during treatment lead to the delivery of low-frequency (2 pps) electrical currents via acupuncture needles inserted through the skin (i.e. electroacupuncture). In 1973, Andersson and colleagues reported that low-frequency (2 pps) electroacupuncture of the hands and cheeks at an intensity producing muscle twitching at the site of needle insertion increased pain threshold to experimental tooth pulp stimulation in 18 healthy subjects (Andersson et al., 1973). Larger elevations in pain threshold were obtained in 12 subjects using electroacupuncture via surface electrodes administered using low-frequency single-pulsed currents only when intensities were sufficient to elicit strong muscle contractions suggesting that activation of receptors deep within tissue (e.g. muscle) were essential for hypoalgesia. The onset and offset of hypoalgesia were gradual and lasted up to 30 minutes. Sjölund and colleagues found that electroacupuncture via surface electrodes increased levels of endorphins in the cerebrospinal fluid, although these muscle contractions generated by low-frequency high-intensity TENS using single pulsed current were found to be unpleasant for pain patients. Sjölund and colleagues found that muscle contractions generated by low-frequency bursts of high-frequency trains of pulses (burst mode TENS) were better tolerated by patients and they introduced the term 'acupuncture-like TENS' to describe the technique (Sjölund & Eriksson, 1976; Sjölund et al., 1977). In 1979, they reported that some of the patients who failed to respond to conventional TENS achieved pain relief using acupuncture-like TENS.

In the 1980s research began to focus on the search for optimal electrical settings for TENS by evaluating effects on experimental pain in healthy humans. It was believed that the specific current amplitudes, frequencies, waveforms, durations, and patterns were optimal for certain types of pain, although study findings were inconsistent. An in-depth investigation of long-term users of TENS revealed a 'remarkable lack of correlation between patient, stimulator and outcome variables' (Johnson et al., 1991c, 226). Research evidence suggested that a strong, non-painful TENS sensation within the site of pain was superior to placebo (no current TENS). However, evidence was, and still is, inconclusive for the influence of frequency, waveform, duration, and pattern of currents on treatment outcome (Chapter 4).

Electrophysiological studies conducted in the 1980s and 1990s using animal models of nociception found that high-frequency TENS reduced activity of nociceptive (pain-related) neurones in the spinal cord indicative of 'closing the pain gate'. When TENS was administered at higher intensities, long-lasting inhibition of centrally located nociceptive neurones occurred with some of the neural circuitry mediating the response located in the brain (supra-spinal). In the last decade, research conducted by Sluka and colleagues provided insights into the complexity of the physiology and pharmacology of TENS (Chapter 9). Hypoalgesia produced by low-frequency TENS is mediated via μ-opioid receptors in the spinal cord whereas hypoalgesia produced by high-frequency TENS is mediated via δ-opioid receptors in the rostral ventral medulla of the brainstem. Gamma-amino-butyric acid (GABA) and a variety of other transmitter systems also appear to be involved. However, whether these specific physiological actions translate into clinically meaningful pain relief remains a matter of debate.

The 1990s saw the use of systematic reviews of clinical research trials to evaluate the efficacy of treatments (Chapter 8). The first systematic reviews on TENS were published in 1996 by Reeve and colleagues who found 'little evidence for other than a limited use of TENS [for acute and chronic pain]', and by Carroll and colleagues (1996) who found limited evidence for acute post-operative pain (Reeve et al., 1996; Carroll et al., 1996). The review by Carroll and colleagues demonstrated that non-randomized studies overestimated treatment effects as TENS was superior to placebo (no current) TENS in only 2 out of 17 randomized controlled clinical trials (RCTs) but superior in 17 out of 19 non-randomized trials. The following year the same reviewers found evidence that pain relief during TENS was no different to placebo TENS during childbirth (Carroll et al., 1997b). In 2003, Bjordal et al. conducted the first meta-analysis of RCTs (1350 patients) that included a subgroup analysis of optimal TENS technique and found larger reductions in post-operative analgesic consumption for optimal versus sub-optimal TENS technique (Bjordal et al., 2003). The largest meta-analysis to date included 23 RCTs on TENS for any type of chronic musculoskeletal pain and found that TENS provided approximately three times more pain relief than placebo (no current TENS) (Johnson & Martinson, 2007). However, the proliferation of systematic reviews that took place through the 2000s has not been matched by the publication of methodologically robust RCTs, resulting in one systematic review team concluding that 'Interestingly, we found nearly as many systematic reviews as trials on the topic [osteoarthritis of the knee]' (Rutjes et al., 2009). This situation has been reflected in clinical guidelines.

In 2009, NICE in the UK recommended that TENS should not be offered for persistent non-specific low back pain, and in 2010 the Therapeutics and Technology Assessment Subcommittee of the American Academy of Neurology (AAN) published similar recommendations (National Institute for Health and Clinical Excellence, 2009b; Dubinsky & Miyasaki, 2010). However, in the same year an Updated Report by the American Society of Anesthesiologists Task Force on Chronic Pain Management and the American Society of Regional Anesthesia and Pain Medicine recommended that 'TENS should be used as part of a multimodal approach to pain management for patients with chronic back pain and may be used for other pain conditions (e.g. neck and phantom limb pain)'(American Society of Anesthesiologists, 2010). The polarization of clinical recommendations for TENS is common.

It is remarkable that improvements in research methodologies have not resolved the issue of TENS efficacy and effectiveness. In 2011, Bennett et al. quantified sources of implementation fidelity in RCTs on TENS and revealed inadequate TENS techniques and infrequent treatments of insufficient duration were contributing to under-dosing in many RCTs, creating bias in the outcome towards no differences between active and placebo TENS (Bennett et al., 2011). Nevertheless, in 2012 the Centers for Medicare & Medicaid Services in the USA decided to re-evaluate evidence for TENS for chronic low back pain and concluded that there was inadequate research evidence to support continued Medicare insurance coverage. Medicare insurance coverage is due to expire in the USA on 8 June 2015 unless evidence demonstrating clinically meaningful reductions in pain or improvements in function from a methodologically robust RCT becomes available.

Goal of this textbook

Research findings and scholarly activity on TENS appear to have confused rather than clarified issues of mechanism, optimal technique, including electrode sites and electrical characteristics, and efficacy. Nevertheless, the success of TENS will depend on the practitioner and patient fully understanding the physiological principles that underpin safe and appropriate technique. TENS is readily available to the general public without prescription so patients may arrive at clinics already using TENS devices and seeking further advice. The goal of this textbook is to synthesize research findings to determine efficacy and guide a safe and appropriate TENS technique for clinical practice. In addition, solutions will be offered to improve the design and delivery of future research. This will be achieved by covering:

◆ TENS equipment, techniques, and biophysical principles (Chapter 3)
◆ Appropriate electrode sites and electrical characteristics for TENS (Chapter 4)
◆ Contraindications, precautions, and adverse events (Chapter 5)
◆ Evaluating TENS on a new patient—the supervised trial (Chapter 6)
◆ Practicalities of using TENS for specific conditions and situations (Chapter 7)
◆ Clinical research on the efficacy of TENS (Chapter 8)
◆ The mechanism of action of TENS (Chapter 9)
◆ The use of TENS for non-painful conditions (Chapter 10)
◆ TENS-like devices (Chapter 11)
◆ Future directions (Chapter 12)

The primary use of TENS is to manage pain and this will be the main focus of the textbook. However, it is necessary from the outset to standardize TENS terminology to be used throughout.

TENS terminology

Much confusion has arisen in clinical practice because of the use of inconsistent and loose terminology in TENS literature. This has fuelled mystique about optimal technique and efficacy.

By strict definition TENS is any technique that delivers electricity across the intact surface of the skin to activate underlying nerves. However, only purists tend to use such a broad definition.

The US National Library of Medicine National Institutes of Health (PubMed) has over 22 million citations from biomedical literature from MEDLINE, life science journals, and online books. Before 1990 PubMed indexed TENS under the broad Medical Subject Header (MeSH) *Electric Stimulation* (1966–1983) and *Electric Stimulation Therapy* (1966–1983). In 1990 the Medical Subject Header 'transcutaneous electric nerve stimulation' was introduced to index with more precision research literature on TENS. The MeSH 'transcutaneous electric nerve stimulation' encompasses a range of additional entry terms including various permutations of transcutaneous electrical stimulation, percutaneous electric nerve stimulation, transdermal electrostimulation, electroanalgesia, and analgesic cutaneous electrostimulation. This means that a literature search conducted in PubMed using the MeSH 'transcutaneous electric nerve stimulation' produces a large number of 'hits'. For example, a search conducted on 1 October 2013 returned 6025 hits, although many of these hits may not be directly related to TENS per se.

In PubMed 'transcutaneous electric nerve stimulation' is defined as: *'The use of specifically placed small electrodes to deliver electrical impulses across the SKIN to relieve PAIN. It is used less frequently to produce ANESTHESIA';* see: <http://www.ncbi.nlm.nih.gov/mesh/?term=transcutaneous+electric+nerve+stimulation>. This definition is useful but misleading. TENS is not just used 'to relieve PAIN' or 'to produce ANESTHESIA' but also for a variety of non-painful conditions (Chapter 10). Whether 'small electrodes' are a prerequisite for TENS is also a matter for debate. The term 'small' is subjective, and the size of TENS electrodes varies considerably, from 1 cm-diameter electrodes for acupuncture points to greater than 20 cm in length for post-operative pain. Glove, sock, and belt electrodes are also available with even larger surface areas.

Definitions from professional bodies and learned societies for laypersons tend to be broad. For example, the National Health Service (NHS) in the UK describes TENS as 'A small, battery-operated machine is used to deliver electrical impulses into the body, which should feel like a pleasant tingling sensation. Leads are attached to the skin with reusable sticky plasters. These impulses help block or reduce pain signals going to the spinal cord and brain, potentially reducing or relieving the pain or muscle spasms associated with a wide range of painful conditions. Low frequencies of electric current are also used to stimulate the body to release pain-relieving hormones called endorphins.' (NHS choices; available at: <http://www.nhs.uk/conditions/tens/Pages/Introduction.aspx>; accessed 29 November 2013).

Definitions for practitioners and researchers tend to be more specific. The Canadian Physiotherapy Society's definition for TENS is clear, informative, and not too rigid: '. . . the use of electrical currents to produce analgesia or hypoalgesia. A variety of pulsed waveforms are used, with frequencies typically in the range of 1–100 Hz. Intensities are set to produce sensory stimulation alone or combined with motor stimulation to produce muscle twitches (acupuncture-like TENS)' (Houghton et al., 2010, 9).

The International Association of Pain (IASP) core curriculum defines TENS according to two main TENS techniques (Charlton, 2005, 94). Conventional TENS is defined as 'high-frequency (50–100 Hz), low-intensity (paraesthesia, not painful), small pulse width (50–200 μs)'. Acupuncture-like TENS is defined as 'low-frequency (2–4 Hz), higher intensity (to tolerance threshold), and longer pulse width (100–400 μs)'. The IASP definitions give the impression that the electrical characteristics of the techniques are prescriptive. Interestingly, there is no reference to frequencies between 5 Hz and 49 Hz.

Overall, the variations in definitions are small, and probably have limited impact on clinical practice. However, unclear terminology causes challenges when evaluating and interpreting research findings and clinical practice guidelines. Health-care professionals tend to use the term to describe stimulation of the intact surface of the skin principally to manage pain.

For the purposes of this book, TENS is defined as the delivery of pulsed electrical currents across the intact surface of the skin using a 'standard TENS device' to stimulate peripheral nerves principally for pain relief.

The definition makes reference to the use of TENS to relieve pain because this is the primary purpose of TENS and is the focus of this textbook. However, TENS is also used to manage non-painful conditions (Chapter 10). It is also necessary to reference the use of a 'standard TENS device' (Chapter 3) because a variety of 'TENS-like devices' are commercially available (Johnson, 2001a; Johnson, 2001b) (Chapter 11). Most practitioners and research investigators do not categorize TENS-like devices as 'TENS'.

> A standard TENS device is a portable, battery-powered generator of monophasic or biphasic pulsed electrical current delivered in a repetitive manner, with a maximum peak-to-peak amplitude of approximately 60 milliamperes (mA) into a 1 kilohm load.

A standard TENS device has a combination of dials, buttons, or touch-pad controls to control electrical output characteristics which are typically pulse waveform durations between 50 and 500 µs, pulse rates (frequencies) between 1 and 200 pulses per second (pps), and continuous and intermittent patterns of pulses. Currents are delivered from the standard TENS device via connecting lead wires to electrodes placed on the surface of the skin. In the UK a standard TENS device with a dual-channel output, two connecting lead wires, a pack of four electrodes, batteries, and a storage pouch/belt clip retails between GB£15.00 and GB£100.00.

Summary

1 Electrical stimulation of the skin is an age-old technique to relieve pain.
2 TENS delivers pulsed electrical currents across the intact surface of the skin using a 'standard TENS device' to stimulate peripheral nerves.
3 TENS is predominantly used as a stand-alone treatment or as an adjunct to core treatment for symptomatic relief of any type pain.
4 TENS is popular with patients and practitioners because it is inexpensive, non-invasive, easy to administer, and has few side effects or drug interactions.
5 The publication of Melzack and Wall's *gate control theory of pain* provided a physiological explanation of how stimulating the skin using electricity could relieve pain.

Further reading

- **Gildenberg, P.L.** (2006) History of electrical neuromodulation for chronic pain. *Pain Med*, **7** Suppl 1, S7–S13.
- **Johnson, M.I.** (2008) Transcutaneous Electrical Nerve Stimulation. In Watson, T. (ed.) *Electrotherapy: Evidence based practice*. Churchill Livingstone, Edinburgh, 253–96.

Chapter 2 will discuss challenges practitioners face when managing pain with reference to the role of TENS. TENS equipment and techniques will be described to lay the foundations for later discussions about the principles underpinning clinical practice.

Chapter 2

TENS for pain management

Introduction

Pain is a major health-care problem. A systematic review of 65 surveys conducted in 34 countries (182,019 respondents) estimated that the weighted mean ± standard deviation prevalence of chronic pain in the general adult population worldwide was 30.3 per cent ± 11.7 per cent (Elzahaf, Tashani, et al. 2012). A pan-European epidemiological survey found that 40 per cent of individuals with chronic pain reported that they had inadequate pain management, with 64 per cent of respondents reporting that there were times when drug treatment was not adequate to control their pain (Breivik et al., 2006). Sixty-nine per cent of respondents had used non-drug treatments for their pain including massage, physiotherapy, and acupuncture. However, 40 per cent of respondents were not satisfied with the effectiveness of the pain management that they were receiving for their chronic pain. The most common use for TENS is to relieve pain. The purpose of this chapter is to contextualize the role of TENS in the management of pain by covering:

- The phenomenon of pain
- Challenges of managing pain
- Physiology of the nociceptive system, including states of sensitivity
- Electrophysical techniques for pain and rehabilitation, including invasive electrical stimulation techniques
- Extent of use of TENS
- TENS: clinical experience

The phenomenon of pain

Pain is a psychological state created by the brain—no brain, no pain! There is no objective way of measuring an individual's pain because it is a subjective phenomenon, so if a person reports that they are experiencing pain they should be believed. Individuals learn when to use the word 'pain' through experiences related to their early life.

Pain is defined as:

'An unpleasant sensory and emotional experience associated with actual or potential tissue damage, or described in terms of such damage' (The International Association for the Study of Pain (IASP); available at: <http://www.iasp-pain.org>).

Pain is a sensation associated with stimuli that have the ability to damage tissue, although it may also exist in the absence of actual or potential tissue damage. The sensory–discriminative dimensions of pain include the intensity, location, and quality of the pain, subserved by the nociceptive system. Pain evokes emotions such as unpleasantness and fear generating affective (emotional)-motivational dimensions of pain, subserved by the reticular and limbic systems of the brain. Pain also evokes thoughts such as consideration of the appropriate action to take in response to pain generating cognitive-evaluative dimensions of pain, subserved by the frontal lobe of the brain.

Challenges of managing pain

Pain assessment and management can be challenging because:

♦ It is not possible to prove or disprove that a person is in pain—pain is whatever the person says it is.

♦ Pain sensation is dynamic and fluctuates in quality, intensity, and location on a moment-to-moment basis (Figure 2.1).

♦ Pain often presents with other sensory phenomenon (Table 2.1).

♦ The link between persistent pain, injury, disease, and healing is often tenuous. For example, pain may be:

  • more intense than expected, e.g. when a slither of metal embeds beneath a fingernail

  • less intense than expected, e.g. when seriously injured soldiers do not feel pain (battlefield analgesia)

  • absent in the presence of life-threatening disease, e.g. cancerous tumours

  • persistent without detectable pathology, e.g. mechanical low back pain.

These factors can complicate diagnosis of underlying pathology, and so pain is often categorized according to its duration (Table 2.2).

The most effective pain-management strategies use a biopsychosocial approach that aims to relieve pain and suffering to improve quality of life. Approaches include treatments to relieve pain, education, empowerment of patients, and early access to care to prevent acute pain becoming chronic pain. Analgesic medication remains mainstay treatment and is particularly effective for pain of recent onset, with non-pharmacological treatments used as adjuncts. However, more potent medication is toxic and associated with side effects, tolerance, and dependence. Approaches to empower to self-care are commonly used for people with chronic pain (e.g. see <http://www.paintoolkit.org>). Pain is a stressor and it has deleterious physiological effects including increased blood pressure, changes in blood gases, delayed gastric emptying, urinary retention, and increased secretion of cortisol. Therefore, under-treating pain for fear of masking important pathological symptoms or incurring side effects is detrimental to biological health.

Pharmacological and non-pharmacological pain-relieving treatments act by reducing activity in the nociceptive system, so a working knowledge of the physiology of

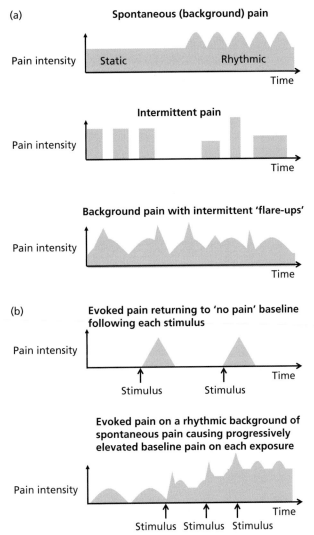

Fig. 2.1 Fluctuations in the intensity of (a) spontaneous and (b) evoked pain. Spontaneous 'background' pain occurs in the absence of provoking stimuli and may present as continuous (static), rhythmic, intermittent (episodic), erratic, in waves or in patterns, and may 'flare up' intermittently. Evoked pain is sensitive to provoking stimuli, including movement, touch, or changes in temperature. The provoking stimuli often produce particularly intense and distressing pain which is out of proportion to the intensity of provoking stimulus (i.e. amplified pain).

Table 2.1 Commonly used pain terms

Term	Definition
Hyperalgesia	Increased pain from a stimulus that normally provokes pain at the site of injury (primary hyperalgesia), or in the healthy tissue surrounding the injury (secondary hyperalgesia)
Allodynia	Pain due to a stimulus that does not normally provoke pain
Hyperpathia	An abnormally painful reaction to a stimulus, especially a repetitive stimulus, as well as an increased threshold
Hypaesthesia (Hypoaesthesia)	Diminished sensitivity to somatosensory stimuli such as touch
Hyperaesthesia	Abnormal increase in sensitivity to somatosensory stimuli (cf, allodynia)
Hypoalgesia	Diminished pain in response to a normally painful stimulus
Paraesthesia	An abnormal sensation, whether spontaneous or evoked
Dysaesthesia	An unpleasant abnormal sensation, whether spontaneous or evoked

Source: data from IASP Taxonomy, updated from H. Merskey and N. Bogduk (eds), Part III: Pain Terms, A Current List with Definitions and Notes on Usage, in *Classification of Chronic Pain*, 2nd edition, IASP Press, Seattle, Copyright © 1994; available from <http://www.iasp-pain.org/Content/NavigationMenu/GeneralResourceLinks/PainDefinitions/default.htm>.

Table 2.2 Broad categories of pain

Category	Attributes
Duration	
Acute pain	◆ Recent onset and probable limited duration ◆ Persists <3 months ◆ Usually has a causal and temporal association with injury and disease
Chronic pain	◆ Long-standing and probable unlimited duration ◆ Persists beyond normal time of healing or because of ongoing disease (≥3 months) ◆ Often no causal link to injury or disease • May be due to changes in nervous system physiology
Pathophysiology	
Nociceptive pain	◆ Arises from actual or potential damage to non-neural tissue ◆ Activation of nociceptors ◆ Often associated with inflammation
Neuropathic pain	◆ Arises from a lesion or disease of the somatosensory nervous system including visceral organs

the nociceptive system is useful. A brief overview is provided in the next section. For a more detailed description, see Johnson (2005).

Physiology of the nociceptive system

The nociceptive system is the part of the nervous system that detects and responds to actual or potential tissue damage

The basic elements of the nociceptive system (Figure 2.2) are:

- Nociceptors, detecting potential or actual tissue damage
- Neural pathways, conducting nerve impulses from nociceptors to the spinal cord and brain
- Processing areas, regulating the flow of nerve impulses in the central nervous system and providing awareness (sensation), meaning (perception), unpleasantness (emotion), and thoughts (cognition) associated with the noxious stimulus

The nociceptive system changes its state of sensitivity according to circumstance (Table 2.3).

Pre-injury state of the nociceptive system

In a pre-injury state, the nociceptive system is primed to detect stimuli causing actual or potential tissue damage. Nociceptors detect noxious stimuli, such as touching a burning hot-cooker ring, and convert the stimuli into nerve impulses (i.e. travelling action potentials).

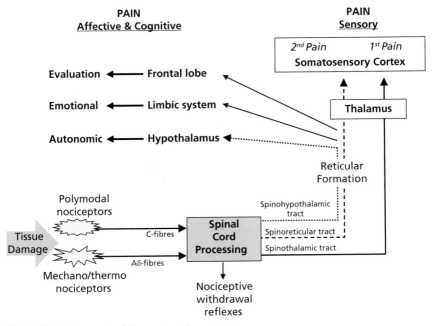

Fig. 2.2 Basic elements of the nociceptive system.

Table 2.3 States of sensitivity of the nociceptive system

State	Status of peripheral tissue	Nociceptive transmission	Low-intensity stimulus	High-intensity stimulus
Pre-injury	Healthy	Normal	Innocuous sensation	Pain
Sensitized	Injured	Amplified	Pain (Allodynia)	Exaggerated pain (Hyperalgesia)
Persistently sensitized	Healthy or injured	Dysfunctional/ amplified	Pain (Allodynia)	Exaggerated pain (Hyperalgesia)
Reorganized	Healthy or injured, especially nerve damage	Abnormal/ amplified	Pain (Allodynia) Dysaethesia	Exaggerated pain (Hyperalgesia) Dysaethesia
Suppressed	Injured or healthy	Diminished	No pain	No pain

> A nociceptor is a high-threshold sensory receptor that detects stimuli that damage or threaten to damage normal tissues and codes this detection by generating nerve impulses

Nociceptors respond to high-intensity thermal and/or mechanical stimuli and to chemicals produced by the body following injury. Nociceptors are 'tissue-damage detectors', not 'pain detectors', because nociceptors may be active without an individual experiencing pain and conversely a person may experience pain without nociceptors being active. Nociceptors are free nerve endings of peripheral neuronal axons that conduct nerve impulses towards the central nervous system (i.e. afferent nerve fibres). Peripheral nociceptive afferents are categorized according to axon structure as either A-δ or C-fibre (Table 2.4), and terminate in superficial layers of the posterior (dorsal) horn of the spinal cord to synapse directly or indirectly (via interneurones) with central nociceptive transmission cells. Glutamate is one of the main excitatory neurotransmitters released at the terminals of nociceptive afferents.

The central nervous system responds to impulses arising in A-δ afferents by producing a rapid, involuntary reflex response to remove the body part from the source of tissue damage (i.e. the withdrawal reflex). This often happens before you experience pain. Protective withdrawal reflexes are mediated via contraction and relaxation of skeletal muscle, and a positive feedback loop may form whereby the reflex muscle contraction causes further activation of nociceptors resulting in a painful muscle spasm. Protective sympathetic reflexes also occur, and they produce vasoconstriction and ischaemia in peripheral tissue and a positive feedback loop whereby nociceptors detect the ischaemia resulting in further enhancement of sympathetic reflexes. Treatments to interrupt these positive feedback loops can help to relieve pain in certain circumstances.

Central nociceptive transmission neurones conduct nociceptive impulses from the spinal cord and brainstem to higher centres of the brain and they are often categorized

Table 2.4 Categories of nociceptive cells

	Properties	Function
Peripheral nociceptor afferent		
A-δ fibre	◆ high threshold ◆ myelinated ◆ large diameter (~1–4 μm) ◆ fast conducting (~5–15 ms^{-1})	◆ responds to extremes of heat, cold, and mechanical stimuli ◆ generates withdrawal reflexes and 'fast/first' pain sensations ◆ associated with the precise location of noxious stimuli on the body
C-fibre (polymodal)	◆ high threshold ◆ unmyelinated ◆ small diameter (~0.1–1 μm) ◆ slow conducting (~0.2–2.0 ms^{-1})	◆ responds to noxious thermal, mechanical, and chemical stimuli that are released during cell damage (e.g. H$^+$, K$^+$, serotonin (5-HT) and bradykinin) ◆ generates 'slow/second' pain sensations ◆ associated with the prevention of further tissue damage
Central nociceptive transmission neurone		
Nociceptive specific neurones	◆ respond to noxious but not non-noxious stimuli ◆ located in lamina I of the posterior horn ◆ conduct impulses in direct, rapidly conducting pathways to the thalamus (spinothalamic tracts) and somatosensory cortex (thalamocortico tracts)	◆ contribute to 'fast/first' pain sensations ◆ associated with sensory-discriminative dimensions of pain (i.e. the intensity, quality, and location of the noxious stimuli)
Wide dynamic range neurones	◆ respond to non-noxious and noxious stimuli ◆ located in lamina V of the posterior horn ◆ conduct impulses in multi-synaptic slower pathways to the reticular formation (spinoreticular tract), limbic system, and cerebral cortex	◆ contribute to 'slow/second' pain sensations ◆ associated with motivational-affective and cognitive aspects of pain

according to their response profile as either nociceptive-specific or wide dynamic range neurones (Table 2.4). Central nociceptive transmission neurones send impulses to many areas of the brain. Following a noxious stimulus, impulses arrive at the somatosensory areas of the cerebral cortex and are processed to create a sharp, intense, localized, 'fast/first' pain followed by a dull, aching, spreading, 'slower/second' pain, both of which help an individual to remember to avoid such stimuli in the future. However, there is no single 'pain centre' but rather a matrix of cerebral structures that process noxious information creating different patterns of brain activity in different circumstances. Areas commonly involved in pain processing are the somatosensory cortex (sensory-discriminative dimensions of pain), the cingulate gyrus and insula (affective-motivational dimensions of pain), and prefrontal cortex (cognitive dimensions of pain). Impulses also arrive at the hypothalamus via spinohypothalamic tracts to elicit autonomic responses associated with pain.

Referred pain

Cutaneous nociceptors are specialized to detect stimuli in the external environment resulting in discrete localized sensations. Nociceptors in visceral and skeletal muscle nociceptors are specialized to detect stimuli in the internal environment and they generate pain sensations that are dull and less well localized because there are fewer central nociceptive transmission neurones dedicated to visceral tissue. Visceral tissue is sensitive to twisting, distension, and chemical irritants (e.g. stomach acid), and less sensitive to cutting, heat, or pinching. Skeletal muscle is sensitive to contraction in the presence of ischaemia, generating a deep, aching pain which can have both nociceptive and neuropathic pain elements. Damage in visceral and skeletal muscle structures often produces patterns of pain and sensitivity on the skin because their afferents are bundled in nerves that also innervate cutaneous tissue. Pain referred to cutaneous areas innervated by the same spinal segment (dermatome) as visceral and skeletal muscle structures occurs because visceral and cutaneous afferents supply the same central nociceptive transmission neurone. The brain interprets the afferent input as arising from cutaneous structures because of the higher proportion of cutaneous afferents converging on central nociceptive transmission neurones (Figure 2.3). This 'referred pain' may be experienced at sites that are distant from tissue damage and pathology and can confuse the clinician and the patient (Figure 2.4).

If minimal tissue damage occurs from a noxious stimulus the nociceptive system usually returns to a pre-injury 'control' state. If, however, tissue damage occurs then the nociceptive system becomes 'sensitized' so that the response to additional non-noxious and/or noxious stimuli is amplified. This sensitized state occurs in cutaneous, visceral, and skeletal muscle tissue and it helps to protect the tissue from further damage.

Sensitized state of the nociceptive system

The peripheral and central components of nervous system become 'sensitized' in the presence of tissue damage, resulting in an increased responsiveness of nociceptive neurones to their normal noxious input and to neurones that normally respond to non-noxious stimuli. Sensitization helps to protect injuries by reducing the threshold of activation of peripheral and central nociceptive cells and by increasing their receptive field size.

Peripheral sensitization

Peripheral sensitization occurs at the site of nociceptors in response to chemical substances that accumulate in the extracellular fluid in response to tissue damage, including bradykinin, 5-HT, H^+, and K^+, prostaglandins, leukotrienes, noradrenaline, adenosine, adenosine 5-triphosphate (ATP), and nitric oxide. This causes the threshold of activation of nociceptors to lower. Nociceptive impulses also invade the distal branches of

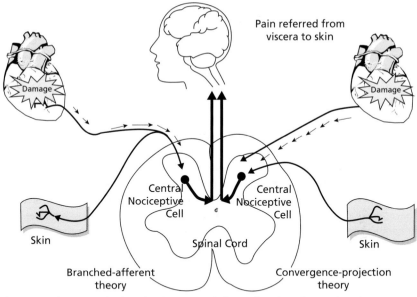

Fig. 2.3 Mechanisms of referred pain. Arrows indicate direction of nerve impulses.

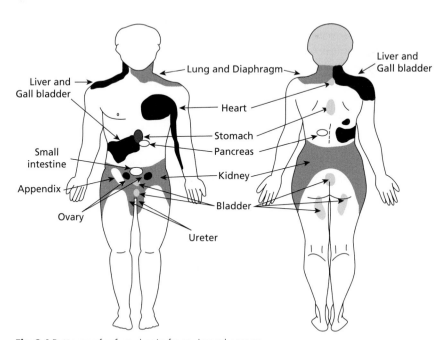

Fig. 2.4 Patterns of referred pain from visceral organs.

nociceptor free nerve endings causing release of substance P and other trophic chemicals contributing further to vasodilation, increased blood flow, increased permeability of blood vessels, and plasma extravasation associated with inflammation (i.e. redness, heat, and swelling). Non-steroidal anti-inflammatory drugs (e.g. ibuprofen, diclofenac) reduce inflammation and peripheral sensitization by inhibiting cyclo-oxygenase (Cox), an enzyme that catalyses the formation of prostaglandins from arachidonic acid.

Central sensitization

Central sensitization occurs at the site of central nociceptive transmission cells in response to repetitive C-fibre nociceptor activity ('wind-up'). The central nociceptive transmission neurones become sensitized and hyperexcitable, and they generate nerve impulses in the absence of evoking stimuli (spontaneous pain), amplify their response to high-intensity stimuli (hyperalgesia), and respond more vigorously to low-intensity, non-noxious stimuli resulting in pain (allodynia). Glutamate and substance P are excitatory neurotransmitters released by peripheral nociceptive afferents that contribute to central sensitization via actions on membrane receptors such as NMDA and neurokinin receptors respectively. Other neurotransmitters involved in central sensitization are calcitonin-gene-related peptide (CGRP), somatostatin, vasoactive intestinal polypeptide (VIP), nerve growth factor, and nitric oxide. Descending pain facilitatory pathways that originate in the brain and terminate in the spinal cord may also reduce the threshold of central nociceptive transmission cells to peripheral input.

Repetitive C-fibre input from noxious stimuli also causes reorganization of neuronal circuitry (central neuroplasticity), whereby central nociceptive transmission neurones expand their receptive fields so that they respond to stimuli applied to sites that do not normally activate the neurone. Central neuroplasticity is particularly prevalent following nerve damage. In most circumstances, central sensitization and the resultant spontaneous pain, allodynia, and hyperalgesia disappear when damaged tissue heals and the nociceptive system returns to its pre-injury state. However, sometimes the nervous system remains in a persistent state of sensitization.

Persistently sensitized state—dysfunctional state

Persistent ischaemia, inflammation, or progressive nerve damage will create ongoing activation of the nociceptive system, and the nociceptive system may remain persistently sensitized. Sometimes the original injury heals but the nociceptive system remains sensitized and does not reset to its original pre-injury state. In this circumstance the nociceptive system itself has become dysfunctional and the chronic pain is considered to be a disease entity in its own right, with a limited useful purpose. This is a common phenomenon following nerve damage (neuropathic pain). Nerve lesions affect sensory, motor, and autonomic fibre integrity, and the resultant persistent central sensitization may be due to various factors including hypersensitive central nociceptive cells, abnormal inputs to central nociceptive cells, reflex muscle spasm, ectopic impulse generation, loss of large-diameter afferent inhibition, sympathetic hyperactivity, and persistent activity in descending pain facilitatory pathways. The exact mechanisms contributing to persistent central sensitization and to the inability of the nociceptive system to reset to its original pre-injury state have not been elucidated as yet.

Suppressed state of the nociceptive system

The intensity of pain can be lower than expected (hypoalgesia) as described by the gate control theory of pain. The 'pain gate' is a metaphor to explain how nociceptive information can be regulated en route to the brain to influence the final experience of pain. From a physiological perspective, the 'pain gate' comprises excitatory and inhibitory synapses that regulate the flow of neural activity within the central nervous system. The 'pain gate' is opened by activity in peripheral nociceptor transmission pathways which form excitatory synapses with central nociceptive transmission cells resulting in onward transmission of noxious information to the brain leading to increased pain sensation. When the 'pain gate' is closed there is a reduction in central nociceptive transmission cell activity resulting in a diminished pain sensation. The pain gate is closed by synaptic inhibition of central nociceptive transmission by:

- increasing activity in low-threshold (innocuous) mechano and thermal afferents (spinal modulation)
- descending pain-inhibitory pathways arising from the brain (supra-spinal modulation).

Synaptic inhibition is generated via interneurones that release inhibitory neurotransmitters onto the terminals of peripheral afferents (pre-synpatic inhibition) or the dendrites of central nociceptive cells (post-synaptic inhibition). Inhibitory neurotransmitters include gamma-amino-butyric acid (GABA), glycine, and met-enkephalin. Opioid peptides, serotonin, and noradrenaline are involved in transmission via descending pain-inhibitory nerve pathways resulting in pre- and post-synaptic inhibition of central nociceptive transmission neurones in the spinal cord and brainstem.

Activity in low-threshold, non-noxious mechanoreceptive afferents can be easily achieved by rubbing healthy skin close to painful or damaged areas of the body—'rubbing pain away'. Conventional TENS utilizes this mechanism by delivering electrical currents through the skin to activate selectively non-noxious peripheral afferents—'electrically rubbing pain away'. Activity in descending pain-inhibitory nerve pathways can be achieved via motivational and distraction techniques. These descending pain-inhibitory nerve pathways arise from the telencephalon and diencephalon, and descend through the brainstem via synapses in the periaqueductal grey and Raphe nuclei terminating in the spinal cord. Acupuncture-like TENS utilizes this mechanism by delivering electrical currents through the skin to stimulate peripheral afferents that activate descending pain-inhibitory nerve pathways. TENS is one of many techniques that utilize electromagnetic or physical energy to create physiological changes in the activity of the nociceptive system to reduce pain.

Electrophysical techniques for pain and rehabilitation

Electrophysical techniques introduce electromagnetic, physical, or light energy into the body to interact with tissue to relieve pain and to promote recovery of injury or function (Watson, 2000) (Table 2.5). Physical therapies activate mechanical and thermal receptors of the somatosensory system (body surface) or stimulate nerve axons directly using therapeutic heat and cold, manipulation, mobilization, massage, traction,

Table 2.5 Examples of electrophysical techniques

Non-invasive electrical stimulation	Invasive electrical stimulation techniques	Thermal techniques	Non-thermal techniques
♦ TENS using a standard TENS device ♦ TENS using TENS-like devices (e.g. Interferential current therapy, microcurrent electrical therapy, transcutaneous piezoelectric current; see Chapter 11) ♦ Transcranial magnetic stimulation of the brain	♦ Peripheral nerve stimulation ♦ Spinal cord stimulation ♦ Deep brain stimulation ♦ Motor cortex stimulation	♦ Shortwave diathermy ♦ Infrared irradiation ♦ Microwave diathermy ♦ Wax therapy ♦ Balneotherapy ♦ Therapeutic ultrasound ♦ Cold therapies (e.g. cryotherapy, ice, topical creams) ♦ Heat therapies (e.g. hot-water bottles, topical creams)	♦ Ultrasound ♦ Low-level laser therapy ♦ Pulsed electro-magnetic fields ♦ Magnetic therapy ♦ Pulsed microwave therapy

Source: data from Tim Watson, *Key Concepts in Electrotherapy*, Copyright © 2012; available from: <http://www.electrotherapy.org/assets/Downloads/Key%20Concepts%20in%20Electrotherapy%20Jan%202012.pdf>.

ultrasound, vibration, and acupuncture. Light therapies use photons generated by devices such as low-level laser therapy that are absorbed by tissue, leading to chemical reactions resulting in increases in ATP, reducing oxidative stress, and improving cell metabolism. Electrical therapies (electrotherapy) influence activity of nerves or tissues for a variety of outcomes including relief of pain. Some non-thermal techniques can generate thermal changes if given at sufficiently high doses, although some of their physiological and therapeutic effects are not dependent on thermal changes in tissues.

Most electrotherapies are claimed to reduce pain, alleviate oedema, and promote tissue repair, although the status of research evidence is a topic of a great deal of debate, resulting in variability in clinical practice which is often based on tradition, clinical experience, and hearsay. Practitioners from different professional backgrounds may be unfamiliar with electrotherapeutic techniques used outside their own professional boundaries or even their local practice.

Invasive electrical stimulation techniques

Invasive electrical stimulation techniques are used to manage intractable pain that is resistant to other treatment, and it is especially useful in managing pain with neuropathic elements. The cost of equipment and staffing tends to be more expensive than non-invasive electrical stimulation techniques. Comprehensive reviews of the various techniques can be found in the textbook by Simpson (2003).

Peripheral nerve stimulation

Peripheral nerve stimulation was developed in the 1960s and uses wire-like electrodes inserted beneath the skin and implanted directly on a nerve using surgical visualization or more commonly, in close proximity to the nerve using percutaneous techniques. The electrode is connected to an external stimulator in the first instance, and if successful, a small electrical pulse generator is implanted under the skin at an appropriate site in the patient's body. A variety of nerve bundles are used as targets to generate different physiological responses for various conditions (see Table 4.1, Chapter 4). When peripheral nerve stimulation is used for pain relief the mechanism of action is similar to TENS via excitation of low-threshold afferents leading to inhibition of onward nociceptive transmission in the spinal cord (Chapter 9, Figure 9.1). Peripheral nerve stimulation generates electrical paraesthesia over the site of pain in a similar manner to TENS. It is used to treat pains where it might be difficult to generate electrical paraesthesia over the pain using other techniques. Peripheral nerve stimulation is effective for neuropathic pain involving one or two peripheral nerves and especially for lesions that are distal to the site of stimulation. When used for the management of other conditions the mechanism of action may be via activation of efferents that regulate autonomic effector organs including the bladder and bowel.

Subcutaneous peripheral field stimulation, also called peripheral field nerve stimulation, is very similar to peripheral nerve stimulation and tends to place electrodes into the painful area itself using percutaneous techniques without naming a target nerve. Stimulation of peripheral nerves can also be achieved using acupuncture needles inserted into the soft tissues or muscles to stimulate either nerve fibres or acupuncture points often at sites related to the location and the potential origin of the pain. Whether this technique differs from electroacupuncture is a matter for debate.

Spinal cord stimulation

Spinal cord stimulation delivers pulsed electrical currents to the spinal cord via implanted electrodes to manage chronic pain or motor dysfunction. Early spinal cord stimulation techniques used radio-frequency stimulation of plate electrodes placed over the dorsal columns. Modern techniques use electrodes that have been implanted in the epidural space and these are powered by a pulse generator implanted subcutaneously usually in the lower abdomen or posterior superior gluteal region. The electrodes are connected to the spinal cord stimulation device and its remote controller. The purpose of spinal cord stimulation is to produce a sensation of electrical paraesthesia within a region of pain. There is a risk of infection although major complications are rare.

The findings of systematic reviews suggest that spinal cord stimulation is effective for refractory neuropathic back and leg pain from failed back surgery syndrome, chronic low back pain, complex regional pain syndrome (CRPS) (type 1), and chronic critical limb ischaemia. Good-quality RCTs provide evidence that spinal cord stimulation is effective for refractory angina pectoris and diabetic neuropathy. Treatment success depends on careful patient selection with decision-analytic modelling showing that two-year cost-effectiveness for patients with failed back surgery syndrome ranged from €30,370 to €63,511 (Taylor & Taylor, 2005). Spinal cord stimulation was more effective and less costly than conventional medical management over the lifetime of failed back surgery syndrome patients. Originally it was thought that spinal cord stimulation inhibited ongoing transmission of nociceptive information in the posterior horn by stimulating A-β fibres in the spinal cord, although recent research suggests that the mechanism is more complex involving descending pain-inhibitory pathways, the autonomic nervous system, and visceral pathways in the posterior columns (Linderoth & Foreman, 2006).

Deep brain stimulation and motor cortex stimulation

Deep brain stimulation has been in used for decades on selected patients and involves the delivery of electrical pulsed currents to stimulate the grey matter of the brain to relieve treatment-resistant chronic pain, movement disorders including Parkinson's disease, essential tremor, and dystonia, and severe depression. Electrodes are implanted stereotactically via a burr hole under local anaesthesia and an electrical pulse generator implanted subcutaneously below the clavicle or in the abdomen. Hazards during electrode insertion include haemorrhage, infection, or seizures. Areas stimulated for nociceptive pain include the periventricular and periaqueductal grey matter, and for neuropathic pain these include the sensory thalamus and internal capsule. Evidence from a meta-analysis of six studies found that deep brain stimulation provided better long-term success for nociceptive pains than neuropathic pain (Bittar et al., 2005). In general, success rates are dependent on appropriate selection of patients.

In recent years motor cortex stimulation has been indicated for the management of intractable neuropathic pain and for patients who do not respond to deep brain stimulation. Electrodes are implanted in the epidural motor cortex electrodes often via a small craniotomy and using intraoperative neuro-navigation and cortical mapping for site targeting on the motor homunculus of the contralateral primary motor cortex. Clinical research evidence on effectiveness is limited although a systematic review with meta-analysis of 22 studies using invasive brain stimulation found that brain stimulation of motor cortex reduced chronic pain, with invasive brain stimulation having a larger effect (Lima & Fregni, 2008).

Non-invasive transcranial magnetic stimulation

Recent developments in technology have resulted in greater use of non-invasive brain stimulating techniques for the management of chronic pain because they are safer to administer, and technological advances have improved spatial resolution enabling more precise targeting of brain areas. Repetitive transcranial magnetic stimulation is a non-invasive technique that uses electromagnetic induction techniques to deliver rapidly changing magnetic fields through the skull to create weak electric currents that stimulate discrete areas of the cerebral cortex in individuals who are awake. Magnetic fields are created by a coil of wire enclosed in plastic casing that is held above the skull and does not come into contact with it. It is claimed that using magnets rather than direct electric current improves comfort during stimulation. Repetitive transcranial magnetic stimulation has been used to treat chronic pain, movement disorders, Parkinson's disease, dystonia, and depression. It is claimed that repetitive transcranial magnetic stimulation causes excitation or inhibition of neural circuits and may also produce changes in cortex architecture at the site of stimulation and at related sites including the spinal cord, and that this leads to pain relief. In 2008, a meta-analysis of 11 studies using various non-invasive brain stimulation techniques found evidence that repetitive transcranial magnetic stimulation of the motor cortex relieved chronic pain (Lima & Fregni, 2008). In 2011 a Cochrane review with a meta-analysis of 19 studies found that single doses of high-frequency repetitive transcranial magnetic stimulation of the motor cortex produced short-term reductions in chronic pain, although this was below the threshold for clinically meaningful effects (O'Connell et al., 2011). Furthermore, low-frequency repetitive transcranial magnetic stimulation did not relieve chronic pain.

Extent of use of TENS

TENS is offered within primary, secondary, and tertiary care by physicians, physiotherapists, nurses, midwives, and other health-care professionals because it has a favourable utility profile compared with medication (Table 2.6). Electrophysical techniques are predominantly used in physiotherapy outpatient departments and private clinics rather than in primary care, with TENS and interferential current therapy proving popular in England, Australia, and Canada (Lindsay et al., 1995; Pope et al., 1995; Robertson & Spurritt, 1998). A postal survey of 3538 registered physiotherapists in Australia by Chipchase and colleagues (2009) found that TENS, interferential therapy, electromyographic and pressure biofeedback, was used on a daily or monthly basis by between 30 per cent and 45 per cent. A postal survey of 83 physiotherapists working in the UK National Health Service utilized exercise supplemented with electrotherapeutic techniques including TENS by 66 per cent practitioners (Walsh & Hurley, 2009). However, the availability of TENS in primary health-care settings, including general practices, remains low. A survey of 129 general practitioners and 77 physiotherapists at 35 primary health-care centres in Uppsala County in Sweden found that few practitioners indicated TENS (Peterson et al., 2005).

There is variation in the use of TENS within and between professions due in part to clinical practices dominated by personal views and experiences of undergraduate courses. Jamtvedt and colleagues (2008) compared evidence from systematic reviews with clinical practice gathered from 297 private physiotherapy practitioners in Norway who collected treatment data of one patient with knee osteoarthritis over 12 treatment sessions. Despite 'moderate' evidence of effectiveness from systematic reviews only 35 per cent of physiotherapists used TENS, or acupuncture, or low-level laser therapy, although 98 per cent used exercise consistent with evidence in support. Physiotherapists used four different treatment modalities for each patient (median) many of which lacked evidence from systematic reviews. Interestingly, severity or co-morbidity did not influence the choice of treatments used to manage knee osteoarthritis by physiotherapists in primary care (Jamtvedt et al., 2010).

TENS expenditure

Patients obtain TENS devices and accessories in a variety of ways depending on local health-care policies and practices. In 2000, the total market for electrotherapy in Norway

Table 2.6 Advantages and disadvantages of TENS

Compared with invasive electrical stimulation techniques

Advantages	Disadvantages

◆ Non-invasive
◆ Better safety profile
◆ Less expensive (equipment, running costs and staffing)
◆ Does not require the expertise of a physician
	◆ Less efficacious for severe intractable neuropathic pain
	◆ Difficulty in stimulating deeper nerves
	◆ Difficulty in achieving stimulation sensation within deep-seated pains
	◆ In the presence of tactile allodynia
	  • Electrodes may irritate skin
	  • Stimulation of cutaneous nerves may worsen pain

Compared with medication

Advantages	Disadvantages
◆ Better safety profile, fewer contraindications, side effects, and drug interactions ◆ Less expensive ◆ No potential for toxicity or addiction ◆ Dosage titrated according to need by patient (empowering patient) ◆ Use as needed ◆ Can be used during activities without affecting alertness ◆ Rapid onset of pain relief	◆ Time and cost associated with training patient-appropriate application technique ◆ Occasional equipment malfunction ◆ Presence of stimulation sensation needed for pain relief ◆ Effort to administer TENS technique reduces adherence ◆ Short post-treatment pain relief

was estimated to be between NOK6 million and NOK7 million (~GB£700,000), with the total public health insurance fee for electrophysical agent services being NOK78.8 million (~GB£8,000,000), although there was no data breakdown for annual expenditure for TENS (Bjordal et al., 2001). The cost of purchasing TENS equipment may be incurred by the patients themselves when buying or renting 'over the counter', the health-care service through health-care taxation, or from charity fundraising and gifts, or via medical insurance . In some countries individuals can claim back the purchase costs of TENS from health-care insurance.

Medicare is the federal health insurance program in the USA. The total number of Medicare beneficiaries purchasing a new TENS device in 2010 was 84,705, a total which had doubled over the preceding five-year period (Jacques et al., 2012). Twice as many women claimed than men with most claimants aged between 65 years and 74 years (n=31,394). Chabal and colleagues (1998) conducted a cost–benefit analysis and found that TENS reduced costs for medications by 55 per cent, and for physical therapy and occupational therapy services TENS reduced costs by 69 per cent. This suggests that TENS could be a potentially cost-effective treatment in resource-limited environments.

TENS in resource-limited environments

There is a case for TENS as a potential treatment where pain management is inadequate because of limited resources, ignorance by health-care professionals, and unavailability of analgesics that are adulterated, or have perished. TENS is available over the counter or via the internet in most resource-limited countries with no restriction on sales, although the cost relative to income is greater in these countries rather than in their wealthier counterparts. Medical practitioners can play a major role by recommending the use of TENS and referring the patient to a physiotherapist or a nurse who educates the patient on how to use TENS.

TENS technology may be more acceptable to individuals who are exposed to technology in their daily life and more acceptable in urban settings than rural, village settings. Most urban dwellers in resource-limited countries are familiar with mobile phones and electronic gadgetry, even if they are from lower socio-economic backgrounds, so TENS is likely to be accepted, especially if health-care services are using a modern, medically based model of health care. In rural settings in resource-limited countries there are likely to be barriers to using TENS because attitudes to pain management may be more traditional and the use of TENS counter-intuitive to beliefs about pain treatment. In hot, dusty climates, carbon–rubber electrodes would be more practical than self-adhering electrodes which will deteriorate if they are not kept in cool, dust-free conditions. In addition, the cost of replacement batteries may also be prohibitive. TENS devices could be lent to in-patients for the duration of their stay in hospital with costs to the clinic being initial outlay for TENS devices, and replacing batteries and self-adhering electrodes. Out-patients could borrow a TENS device from the clinic with a view to buying for themselves, perhaps through a series of monthly instalments. The use of carbon–rubber electrodes that can be cleaned after each patient would reduce costs compared with purchasing self-adhering electrodes for each new patient. For TENS to be more widely accepted in resource-limited countries health promotion authorities need to raise public and heath-care practitioner awareness about the potential role of TENS (Tashani & Johnson, 2009).

Regulation of safety and effectiveness

Most countries have government departments responsible for assuring safety and effectiveness of medical devices that are commercially available. In Europe TENS falls under the European Union core legal framework Directive 93/42/EEC regarding medical devices to ensure protection of human health and safety. Each member state appoints a competent authority to ensure that medical device directives are transposed into national law. In the UK, the Medicines and Healthcare products Regulatory Agency (MHRA) is the competent authority that investigates allegations about non-compliance with regulations, although approval of medical devices is undertaken by 'notified bodies' in the private sector rather than the MHRA itself (see: <http://www.mhra.gov.uk/Howweregulate/Devices/index.htm>). In the UK, TENS is categorized as a Class IIa low-risk medical device and subject to special labelling requirements, mandatory performance standards, and post-market surveillance (Table 2.7).

Table 2.7 Categories of medical device

Class	Level of risk and control	Examples
Class I	Low: non-invasive devices Least regulatory control	Elastic bandages, examination gloves, and hand-held surgical instruments
Class IIa	Medium: active therapeutic devices administering or exchanging energy General controls with special controls	TENS devices Muscle stimulators and electro-acupuncture External bone growth stimulators
Class IIb	Medium: potentially hazardous active therapeutic devices, i.e. intended for wounds that breach dermis or supply ionizing radiation General controls with special controls	Electroconvulsive therapy High-frequency electrosurgical generators External pacemakers/defibrillators Electrocautery equipment
Class III	High: implantable devices General controls and pre-market approval	Implantable electrical pulse generators Internal pacemakers and automated external defibrillators

All medical devices must be identified with the CE mark declaring conformity of the product with requirements of the European Commission directives that it is safe and functions for the intended purpose as described by the manufacturer. Thus, a CE-marked TENS device is a declaration from the manufacturer that the device intends to relieve pain safely; the mark is similar in function to a medicine license. Compliance with these requirements is proved within a certified quality management system according to ISO 9000 and therefore TENS devices from the UK should have a National Accreditation and Certification Board tick and Crown logo printed in the manufacturer's literature.

Similar systems are found in the USA, Canada, and Australia. In the USA, the Center for Devices and Radiological Health of the Food and Drug Administration (FDA) is responsible for assuring access to safe, effective, and high-quality medical devices. In the USA, market approval for TENS was 'grandfathered' because it was marketed before the introduction of the 1976 Medical Device Amendments to the Federal Food, Drug, and Cosmetic Act. 'New' TENS devices are approved by assessing whether the device is equivalent to devices commercially available (i.e. substantial equivalence). Assessments are made against any changes or modifications to the design, material, chemical composition, energy source, manufacturing process, or intended use. Hence, TENS as a treatment modality for pain relief is cleared under 510(k) guidelines and has never undergone a recent, full, pre-market approval process. This has started to raise doubts about whether there is reasonable assurance of safety and effectiveness. In 2010, the Center for Devices and Radiological Health issued guidance for industry and FDA staff which required that any submissions for 510(k) clearance for a TENS device for pain relief must meet the requirements of 21 CFR 807.87, and also must comply with special controls to assure safety and effectiveness.

On 8 June 2012, the Centers for Medicare & Medicaid Services in the USA revised its coverage for TENS for chronic low back pain of three months or longer that does not result from a primary disease entity (Jacques et al., 2012). An analysis of research by the Centers for Medicare & Medicaid Services concluded that there was inadequate research evidence to support TENS for chronic low back pain. Objections from TENS advocates (Sluka et al., 2013) and the general public were overruled by the Centers for Medicare & Medicaid Services because available evidence was not sufficient to conclude that TENS is reasonable and necessary for chronic low back pain. It was decided that Medicare insurance coverage would only continue for individuals enrolled in an approved randomized, controlled clinical study that addresses the following:

- Does the use of TENS provide clinically meaningful reduction in pain in Medicare beneficiaries with chronic low back pain?
- Does the use of TENS provide a clinically meaningful improvement of function in Medicare beneficiaries with chronic low back pain?
- Does the use of TENS impact the utilization of other medical treatments or services used in the medical management of chronic low back pain?

This period of evidence development and associated insurance coverage is due to expire on 8 June 2015. Clearly, the uncertainty about effectiveness also raises questions about how TENS is advertised to the general public.

Regulation of advertising

In the UK, the Advertising Standards Authority, a non-statutory organization funded by a levy on the advertising industry, is responsible for regulating the content of advertisements, sales promotions, and direct marketing of products. Its sister organization, the Committee of Advertising Practice, is responsible for revising and updating the British Code of Advertising, Direct Marketing and Sales Promotion. The Committee of Advertising Practice takes a position that research evidence for TENS effectiveness is inconclusive and allows commercial companies to make claims about the ability of TENS to provide temporary relief of minor aches and pains, but not to make claims for chronic or serious conditions unless robust randomized controlled clinical trials are forthcoming (Committee of Advertising Practice, 2010). Studies on animals, dorsal horn cells, or in vitro are usually not acceptable to make claims about clinical effectiveness. A detailed discussion of the reliability and validity of clinic research evidence is provided in Chapter 8 (150–171), although it should be remembered that evidence-based practice combines knowledge from clinical research with that from clinical experience.

TENS: clinical experience

Case series, surveys, and audits suggest that 50–80 per cent of individuals who try TENS report meaningful pain relief, with some individuals continuing to use TENS for many years reporting improvements in pain interference, activity level, and use of non-pharmacological and pharmacological therapies (Johnson et al., 1992a; Fishbain et al., 1996). The first case series on the success of TENS was published by Long (1974) and there has been a continuous stream of case series ever since. Loeser and colleagues (1975) reported that 68 per cent of 198 chronic patients achieved short-term pain relief with TENS declining to 12.5 per cent in the long term. Bates and Nathan (1980) reported the results of seven-years' experience of treating 74 patients with post-herpetic neuralgia, and 161 patients with various chronic pains, and found that half of the patients returned their stimulators after one month, but one-quarter of patients were still using TENS after two years. Eriksson and colleagues (1979) found that initially 75 per cent of patients reported more than 50 per cent pain relief and that 55 per cent continued using TENS after three months, 41 per cent at 12 months, and 31 per cent at 24 months. However, approximately 30 per cent of patients required AL-TENS to get meaningful pain relief. In a later study, Eriksson and colleagues (1984) found that 45 per cent of patients with atypical facial pain reported satisfactory pain relief from conventional or AL-TENS at two-year follow-up. A study of long-term use of TENS at a pain clinic in the UK found that 58.6 per cent of 1,582 patients who tried TENS continued to use it for several years (Johnson et al., 1992c), although 32 per cent of long-term TENS users reported a decline in the efficacy of TENS since the time of issue (Johnson et al., 1991c).

A similar proportion of respondents have been found in randomized controlled clinical trials (RCTs). Koke and colleagues (2004) found that 56 per cent of participants with chronic pain continued to use high-frequency, low-intensity conventional TENS at two-week follow-up and 42 per cent continuing to use TENS at six-month follow-up. Likewise, an RCT by Oosterhof and colleagues (2008) found that 58 per cent patients receiving TENS were satisfied with treatment. However, 42.7 per cent of patients were also satisfied with placebo TENS suggesting that non-specific treatment effects associated with the act of receiving a treatment rather than the active ingredient of the treatment (i.e. electrical currents) were contributing to self-report of satisfaction. It is for this reason that RCTs are needed to evaluate the efficacy of TENS (see Chapter 8). Oosterhof and colleagues (2008) also found that patients diagnosed with osteoarthritis or peripheral neuropathic pain were less satisfied with high-frequency TENS than were patients with injury of bone and soft tissue (especially post-surgical pain), suggesting that TENS parameters and type of pain may affect outcome (Chapter 4, 78–85).

Overall, long-term, follow-up data are variable but suggest that use of TENS declines over time although up to 50 per cent of patients given a trial of TENS may achieve meaningful pain relief after one year. However, the evidence is not consistent with reports that some patients find repeated application of TENS improves the pain relief (cumulative response). For example, Marchand and colleagues (1993) found that over time, repeated treatment sessions of TENS reduced the intensity of chronic low back pain, and Oosterhof and colleagues (2006) found that repeated treatment sessions of TENS reduced the intensity of pain in a mixed population of chronic pain patients referred to a pain centre. One problem has been obtaining reliable data about usage. Recently, Pallett and colleagues (2013) used electronic data-logging devices to time-link pain report to TENS use, and found that 42 per cent of individuals with non-specific chronic low back pain achieved ≥30 per cent reduction in pain score during TENS in the short term. Capturing data in this way over a longer time period would be useful. The decline in the effect of TENS over time may be due to a variety of factors including placebo response, worsening pain condition, physiological tolerance, and nervous system habituation, and too much effort required to administer TENS regularly.

Summary

1   TENS modulates activity and sensitivity of the nociceptive system.

2   TENS has a favourable utility profile compared with medication.

3   TENS is categorized as a Class IIa medical device and subject to special labelling requirements, mandatory performance standards, and post-market surveillance.

4   50–80 per cent of individuals who try TENS report improvements in pain symptoms and activity levels in the short term although benefits may decline over time.

5   Some patients continue to use TENS for many years.

Further reading

+ Johnson, M.I. (2005) Physiology of chronic pain. In Banks, C., and Mackrodt, K. (eds) *Chronic Pain Management*. Whurr Publishers Ltd, London, 36–74.

+ Johnson, M.I., Ashton, C.H., and Thompson, J.W. (1991) An in-depth study of long-term users of transcutaneous electrical nerve stimulation (TENS). Implications for clinical use of TENS. *Pain*, **44**, 221–9.

+ Simpson, B.A. (ed.) (2003) *Electrical Stimulation and the Relief of Pain*. Elsevier, Amsterdam.

+ Walsh, D. (1997) *TENS. Clinical applications and related theory*. Churchill Livingstone, New York.

+ Electrotherapy resources for practitioners, students, and educators. See: <http://www.electrotherapy.org>.

Chapter 3 will review the biophysical principles of TENS prior to provide foundation knowledge to underpin safe and appropriate use of TENS.

Chapter 3

TENS equipment, techniques, and biophysical principles

Introduction

Over the decades there has been much debate about the most appropriate way to administer TENS arising in part from the array of possible combinations of electrical characteristics attainable from a standard TENS device. This has resulted in uncertainty about optimal technique for TENS, leading to the use of irrational treatment protocols in some circumstances. The purpose of TENS is to provide an electrical stimulus of sufficient amplitude to depolarize the axonal membrane and to generate nerve impulses that modulate the flow of nociceptive information and reduce pain. A variety of factors influence the ability of electrical currents to depolarize the axonal membrane, including the electrical characteristics of the currents (i.e. stimulating parameters) and physiology at the electrode–skin interface. The purpose of this chapter is to provide an overview of the biophysical principles of TENS and to explain how these principles have been used to inform clinical practice. It covers:

◆ TENS equipment and the standard TENS device
◆ The electrical characteristics of currents produced by a standard TENS device
◆ Lead wires and electrodes
◆ Physiology at the electrode–skin interface, including nerve fibre activation by TENS
◆ TENS techniques used in clinical practice including conventional TENS and acupuncture-like TENS (AL-TENS)

TENS equipment

The manufacture of TENS equipment is a profitable exercise so equipment is frequently launched on the market with a bewildering array of purchase possibilities. It is worth piloting different TENS devices and accessories to determine how effective, reliable, and economical they are from the point of view of the patients and staff who will be using the equipment. For the purposes of this book TENS devices are categorized as either a standard TENS device or a TENS-like device, according to their technical output characteristics.

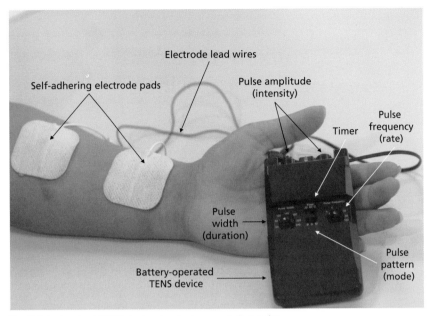

Fig. 3.1 A standard TENS device, lead wires, and electrodes.

TENS equipment consists of:

- a standard TENS device (stimulator)
- electrodes
- connecting lead wires (Figure 3.1)

Standard TENS device

Standard TENS devices are portable, battery-powered, electrical pulse generators that produce monophasic or biphasic waveforms of pulsed electrical currents in a repetitive manner (Figure 3.2). The main components of a standard TENS device are:

- A power source to generate electrical currents, usually a 9V PP3 or 2 × AA 1.5V batteries.
- DC oscillators to transform direct current (DC) from batteries to a pulsed output, and to determine the rate (pulses per second, pps) and pattern (mode) of pulses.
- An amplifier to amplify battery power to maximum peak-to-peak amplitude of approximately 60 milliamperes (mA) into a 1 kilohm load.

Most standard TENS devices enable adjustment of pulse amplitude, frequency, duration, and pattern (Figure 3.3). There are variations in the design between manufacturers, with the incorporation of additional features tending to increase the cost of the device. Often manufacturers rebrand standard TENS devices following cosmetic or minor technical modifications such as redesigning the outer casing, adding preset combinations of TENS parameters, or providing add-on accessories such as a hand-held

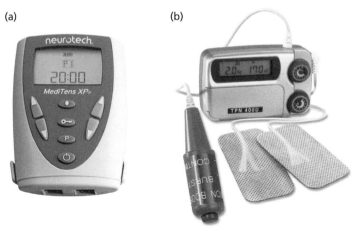

Fig. 3.2 Standard TENS devices with digital displays: (a) touchpad controls and (b) obstetric TENS used for labour pain with a 'boost button' control for contraction pain.

Images courtesy of Patterson Medical Ltd, www.pattersonmedical.co.uk

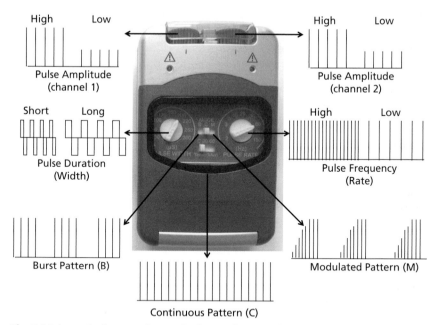

Fig. 3.3 Schematic diagram of a standard TENS device and output characteristics.

intensity 'boost' button for use in treating contraction pain during childbirth. In these instances the technical output specifications do not differ substantially from a standard TENS device (Table 3.1). Battery usage increases by using higher pulse amplitudes and frequencies, longer pulse durations, and continuous patterns of pulse delivery. For individuals who are using TENS frequently and for prolonged periods of time, it may be worth purchasing rechargeable batteries. A packet of four rechargeable batteries that can be charged hundreds of times costs approximately GB£20.00, and this could equate to a saving of hundreds of pounds over time.

Characteristics of currents from a standard TENS device

Principles of electricity

Electric current is the flow of electric charge through a medium. Electric charge can be carried in a metallic solid (e.g. a wire) by negatively charged electrons moving through a conductor or in other conductive media (e.g. water) by the movement of any type of charged particles. For example, electric currents in liquid electrolytes, such as body fluids, are generated by streams of positively and negatively charged ions. The rate of flow of electric charge (i.e. electric current) is measured in amperes. The driving force to move an electric charge across a resistance is voltage (V). Voltage refers to the difference in electric potential between two points (e.g. in space, a material, or an electric circuit). Resistance is a material's opposition to the flow of direct electric current. Direct current (DC) describes the flow of electric charge that is in one direction. Alternating current (AC) describes the flow of electric charge that periodically reverses direction, i.e. from positive to negative or vice versa. The relationship between voltage and current is described by Ohms law where Voltage (V) = Current (I) × Resistance (R).

Resistance is any force that opposes the flow of DC and is similar to friction, which is encountered in mechanical forces. The converse of resistance is electrical conductance (measured in Siemens) which is the ease with which an electric current passes through a material. Impedance is the opposition to the flow of an AC through a material and considers the magnitude and the phase of the current. Resistance only considers the magnitude of current because there is no phase in DC. There is no distinction between impedance and resistance during DC because the impedance would have a zero-phase angle. The term 'impedance' is more appropriate in discussions about TENS because TENS uses pulsed currents that have magnitude and phase. Impedance is encountered at the electrode–skin interface where the opposition to the flow of current between electrode and biological tissue is at its greatest; thus, good electrical contact between electrode and skin is necessary to reduce impedance and to improve conductance.

Waveform

Waveform is the shape of a current and is represented by plotting amplitude against time (Figure 3.4).

Direct current flows continuously over time in one direction and AC flows continuously over time in a bidirectional manner (Robertson et al., 2006). A standard TENS device produces pulsed currents where the flow of current periodically ceases and may produce single polarity (monophasic) or polarity that is positive in one phase of the wave and negative in the other (biphasic). Biphasic waveforms may be symmetrical, where the first phase of the wave is a mirror image with opposite polarity to the second phase of the wave, or asymmetrical where it is not. Human skin exhibits a non-linear relationship with stimulation current and this will distort a monophasic rectangular waveform into an asymmetrical waveform when applied via TENS electrodes (Figure 3.4e).

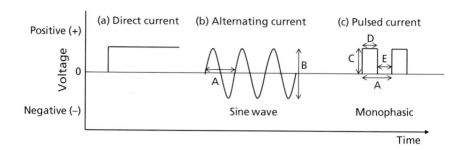

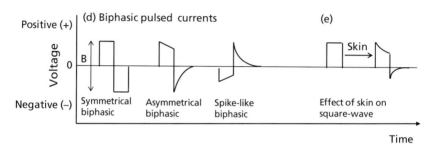

Fig. 3.4 Waveforms of electrical current. (a) DC, (b) AC sine, (c) monophasic pulsed square wave, (d) biphasic pulsed square wave, and (e) effect of skin on monophasic pulsed wave. Key: A = duration of one cycle (period); B = peak-to-peak amplitude; C = pulse amplitude (monophasic); D = pulse duration, often measured at 50 per cent of pulse amplitude for non-square waveforms; E = inter-pulse interval. Frequency is calculated as the number of cycles or pulses in 1 second. second per period.

By convention the direction of electric current is opposite to the direction of the flow of electrons, so rather confusingly electrons flow into the TENS device whilst flowing out of the electrical circuit made by the patient. For monophasic pulsed waves the cathode (negative) is the electrode through which electric current flows out of a device (Cathode Current Departs, or CID) and the anode (positive) where current flows in (Anode Current into Device, or ACID). The cathode excites the axonal membrane leading to an action potential (Figure 3.5). Most modern TENS devices use biphasic waveforms because monophasic waveforms may cause an accumulation of ions, resulting in polar concentrations beneath the electrodes that may cause reactions in underlying tissue.

Devices that utilize symmetrical biphasic waveforms where the cathode and anode alternate between each electrode for the same period of time, result in zero net current flow and no build-up of ion concentrations beneath electrodes. Devices that utilize asymmetric biphasic waveforms, where current flow is slightly unequal in both directions act more like monophasic waveforms, so placement of the cathode and anode may affect excitation of underlying tissue. Thus, for devices using monophasic pulsed waves or asymmetric biphasic waveforms, the cathode is placed directly over the nerve and proximal to the anode to prevent block of nerve transmission due to

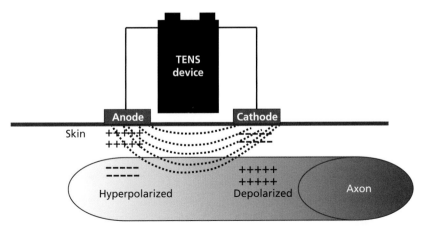

Fig. 3.5 A build-up of negative charge beneath the cathode creates a membrane potential that depolarizes the axon.

hyperpolarization of the underlying tissue at the anode, although this tends not to be an issue when using surface electrodes. By convention the cathode is the black lead.

Pulse amplitude

Pulse amplitude refers to the magnitude of current (mA) or voltage (V) delivered (Figure 3.5). As current activates the nerve axon, current amplitude is the key parameter. Amplitude should be distinguished from intensity which is the subjective phenomenon experienced by an individual when amplitude is changed, i.e. the magnitude of the resultant sensation. Peak amplitude refers to the maximum value of the electrical current waveform from zero whereas peak-to-peak amplitude refers to the peak of the positive phase of the electrical current waveform to the peak of the negative phase.

Increasing pulse amplitude whilst maintaining pulse frequency, duration, and pattern at the same setting produces a more intense (stronger) TENS sensation. Research evidence suggests that hypoalgesia occurs when pulse amplitude, and subsequently TENS intensity, is above sensory-detection threshold, with a positive correlation between pulse amplitude, intensity, and hypoalgesia (Moran et al., 2011). The intensity of TENS subsides over time despite a constant pulse amplitude and therefore it is necessary to increase pulse amplitude during TENS to maintain TENS intensity and hypoalgesia (Pantaleao et al., 2011) (Chapter 4, 79–81).

Pulse duration (width)

Pulse duration is the time interval between the leading and trailing edge of a pulsed current, normally measured at 50 per cent of the positive peak amplitude although sometimes as the sum of the duration of the positive and negative phases. Increasing pulse duration produces more intense TENS sensations because of the high impedance of the skin to long pulses resulting in limited penetration of tissue and activation of cutaneous fibres. There is a negative correlation between pulse duration and pulse frequency at constant TENS intensity (Szeto, 1985).

Pulse frequency (rate)

Pulse frequency—labelled 'rate' on some TENS devices—is the number of pulsed currents per unit time and measured as pulses per second (pps), although hertz (Hz, cycles per second) are also used.

Increasing pulse frequency causes TENS sensations to feel more rapid from slow pulsate sensations at low frequencies, rapid pulsate sensations at intermediate frequencies (10 to ~ 60 pps), and electrical paraesthesiae with kinaesthetic sensations of body movement at high frequencies (>60 pps) (Geng et al., 2012). Furthermore, increasing pulse frequency increases the intensity of TENS sensation and lowers perception thresholds (Jelinek & McIntyre, 2010).

Pulse pattern (mode)

A continuous pattern of pulses—labelled 'normal' on some TENS devices—refers to the delivery of uninterrupted pulses (Figure 3.3). Adjustments to amplitude, frequency, and duration are more easily perceived during continuous patterns so it is the mode of choice when using TENS on a patient for the first time. Burst patterns deliver trains of pulses interrupted by periods of no current output (Figure 3.3). The frequency of the burst is usually preset in TENS devices at 2–4 bursts per second (bps), although the frequency of pulses contained within each burst (the internal pulse frequency) can be adjusted according to the upper and lower limits of the device. When burst patterns are used to induce phasic muscle contractions the internal pulse frequency should be set above the fusion frequency of skeletal muscle (i.e. between 20 pps and 50 pps) to achieve tetanic contraction of muscle within the phasic twitch. Nervous system processing of single rectangular pulses may differ from bursts of pulses, with burst stimulation less dependent on stimulus location (van der Heide et al., 2009). Whenever a user switches between patterns it is important to decrease pulse amplitude to reduce the chance of sudden discomfort.

Modulated patterns refer to pre-programmed fluctuations in one or more electrical characteristic by, say, ± 25 per cent of the dial setting (Figure 3.6). Amplitude modulation varies the amplitude of pulses between upper and lower limits over a fixed unit of time (e.g. 0.0–25 mA over three seconds followed by a two-second period of no current), frequency modulation varies frequency (e.g. 20–100 pps and back over 12 seconds), and duration modulation varies pulse duration (e.g. 50–250 μs and back over 12 seconds). Alternating patterns switch a variable, usually frequency, duration, or pattern at fixed time points (e.g. 2 pps for three seconds followed by 110 pps for three seconds).

Preset combinations of characteristics

Many modern devices, especially those with digital displays and touchpad facilities, offer preset combinations of electrical characteristics TENS which enables users to switch between different combinations of settings easily (see examples in Table 3.1). This may add to the cost of the device. Claims that certain preset parameters are efficacious for different painful conditions are not supported by available research evidence.

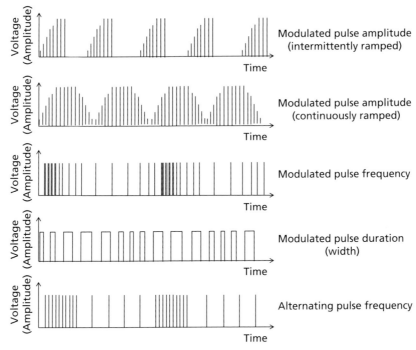

Fig. 3.6 Modulated pulse patterns.

Table 3.1 Output specifications of the majority of the commercially available standard TENS devices

Characteristic	Specification	Considerations
Electrical output		
Pulse waveform	◆ Biphasic (symmetrical or asymmetrical) or monophasic	◆ Usually fixed by manufacturer
Pulse amplitude	◆ Peak-to-peak voltage of 1–60 V with 1–60 mA into a 1 kilohm load (adjustable) ◆ Most are constant current	◆ Can a sufficiently strong TENS sensation be produced? ◆ Constant current devices prevent intensity surges
Pulse frequency (rate)	◆ 1–200 pps (adjustable)	◆ Can all frequencies be easily obtained? Is there a linear relationship between frequency and dial? ◆ Step-wise control may be helpful
Pulse duration (width)	◆ 50–500 µs (adjustable)	◆ As above

Table 3.1 (continued) Output specifications of the majority of the commercially available standard TENS devices

Characteristic	Specification	Considerations
Pulse pattern (mode)	◆ Continuous ◆ Burst (intermittent trains of pulses) ◆ Modulated amplitude ◆ Modulated frequency ◆ Modulated duration ◆ Random frequency	◆ Continuous and burst essential ◆ Is the internal frequency of the pulses adjustable? ◆ The frequency of burst patterns are usually permanent ◆ Modulation highly desirable but will increase cost
Channels	◆ One (single) or two (dual)	◆ Two channels essential for widespread pain or to treat more than one pain simultaneously ◆ Independent control of amplitude of each channel essential ◆ Desirable to have independent control of frequency and pattern but will increase cost
Additional features		
Pre-programmed settings (examples)	◆ Continuous, 110 pps, 50 µs ◆ Continuous, 4 pps, 200 µs ◆ Burst, 2 bps, 100 pps, 200 µs ◆ Modulated frequency, 20–110 pps, 200 µs ◆ Alternating frequency 2 pps/110 pps, 200 µs ◆ Modulated amplitude and duration, 110 pps, 50–250 µs	◆ Useful for individuals who have difficulty adjusting other settings ◆ There is no strong evidence that certain pre-programmed settings are better for specific types of pain
Timer	◆ 30 and 60 minutes	◆ Useful to assist sleep
Dials, touchpads, and switches	◆ Dials for continuous increments ◆ Touch pads for step-wise increments ◆ Switches for patterns and timer	◆ On–off switch and amplitude dial/pad should be easy to adjust ◆ Cover to protect accidental knocking or disturbance ◆ Larger dials, touch pads and switches for dexterity-challenged individuals (e.g. arthritic hands)
Output display	◆ Digital or analogue	◆ Easy to read
Cost	◆ GB£15.00–GB£100.00	◆ Additional features will increase cost

Table 3.1 (continued) Output specifications of the majority of the commercially available standard TENS devices

Characteristic	Specification	Considerations
Dimensions and weight	◆ Small device = 6 cm × 5 cm × 2 cm ◆ Large device = 12 cm × 9 cm × 4 cm (50–250 g)	◆ Compact, lightweight, and convenient shape so that comfortable to wear and handle ◆ Larger devices for dexterity-challenged individuals ◆ Colour to match favourite clothes ◆ Belt clip easily attachable to belt or pocket ◆ Inclusion of a carrying case
Batteries	◆ PP3 (9 V) or AA (2 × 1.5 V = 3 V)	◆ Standard batteries to ease replacement ◆ For intensive use consider rechargeable batteries
After-purchase support	◆ Instruction manual with DVD ◆ Web-support materials ◆ Manufacturers guarantee, helpline, and maintenance/ replacement service	◆ A simple and well-illustrated instruction manual is essential

Lead wires and electrodes

Lead wires

Lead wires take the currents from the TENS device to electrode pads attached to the intact surface of the skin and wires are thin, flexible, and durable so that they can run underneath clothes without irritating the skin (Figure 3.7). They are approximately 1 metre in length, and made of braided tinsel wire with a jack plug connector encased in a plastic sheath for an electrically safe attachment to the TENS device. The other end of the lead wire connects to the electrode and most, but not all, electrode systems use 2 mm-diameter pin (DIN42802) compatible with the international standard. Most electrodes are pre-wired with a lead connector to enable easy attachment of the lead wire pin although it is important to check compatibility before purchase of electrodes. Some electrodes use press-stud fastenings, ideal for patients who find lead wires inconvenient, although these may concentrate current under the stud unless they have some kind of compensation built into the system. Some press-stud fastenings can be difficult to source if replacements are required. In the past standard metal jack plugs, similar to those found in headphones and portable speakers, were used as the connector to the TENS device which enabled a set of portable speakers to be connected to the TENS device so that the patient could listen to the electrical output of the TENS device.

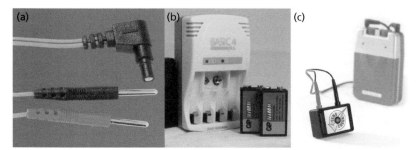

Fig. 3.7 TENS accessories. (a) Lead wire with 2 mm pin and jack plug connector, (b) battery recharger, and (c) TENS output and battery checker.

Images courtesy of Patterson Medical Ltd, www.pattersonmedical.co.uk

Electrodes

The function of the electrode is to provide an electrical conductivity medium to aid passage of currents through skin. There needs to be good contact between the electrode and the skin as current density decreases with poor contact. Electrodes that are deteriorating, inflexible, or 'dry' will cause pockets of increased current density ('hot spots') because of uneven electrical contact points with the skin. This will produce prickling sensations, skin irritation, and even mild skin burns.

Various types of electrodes have been used over the years (Figure 3.8). Carbon–rubber electrodes with wet-gel and adhesive tape were used from the outset of TENS in the late 1960s. Replaceable self-adhesive gel patches were introduced in the 1980s to improve conductivity and reduce messiness associated with the use of wet-gels in the carbon–rubber electrode systems. Nowadays, various types of self-adhesive electrodes with water-based gels using a carbon film or woven knitted stainless steel lattice to conduct currents. Carbon–rubber electrodes with wet-gel and adhesive-tape systems are still used in resource-limited settings.

Carbon–rubber electrodes with wet-gel and adhesive tape

Carbon–rubber electrodes with wet-gel and adhesive tape was the electrode system of choice for decades and is still popular in resource-limited countries because it is less expensive to replace gel and adhesive tape regularly than to replace new self-adhesive gel electrodes (Figure 3.8). Carbon–rubber electrodes need to be cleaned with soap and water after each use to remove conductive wet-gel. They are moulded from an elastomer such as silicone rubber or ethylene vinyl acetate and are impregnated with electrically conductive, finely divided carbon particles. They are used in conjunction with ion-containing conductive hydrogel made of water, thickening agents, and bactericides and fungicides. The ions contained within the conductive gel need to be compatible with tissue fluids and sweat to reduce skin irritation, and the electrolyte salt concentration should not be too high otherwise current may drive ions into skin via electrophoresis causing skin irritation. Carbon–rubber electrodes are generally flexible enough to follow body contours, and the conductive gel fills up troughs between the electrode and

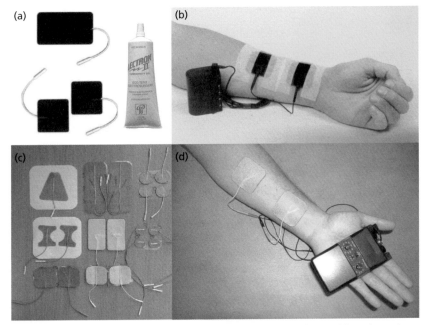

Fig. 3.8 TENS electrodes. (a) Carbon–rubber requiring gel, (b) carbon–rubber electrode system in situ, (c) self-adhesive re-usable electrodes, and (d) self-adhesive re-usable electrodes in situ.

Figure (a) courtesy of Patterson Medical Ltd. <http://www.pattersonmedical.co.uk>.

skin providing good contact as long as gel is spread evenly. The gel is wet and messy, and if the adhesive tape is not applied firmly then the electrodes can move across the surface of the skin shifting current distribution. Current hot spots will develop if gel dries out so regular replenishment is necessary if TENS is to be used for prolonged periods of time. Surgical microporous adhesive tape identical to that used to secure bandages and wound dressings to the skin is used to secure electrodes in position. Nowadays surgical tape uses hypoallergenic adhesive and microporous materials that enables exchange of gases but prevents airborne contaminants from getting to the skin.

Self-adhesive reusable electrodes
Reusable self-adhesive electrodes with hypoallergenic gel bonded into conducting materials such as a carbon film have replaced carbon–rubber electrodes and forgo the need for separate conductive gel and adhesive tape, making them more convenient to reposition (Table 3.2, Figure 3.8). The conductive fibres from the lead wire are woven into the conductive pad to provide an even distribution of current across the surface of the electrode. Self-adhesive electrodes become less sticky with each application and this may cause peeling of the electrodes from the skin and uneven distribution of currents (Barkana et al., 2010). Hydrating self-adhering electrodes by smearing an even film of water over the electrode helps to maintain stickiness.

Table 3.2 Main types of TENS electrodes

Characteristic	Specification	Considerations
Self-adhering electrodes	◆ Most common are square electrodes 5 cm × 5 cm ◆ Various size, shapes and colours available	◆ Self-adhesive gel is strong enough to keep the electrodes in place but easy to remove ◆ Electrodes are lightweight and flexible to follow contours of the skin and distribute currents evenly to prevent irritation or discomfort ◆ Match size, shape, and colour to body part to be stimulated ◆ Large rectangular electrodes for large areas of stimulation (e.g. post surgical pain) ◆ Small circular electrodes for acupuncture points ◆ Butterfly electrodes of skin creases ◆ Skin-tone coloured electrodes for exposed skin
◆ Carbon–rubber electrodes	◆ Require wet-gel and adhesive tape	◆ Easy to clean ◆ Re-useable with less deterioration than self-adhesive electrodes ◆ Useful in resource-limited environments ◆ Need supplier for gel and tape
◆ Garment electrodes	◆ Glove, sock, and sleeve	◆ Useful to keep body warm ◆ Check garment does not irritate skin (e.g. tactile allodynia)
◆ Specialized electrodes	◆ Knee brace, lower-back belt, and slipper electrode	◆ May provide postural support

Self-adhesive electrodes retail at around GB£5.00 per pack of four electrodes and are available in various shapes, sizes, and colours. Larger electrodes generate lower current density at the electrode–skin interface resulting in more comfortable TENS sensations, although they require more current to generate non-painful TENS sensations (Alon et al., 1994). Electrodes that are 50 mm × 50 mm are commonly used with larger rectangular strip-like electrodes (100 mm × 50 mm) useful when large areas need to be stimulated (e.g. post-surgical and maternity pain). Butterfly electrodes are useful for skin creases around small joints (e.g. groin, elbow crease), and small circular electrodes are useful to stimulate discrete points (e.g. acupuncture or trigger points) (Figure 3.8c). There is tentative evidence that small electrodes (8 mm × 8 mm) are more comfortable for stimulating superficial nerves lying at depths of 1 mm in the skin, and larger electrodes (41 mm × 41 mm) for stimulating nerves at depths of 11 mm (Kuhn et al., 2010). If two electrodes of different sizes were used simultaneously then the current density and strength of sensation would be higher beneath the smaller electrode.

The non-conductive backing side of the electrode is usually made of a woven cloth lace-fabric backing available in different colours including skin-tone, grey, white, and blue. Sometimes thin plastic foam, polyurethane film, or semi-rigid plastics are used. The conductive side of the electrode uses a self-adhesive conductive gel which is viscous (solid-like) and hydrophilic so it does not hydrate the skin (Figure 3.9). It may even absorb water from the skin. These viscous gels have higher resistive properties than the old-fashioned wet-like gels and therefore they may cause minor irritation of the skin. Stainless steel is often used as the conductive material because it has good conductivity and is chemically inert thus reducing the potential for chemical reactions leading to toxicity. Grid patterns are often used for the conductive material to spread electrical current evenly over the surface of the electrode. A non-conductive border around the face of the electrode provides a drop-off to current to prevent increased

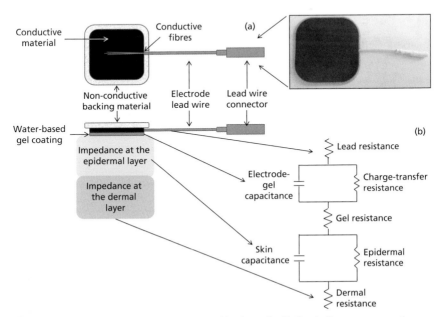

Fig. 3.9 (a) Composition of a self-adhesive re-usable electrode. (b) Circuit diagram repre-senting impedance at the electrode–gel and skin interfaces.

current densities that may be amplified at the edges and causing 'edge biting and sting-ing'. Some electrodes use flood-coated silver to reduce edge biting.

Electrode garments

Conductive garments are available as gloves, socks, and sleeves for legs (knee) and arms (elbow) (Figure 3.10). The garment is usually made of woven silver nylon that conducts currents across the entire surface of the garment. Most garments are de-signed to be used with most types of TENS device although it is worth checking com-patibility prior to purchase. One lead wire connects to a standard electrode placed on the skin and the other to the garment using a stud connector. Stud adaptors are available for compatibility. Garments stretch so that one size fits all and can be hand-washed in warm water and dried naturally, although they are not recommended for machine washing. Manufacturers claim that conductive garments provide a larger surface area of contact with the skin and can be useful for arthritis in the hand or foot, tendonitis, carpal tunnel syndrome, repetitive strain injury, Raynaud's syndrome, post-operative swelling, plantar fasciitis, and diabetic neuropathy. In a study using 56 healthy individuals, Cowan and colleagues (2009) found that there were no dif-ferences in blunt-pressure pain threshold in strong but comfortable high-frequency TENS (100 pps, continuous pulse pattern) between a standard electrode system and a glove electrode system, although both were superior to inactive TENS controls. Clinical experience suggests that stronger TENS sensations are achieved in the hand and feet using two self-adhesive electrodes placed over peripheral nerves when com-pared with glove and sock electrodes.

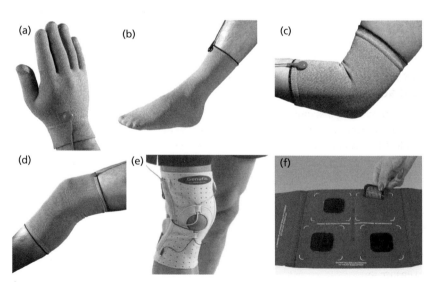

Fig. 3.10 Garment electrodes. (a) Glove, (b) sock, (c) elbow sleeve, (d) knee sleeve, (e) knee brace, and (f) back belt.

Images courtesy of Patterson Medical Ltd. see: <http://www.pattersonmedical.co.uk>.

TENS belts are available for low back pain. Some use re-usable self-adhesive electrodes attached to the inner surface of the belt using press-stud connectors, and others use electrodes integrated into the belt itself that do not need replacing (e.g. Beurer EM 38 Back Pain TENS Belt, ~ GB£35.00; see: <http://www.youtube.com/watch?v=q3vPqYhHnUU>). The skin is moistened with water or conductive gel prior to treatment and the TENS device is placed into a pouch on the belt itself. Conductive knee braces with electrodes integrated into the brace using conductive fabric strips are available for knee pain, including osteoarthritis of the knee (e.g. TENSPros E-Knee+ Plus Conductive Stimulation Knee Brace, ~ US$70.00; see <http://www.tenspros.com/TENSPros-E-Knee-Plus-Conductive-Knee-Brace_p_208.html>). Knee braces reduce entangled lead wires around the knee joint and provide additional knee support. TENS slippers that deliver pulsed currents through the soles of the feet in combination with foot massage have been developed for use with a 'digital therapy machine', to relieve pain, numbness, and fatigue of feet and legs (see: <http://www.digitaltherapymachine.net> and <http://www.dhgate.com/store/product/topsale-1-pair-digital-therapy-machine-slippers/14281507-117327932.html>).

Skin preparation cream

Pre-TENS skin preparation cream is available to improve adhesion and electrode conductivity and to reduce skin irritation and prevent electrode slippage caused by perspiration (e.g. Pre-TENS® Skin Prep, ~ GB£5.00 per 56.80 ml bottle). Oil-free, hypoallergenic, post-TENS skin creams are available to moisturize and soothe tender and irritated skin after each treatment (e.g. After-TENS cream, ~ GB£7.00 for 60 ml tube). They will not affect electrode–skin conductivity or harm electrodes provided manufacturers' instructions are followed.

Considerations when purchasing a standard TENS device and accessories

When purchasing a standard TENS device it is wise to survey the field first as there can be differences in the strength and quality of TENS sensations between devices (Table 3.1). Do not assume that the electrodes supplied with the TENS device are the best. Clinics should stock different types of device and accessories for demonstration so that patients can see the range of models available. Some clinics have sufficient resource to offer indefinite loans of TENS devices until the patient no longer requires the device, although in practice devices may never be returned. More commonly, clinics allow patients to borrow a device for a short period of time to help them decide whether to invest in purchasing their own device. For clinics that require a regular supply of TENS devices and accessories it is important to consider the choice of TENS supplier to ensure immediate delivery, plentiful supply of accessories, good after-sales support, rent-to-buy offers, and 30-day money-back offers. For patients new to TENS it is wise to start using a device with a simple design, progressing to more complex devices if necessary.

Physiology at the electrode–skin interface

Electrodes provide the conductive interface between electrical currents generated by the TENS device and the patient's skin. The type and number of nerve bundles and their respective nerve fibres that are excited during TENS will depend on the depth and distribution of currents and nerves in the skin and tissue underneath the electrodes. Current is carried by electrons generated by the TENS device to the electrodes and then by ions in the electrode gel and the patient's body. This transfer in charge from electrons to ions requires good electrical contact between the electrode and the skin and can be represented as a charge-transfer resistance and a double-layer capacitance connected in parallel (Figure 3.9b). Impedance of a capacitor is inversely proportional to the frequency of the current so that increasing frequency reduces impedance, making it easier for the currents to enter the skin. Impedance at the electrode–gel interface is lower and of less importance than the impedance presented by the skin.

There has been very little empirical research on the depth of penetration of currents during TENS in situ. Thompson and Cummings (2008) used an oscillographic method (model 3425 PicoScope™, Pico Technology Ltd), to visualize electrical currents passing through the skin during electroacupuncture. They found no appreciable spread of currents when needles were placed close together, yet when needles were placed on opposite arms currents distributed into pectoral muscles. Demmink (1995) found that the amplitude-modulated wave of interferential currents was reproduced in water but not when delivered transcutaneously in pork tissue. Thus, the complex and non-homogeneous impedance of tissue underlying electrodes is likely to influence the distribution of currents. Moment-to-moment fluctuations in moisture (sweat), temperature, and movement will also affect impedance and current distribution. Most TENS devices on the market are designed with constant current output despite fluctuations in impedance, i.e. voltage is automatically adjusted by the device to accommodate fluctuations in impedance. Thus, if impedance rises, then the voltage is automatically increased to maintain a constant current without the need for adjusting the amplitude dial.

Properties of the skin

The skin and accessory structures including blood vessels, sensory receptors, nerves, hair follicles, and sweat and sebaceous glands form the integumentary system which protects the internal body from the hostile external environment, and which detects stimuli in the external environment mediating protective responses. The skin is a solid, elastic, self-repairing, cutaneous membrane. The outermost layer of the skin is the epidermis consisting of superficial stratified squamous epithelium with an outer stratum corneum of keratinized cells (15 micrometres), and up to five basal layers (100 micrometres); stratum basale (innermost), stratum spinosum, stratum granulosum, stratum lucidum, and stratum croneum. In thin skin which covers most of the body, the stratum lucidum is absent. Basal layer cells multiply and are pushed upwards whilst hardening from keratin (corneocytes), finally morphing into dry and dead cells of stratum corneum that increase impedance to electrical currents. The underlying connective tissue which supports the epidermis is called the dermis (2 mm in depth) and consists of a superficial papillary layer containing capillaries, lymphatics, and sensory neurones, and a deeper reticular layer containing a dense irregular mesh of collagen and elastic fibres. The hypodermis is a subcutaneous layer that is not part of the integument but connects with the reticular layer of the dermis to stabilize the position of the skin with other organs. The epidermis is avascular and relies on diffusion of oxygen and nutrients from dermal capillaries. Blood supply to the dermis is from arteries forming the cutaneous plexus in the hypodermis and reticular layer and capillaries empty into small veins connected to a large venous plexus in the hypodermis. Trauma to the skin results in rupture of blood vessels and leakage of blood into the dermis resulting in a bruise.

The stratum corneum can be represented by a parallel resistance circuit with capacitance properties in the stratum corneum (0.02–0.06 microF/cm^2). Washing the skin with soapy water, hydration using good-quality electrodes, and larger electrode surface area will decrease impedance. Mild abrasive creams such as Pre-TENS® Skin Prep may also be useful. Repeatedly applying and removing adhesive strips is not recommended because it can lead to skin irritation. Alcohol washes can dehydrate skin.

Neural innervation

The integument contains the axons and axon terminals of efferent neurones that innervate skeletal and autonomic effectors regulating a wide range of physiological responses. The integument also contains sensory receptors and axons of afferent neurones that are part of the somatosensory system providing information about the condition of the body surface, and often leading to body sensations (Table 3.3). The response of sensory receptors to stimuli varies according to type. Peripheral adaptation is a reduction in the response of a neurone to a constant stimulus which may be rapid (fast-adapting receptors) or slow (slow-adapting receptors). A similar phenomenon occurs in the central nervous system whereby activity in neural pathways decline in response to ongoing peripheral input (habituation). Interestingly, the sensitivity of peripheral nociceptors increases in the presence of tissue damage (peripheral sensitisation), and activity of neurones in the central nervous system increases during repetitive noxious stimuli (wind-up) contributing to central sensitisation.

Whether nerve fibres are close to electrodes is critical for activation (Sang et al., 2003). Current density is highest at the electrode–skin interface so axons of superficial, fine-touch tactile receptors will be excited before those from deep, crude-touch receptors. Increasing current amplitude to stimulate axons of receptors in deeper layers is compromised by concurrent activation of higher threshold nociceptive fibres located in superficial tissue. Furthermore, skin offers high impedance at pulse frequencies used by TENS so currents will tend to remain superficial within cutaneous rather than deep-seated visceral and muscle tissue.

The distribution and density of receptors varies according to body site, with tactile receptors densely populated on body parts sensitive to touch such as the fingers, hands, lips, and face, consistent with the somatosensory homunculus (Davey et al., 2001). There is a positive correlation between sensitive body and lower sensory-detection thresholds (the point where a user perceives the first sensation of TENS) and temporal-discrimination thresholds for pairs of electrical stimuli, in line with that expected for the somatosensory homunculus (Hoshiyama et al., 2004). A study using 30 healthy participants that measured the perception of comfort of TENS sensations at different

Table 3.3 Sensory receptors: structure and properties

Sensory receptor	Stimulus	Structure	Associated afferent fibre	Location	Associated sensation
Nociceptors					
Mechano-thermal nociceptors	Potential tissue damage associated with extremes of mechanical and thermal stimuli	Free nerve endings	A-δ	Superficial layers of dermis	Sharp, pricking 'fast' pain
Polymodal nociceptors	Actual tissue damage associated with harmful exogenous and endogenous chemicals (i.e. chemical nociceptors) as well as extremes of temperature and mechanical damage (hence polymodal)	Free nerve endings	C	Superficial layers of dermis	Dull, burning, sickening 'slow' pain
Thermoreceptors					
Cold-sensitive thermoreceptors	Decreasing temperature	Free nerve endings (three to four times more numerous than heat-sensitive thermoreceptors)	A-δ and C	Dermis	Cold
Heat-sensitive thermoreceptors	Increasing temperature	Free nerve endings (no structural differences between heat and cold-sensitive thermoreceptors)	C	Dermis	Warmth

Table 3.3 (continued) Sensory receptors: structure and properties

Sensory receptor	Stimulus	Structure	Associated afferent fibre	Location	Associated sensation
Mechanoreceptors					
Tactile receptors	Distortion of cell membranes	Fine touch and pressure a) free nerve endings b) Merkel's tactile disc (cutaneous) c) Meissner's tactile corpuscles (cutaneous) d) root-hair plexus receptors (cutaneous) e) Pacinian laminated corpuscles (cutaneous/joint) f) Ruffini corpuscles (cutaneous/joint)	A-β	a) superficial layers of skin and between cells in epidermis b) stratum basale of the epidermis c) dermis d) hair shafts in dermis e) dermis f) reticular dermis	a) light touch b) skin indentation, touch-pressure c) Touch-flutter, vibration, tickle, motion d) touch, vibration e) Vibration f) Skin indentation, touch-pressure
Proprioceptors	Stretch and movement of joints, skeletal muscle and associated structures	Free nerve endings Secondary muscle spindle (skeletal muscle)	A-α, A-β, A-δ	Joint capsules, tendons, ligaments, and skeletal muscle	Pressure and proprioception Position of body parts in space
Baroreceptors	Stretch during pressure rise	Free nerve endings that branch within the wall of a distensible organ	A and C	Blood vessels, the digestive and urinary tracts and lungs	Pain at extremes of stretch

body sites found that TENS was most comfortable and easiest to titrate to a strong, non-painful intensity when applied over areas of muscle and soft tissue (Hughes et al., 2013). In general a strong, non-painful TENS sensation was achieved when current amplitudes were ~ 80 per cent of a current window calculated as the difference in mA between sensory-detection threshold and pain threshold. Titrating current will be more precise for current windows that are large, such as the lower back (skeletal muscle) and knee joint (connective tissue), compared with those that are small, such as the tibia (bone) and forearm (nerve). The relationship between body site and current window was not independent of body mass index suggesting that individuals with low body fat may have narrow current windows. There has been little research on skinfold thickness and response to TENS. Miller and colleagues (2008) found higher pulse amplitudes were necessary to achieve 30 per cent of maximal voluntary isometric contractions of the quadriceps using a transcutaneous neuromuscular electrical stimulator for individuals with thicker skinfold.

Current takes the path of least impedance via sweat glands and between cells. The palms of the hands and soles of feet have a high density of sweat glands and distal endings of afferent neurones so TENS of these areas may result in TENS sensations more 'evenly' distributed between electrodes. In contrast, TENS sensation may be more localized to beneath electrodes themselves when the density of sweat glands, and sensory receptors are low (e.g. on the forearm), unless electrodes are over superficial nerve bundles.

The ability of TENS to excite sensory receptors and their afferent fibres depends on the type and sensitivity of receptors and their afferents beneath the electrodes. However, the complex structure of human skin coupled with the crudeness of delivering currents transcutaneously using electrodes with large surface areas means current distribution and depth is likely to be relatively imprecise. More specific targeting of nerves is possible using invasive peripheral nerve stimulation techniques which are more costly and associated with greater hazards. Nevertheless, using appropriate techniques it is possible to use TENS to selectively activate different types of nerve fibres.

Nerve fibre activation by TENS

Pulsed electrical currents excite neural tissue and the characteristics of current influences which neurone becomes active. Large-diameter myelinated axons have lower thresholds of excitation and faster conduction velocities of impulses than small-diameter unmyelinated axons. Large-diameter myelinated afferent axons transmit neural information related to activation of mechanoreceptors resulting in sensations of touch and pressure (Table 3.4). Small-diameter unmyelinated afferent axons transmit neural information related to activation of nociceptors resulting in sensations of pain.

When the pulse amplitude of TENS is increased large-diameter myelinated afferent axons are activated first and the user experiences a non-painful tingling sensation under the electrodes. Electrical paraesthesiae (tingling sensations) are experienced rather than touch and pressure due to an abnormal pattern of impulses generated during TENS because mechanoreceptors have evolved to transduce mechanical stimuli

Table 3.4 Structure and properties of different types of nerve fibre (axons) categorized using the Erlanger Gasser system (Lloyd system categorization approximation in brackets)

Name	Structure	Conduction velocity	Afferent role	Efferent role
A-α (Group Ia and Ib)	Myelinated, large diameter, 22–13 µm	120–70 ms⁻¹	Muscle spindle (primary endings) Golgi tendon organs Mechanoreceptors	Contraction of slow and fast skeletal muscle fibres (extrafusal)
A-β (Group II)	Myelinated, large diameter, 8–13 µm	40–70 ms⁻¹	Mechanoreceptors Proprioceptors Muscle spindles (secondary endings)	Contraction of muscle spindle fibres (intrafusal)
A-γ (Group II/III)	Myelinated, medium diameter, 4–8 µm	15–40 ms⁻¹	Mechanoreceptors	Contraction of muscle spindle fibres (intrafusal)
A-δ (Group III)	Myelinated small diameter, 1–4 µm	5–15 ms⁻¹	Nociceptors Mechanoreceptors (crude touch) Cold-sensitive temperature	
B	Myelinated, small diameter, 1–3 µm	3–14 ms⁻¹		Pre-ganglionic autonomic
C (Group IV)	Unmyelinated, small diameter, 0.1–1 µm	0.2–2.0 ms⁻¹	Nociceptors Mechanoreceptors Cold-sensitive and heat-sensitive thermoreceptors	Post-ganglionic autonomic

rather than 'unnatural' electrical currents. Also, currents activate the nerve fibre rather than the mechanoreceptor. If the pulse amplitude of TENS is increased further, high-threshold, small-diameter nociceptive axons (A-δ and C) become active and the user experiences a painful tingling under the electrodes (Figure 3.11).

It is the leading edge of the pulsed current that excites the nerve fibre and the resultant action potential travels in both directions from its point of origin. Impulses travelling in their 'normal' direction towards the axon terminal are termed 'orthodromic', and those travelling opposite to normal, towards the neuronal cell body, are termed 'antidromic'. In afferent axons antidromic impulses travel towards the sensory receptor in the periphery and orthodromic impulses travel towards the central nervous system. In efferent axons antidromic impulses travel towards the neuronal cell body in the central nervous system and orthodromic impulses travel towards the axon terminal in

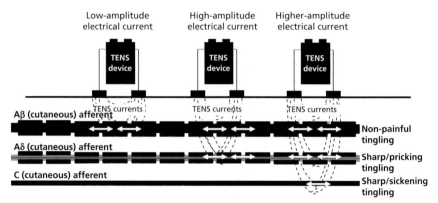

Fig. 3.11 Excitation of different axons by increasing amplitude of TENS. White arrows indicate depolarization of the axon and direction of nerve impulses.

the periphery. Thus, TENS may cause peripheral blockade of afferent impulses arising from sensory receptor activation during injury (Chapter 9).

The shape of the leading edge of the waveform may influence depolarization with a vertical edge being more efficient than a shallow sloping edge. If the leading edge is prolonged the axon may accommodate, although this is less likely when pulse durations are less than 300 μs, as used during TENS. Pulsed electrical currents with short pulse durations require larger amplitude currents to achieve sensory threshold and pain threshold related to excitation of A-β and A-δ axons respectively (Figure 3.12)

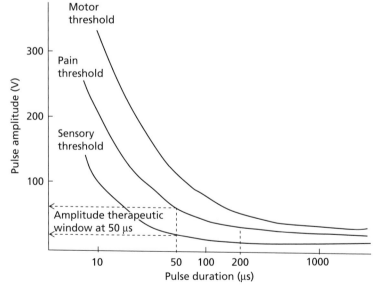

Fig. 3.12 Strength–duration curve showing the amplitude and duration of electrical pulsed stimuli to reach sensory, pain, and motor thresholds.

(Howson, 1978). The largest separation of pulse amplitudes between sensory threshold and pain threshold is observed using short pulse durations, although markedly higher pulse amplitudes are necessary. Pulse durations above 500 µs are likely to activate nociceptive fibres at lower pulse amplitudes with small differences in the current amplitude window between sensory and pain thresholds. Thus, optimal pulse durations to activate large-diameter sensory fibres (A-β) without simultaneously activating small-diameter nociceptive fibres (A-δ and C) and causing pain are low-amplitude (i.e. low-intensity), pulsed currents between 50 µs and 500 µs. That is to say that pulse durations between 50 µs and 500 µs provide greatest sensitivity when titrating pulse amplitude to achieve a non-painful TENS sensation.

The number of nerve impulses generated in response to TENS increases according to the frequency of the pulsed currents. This number of nerve impulses will be limited by the absolute and relative refractory periods for the axon. Action potentials generated in large-diameter fibres have short refractory periods and therefore nerve impulses can be produced at higher rates. Thus, higher frequency currents will result in more nerve impulses reaching the central nervous system per second generating more powerful effects, although there is a maximum frequency above which the nerve axon is unable to generate more nerve impulses because the TENS pulse falls within the refractory period. For this reason the frequency output of many standard TENS devices is not above 200 pulses per second.

TENS techniques used in clinical practice

Two main TENS techniques have developed from the theoretical biophysical actions of pulsed electrical currents at the skin electrode interface. It is important that the practitioner is familiar with the physiological principles and operational procedures associated with these techniques (Table 3.5).

Table 3.5 Comparison of effects of conventional and acupuncture-like TENS

Characteristic	Conventional TENS	Acupuncture-like TENS
Intention of stimulation	◆ Activate low-threshold, large-diameter cutaneous afferents (A-β)	◆ Activate higher threshold smaller diameter, deep muscle afferents and possibly cutaneous afferents (A-δ)
Intensity and TENS sensation	◆ Low intensity, producing strong, non-painful tingling TENS sensation with minimal muscle activity	◆ Higher intensity, producing muscle twitching and/or non-painful pulsating TENS sensation
Pulse amplitude	◆ Usually <60 mA	◆ Usually <60mA
Pulse pattern (mode)	◆ Continuous in first instance but subsequently determined by patient preference	◆ Burst or amplitude-modulated in first instance ◆ Use continuous if delivering low-frequency, single pulsed currents

Table 3.5 (continued) Comparison of effects of conventional and acupuncture-like TENS

Characteristic	Conventional TENS	Acupuncture-like TENS
Pulse frequency (rate)	◆ High-frequency ◆ 10–200 pulses per second ◆ Determined by patient	◆ Low-frequency bursts of high-frequency pulses ◆ Usually 2–4 bursts (trains) per second of high frequency pulses (>10 pps and determined by patient) ◆ Low-frequency single pulses at <5 pulses per second
Pulse width (duration)	◆ Between 50 µs and 200 µs ◆ Determined by patient	◆ Between 100 µs and 200 µs. Shorter pulse duration will generate a weaker TENS sensation yet still create muscle twitching
Electrode positions	◆ Dermatomal ◆ Straddle site of pain ◆ Over main nerve bundle ◆ Contralateral 'mirror' site when hyper- or hypo-sensitive skin	◆ Myotomal ◆ Over motor point or muscle belly at site of pain ◆ Over main motor nerve ◆ Contralateral 'mirror' site when hyper- or hypo-sensitive skin ◆ Trigger points or acupuncture points sometimes used
Dose	◆ Stimulate whenever pain relief required and use throughout day with regular breaks if necessary, for example for 1–2 hours of stimulation with a 15–30 minute rest	◆ Stimulate for 30–45 minutes a few times each day ◆ Excessive stimulation over large muscle masses may generate muscle fatigue and delayed onset muscle soreness the following day
Profile of pain relief	◆ Rapid in onset and offset ◆ Localized pain relief from segmental action (i.e. spinal gating)	◆ Rapid onset and delayed in offset ◆ More widespread pain relief from segmental (i.e. spinal gating) and extrasegmental actions (i.e. descending pain inhibitory pathways)

Conventional TENS

The International Association of Pain (IASP) defines conventional TENS as 'high frequency (50–100 Hz), low intensity (paraesthesia, not painful), small pulse width (50–200 µs)' (Charlton, 2005, 94).

However, the definition focuses on the technical output characteristics of the TENS device and is restrictive with respect to pulse frequencies and pulse durations (widths). It would

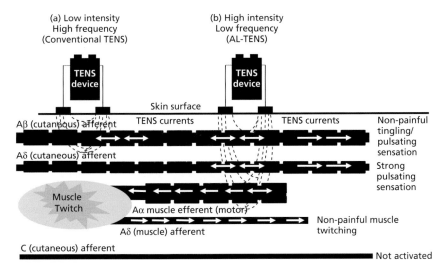

Fig. 3.13 Selective activation of peripheral afferents by (a) conventional TENS and (b) acupuncture-like TENS (AL-TENS). White arrows indicate direction of nerve impulses.

be more appropriate to define TENS techniques according to their physiological intention. The physiological intention of using conventional TENS is to activate low-threshold, large-diameter afferent nerve fibres in the skin without concurrently activating higher threshold, small-diameter afferent nerve fibres (A-δ and C-fibres) in the skin (pain-related) or afferent or efferent nerve fibres in skeletal muscle (Figure 3.13a). Users will recognize this when they experience a strong, non-painful TENS sensation often described as tingling, buzzing, or pleasant pins-and-needles (i.e. electrical paraesthesia) without concurrent muscle contraction. TENS-induced low-threshold afferent activity inhibits ongoing transmission of nociceptive information and reduces central sensitization at segments in the spinal cord via neural mechanisms which are rapid in onset and offset (Chapter 9). Thus, conventional TENS is administered at the site of pain or at dermatomes related to the origin of the pain (Chapter 4), and is the focus of the majority of this textbook.

> Conventional TENS is the use of electrical pulsed currents generated by a standard TENS device and delivered across the intact surface of the skin to generate a strong, non-painful TENS sensation indicative of selective activation of low-threshold peripheral afferents.

Acupuncture-like TENS (AL-TENS)

The International Association of Pain (IASP) defines acupuncture-like TENS (AL-TENS) as hyperstimulation using currents that are low frequency (2–4 Hz), higher intensity (to tolerance threshold), [and] longer pulse width (100–400 μs)' (Charlton, 2005, 94).

The definition not only focuses on the technical output characteristics of the TENS device and is restrictive with respect to pulse frequencies and pulse durations (widths), but it also uses a vague endpoint for TENS intensity as 'to tolerance threshold'. This endpoint does not specify whether 'tolerance threshold' means at, above, or below pain threshold. Moreover, some opinion leaders consider the induction of forceful but non-painful phasic muscle contractions at myotomes related to the origin of the pain important to achieve pain relief during AL-TENS. Most research reports describe AL-TENS as low-frequency, high-intensity TENS without any reference to the presence or absence of muscle contractions (see Francis & Johnson, 2011, for review). TENS over acupuncture points irrespective of muscle activity has also been described as AL-TENS, although this technique has also been described as acu-TENS or transcutaneous electrical acupoint stimulation (TEAS) (see Walsh, 1996; Brown et al., 2009, for reviews). Whether there are differences in physiological action when TENS is applied over acupuncture points in the presence or absence of muscle contractions is uncertain.

Generally, it is accepted that the physiological intention of using AL-TENS is to generate nerve impulses in deep-seated, small-diameter afferents (i.e. A-δ). However, large amplitude currents would be necessary for direct stimulation of high-threshold, deep-seated skeletal muscle afferents and these large amplitude currents would also excite small-diameter cutaneous afferents generating sensations of sharp, pricking pain which would not be acceptable to the patient. One way to overcome this problem would be to stimulate low-threshold, A-α motor efferents using small amplitude currents to produce forceful but non-painful muscle twitches. These muscle twitches would set up activity, indirectly, in skeletal muscle afferents that provide feedback from working muscles and do not generate sensations of pain (Figure 3.13b). Thus, AL-TENS is applied over large peripheral nerves or motor points using higher amplitudes of current than conventional TENS although the intensity of AL-TENS is non-painful. Low-frequency pulses (~1–10 pps) or low-frequency bursts of pulses (~2–5 bursts per second of 100 pps) are used, with the latter tending to be more comfortable for the patient. The pulse frequency within each burst, called the internal pulse frequency, can be adjusted by the user within a range corresponding to the frequency output of the device (usually 1–200 pps). In order to mirror physiological contraction of muscle it is necessary for the internal pulse frequency to be above the fusion frequency of skeletal muscle, normally above 40 pps. During AL-TENS low-threshold, A-β cutaneous afferents will also be excited as described for conventional TENS, although the resultant pattern of impulses will be different (i.e. low frequency rather than high frequency).

> Acupuncture-like TENS is the use of low-frequency, electrical pulsed currents generated by a standard TENS device and delivered across the intact surface of the skin to generate strong, non-painful skeletal muscle twitching in order to activate deep-seated peripheral afferents. Some practitioners deliver acupuncture-like TENS to produce strong, nearly painful, pulsating TENS sensations indicative of activity in high-threshold cutaneous afferents.

Milestones in the development of AL-TENS

AL-TENS was developed following observations of acupuncturists who manually twirled acupuncture needles at low frequencies and/or delivered low-frequency electrical currents through the needles (electroacupuncture) to relieve pain (Table 3.6).

Table 3.6 Milestones in the development of AL-TENS

Date	Source	Discovery
1973	Editorial (1973)	Observations of acupuncturists who manually twirled acupuncture needles at low frequencies and/or delivered low-frequency electrical currents through the needles (electroacupuncture) to relieve pain
1973	Chiang et al., (1973)	Pain relief achieved from acupuncture decreased when activity in deep-seated nerves was blocked using local anaesthetic but not when nerves innervating the skin were blocked
1973	Andersson et al., (1973)	'Electroacupuncture via surface electrodes' using low-frequency, high-intensity single pulsed current producing strong muscle contractions in related myotomes increased pain threshold in healthy humans
1976	Andersson et al., (1976)	Low-frequency single pulsed currents over nerve bundles with muscle twitching was less effective at relieving chronic pain than fasciculatory muscle contractions elicited using high-frequency pulsed currents
1976	Eriksson & Sjölund (1976)	Strong muscle contractions generated by low-frequency, high-intensity TENS using bursts of low-frequency trains of pulses was tolerated much better by patients than low-frequency, high-intensity TENS using single pulsed current—the term 'acupuncture-like TENS' was introduced to describe the technique
		Chronic pain not responding to conventional TENS was relieved when low-frequency trains (bursts) of high-frequency pulses were used. Opioids were implicated in the mechanism of action
1977	Sjölund et al., (1977)	AL-TENS elevated endorphin levels in cerebrospinal fluid
1979	Sjölund et al., (1977) Sjölund & Eriksson (1979)	Pain relief during AL-TENS but not conventional TENS was naloxone reversible
1979	Eriksson et al., (1979)	Acupuncture-like TENS was efficacious in patients who did not respond to conventional TENS

In 1973, Andersson and colleagues found that low-frequency TENS eliciting strong muscle contractions in related myotomes reduced experimental pain and they concluded that activation of sensory receptors within skeletal muscle was necessary for hypoalgesia during 'electroacupuncture via surface electrodes' (Andersson et al., 1973). However, muscle contractions elicited using low-frequency, single pulsed currents were uncomfortable, so low-frequency trains (bursts) of high-frequency pulses were used and it was found that this technique relieved chronic pain in individuals resistant to conventional TENS. The term 'acupuncture-like TENS' (AL-TENS) was introduced to describe the technique, and manufacturers incorporated burst patterns of pulse delivery into stimulator design. Evidence accumulated that AL-TENS, but not conventional TENS, mediated pain relief via endogenous opioids, catalysing investigations into optimal parameters for TENS, the findings of which have remained largely inconclusive. Despite a proliferation in systematic reviews and meta-analysis of clinical trials, attempts to compare the effectiveness of conventional TENS with AL-TENS have been compromised by the lack of studies to make any meaningful comparison.

To this day, the definition of AL-TENS has remained broad and ambiguous. Evidence from animal studies suggests that inhibition of central nociceptive transmission cells is more prolonged and widespread during AL-TENS compared with conventional TENS with spinal and supraspinal segmental mechanisms including the release of endogenous opioid peptides involved (see Chapter 9). Interestingly, evidence for differing analgesic profiles in humans is less convincing. Levin and Hui-Chan (1993) measured compound action potentials over the median nerve in the cubital fossa during conventional TENS (3 × sensory threshold) and AL-TENS (0.1 pps and trains of 100 pps at 4 Hz at intensities greater than 3 × sensory threshold) to the median nerve at the wrist of 17 healthy volunteers. They found that conventional and AL-TENS activated A-α and A-β afferents suggesting that hypoalgesic effects produced by both techniques were mediated by TENS-induced activity in similar peripheral afferent fibres.

Other TENS techniques

Intense TENS and acu-TENS are used less frequently than conventional and AL-TENS.

Intense TENS

Intense TENS describes high-frequency (<200 pps), high-intensity TENS at, or just above, pain threshold (i.e. it is painful) delivered at the site of pain, close to the site of pain, or at a distant site. Intense TENS acts as a counter-irritant and can only be administered for short periods of time. It is useful during minor painful procedures including wound-dressing changes, suture removal, and venepuncture. Intense TENS excites high-threshold cutaneous A-δ afferents and is likely to block transmission of nociceptive information in peripheral nerves and inhibit central nociceptive transmission cells within and beyond spinal segments with diffuse noxious inhibitory controls (DNIC) playing a role (Chapter 9).

Acu-TENS

Acu-TENS describes TENS of acupuncture points using various electrical parameters, including low- and high-frequency currents at low- and high-intensities (see Walsh, 1996; Brown et al., 2009, for reviews). Other terms that have been used to describe TENS of acupuncture points include 'AL-TENS' and 'transcutaneous electrical acupoint stimulation' (TEAS), creating confusion in the literature. At present, there is no consensus on features that distinguish acu-TENS from AL-TENS or TEAS. The majority of research on acu-TENS has been conducted by Jones and co-workers (see Ngai & Jones, 2012, for a recent example). In studies using healthy volunteers they have found that acu-TENS at BL13 (Feishu) decreased skin impedance of acupoints and reduced sympathetic activity; acu-TENS at PC6 reduced blood pressure in response to head-down tilt and facilitated recovery of resting heart rate after treadmill exercise; and acu-TENS at Lieque (LU7) and Dingchuan (EX-B1) increased post-exercise forced expiratory volume at 1-second (FEV1) and exercise duration, and reduced the decline of FEV1 following exercise training in patients with asthma. Randomized placebo controlled clinical trials by Jones and colleagues have found that acu-TENS bilaterally over Dingchuan (EX-B1) improves functional outcomes in patients with chronic obstructive pulmonary disease including FEV1, FVC, dyspnoea, and physical activity with increased β-endorphin levels facilitating bronchodilation being a possible mechanism. Typical regimens were 45 minutes of acu-TENS administered five days per week for four weeks. Acu-TENS bilaterally over PC6 was also shown to facilitate return of pre-operative blood pressure, heart rate to baseline after acute heart surgery. Other investigators have also found beneficial effects of TENS over acupuncture points, although not described as acu-TENS. For example, Chao et al. (2007) found TENS over LI4 (Hegu) and SP6 (Sanyinjiao) reduced pain in parturients in the active phase of first-stage labour. The delivery of TENS over acupuncture points is discussed further in Chapter 4, 75–76.

Summary

1 A 'standard TENS device' (stimulator) generates monophasic or biphasic waveforms of pulsed electrical currents, and lead wires transfer currents between the TENS device and electrodes that are attached to the surface of the skin.

2 The electrical currents excite neural tissue causing nerve impulses that influence a variety of physiological processes including reducing transmission of pain-related information in the nervous system.

3 The variety of output characteristics available on TENS devices has generated uncertainty about optimal technique for TENS.

4 Conventional TENS is a technique that administers *high-frequency, low-intensity* currents to generate a strong, non-painful TENS sensation indicative of activity of low-threshold peripheral afferents.

5 Acupuncture-like TENS (AL-TENS) is a technique that administers *low-frequency, high-intensity* currents to generate non-painful phasic muscle contractions (twitching) resulting in activity in small-diameter muscle afferents.

Further reading

♦ **Grimnes, A., and Martinsen, O.G.** (2000) *Bioimpedance and bioelectricity.* Academic Press, San Diego, CA.

♦ **Johnson, M.** (1998) Acupuncture-like transcutaneous electrical nerve stimulation (AL-TENS) in the management of pain. *Physical Therapy Reviews,* **3**, 73–93.

♦ **Robertson, V., Ward, A., Low, J., and Reed, A.** (2006) *Electrotherapy Explained: principles and practice.* 4th edn, Butterworth-Heinemann, Oxford.

In Chapter 4, the principles and research findings that underpin safe and appropriate electrode positioning and choice of electrical characteristics for conventional and AL-TENS are reviewed.

Chapter 4

Appropriate electrode sites and electrical characteristics for TENS

Introduction

TENS is used as a stand-alone treatment for mild to moderate pain and, in combination with other analgesic treatments, for moderate to severe pain. Best responses are observed for pains that are highly localized arising from joints, skeleton, muscle, tendons, skin, and peripheral and central nerve damage. TENS is particularly useful as part of a treatment package for chronic pain where long-term analgesic medication tends to produce side effects and diminishing effectiveness. TENS is indicated for acute pain, but is used less often because acute pain can be managed effectively using appropriate analgesic medication. The success of TENS treatment depends on the practitioner being able to select safe and appropriate electrode positions and electrical characteristics for TENS. The purpose of this chapter is to discuss the principles and evidence that underpins the use of safe and appropriate electrode sites and electrical characteristics during TENS by covering:

- Choosing between conventional and AL-TENS
- Appropriate electrode positioning for conventional TENS and AL-TENS including instances where AL-TENS may be more beneficial than conventional TENS
- Appropriate choice of electrical characteristics for stimulation
- Biological, psychological, and social factors influencing response to TENS

Choosing between conventional and AL-TENS

Conventional TENS is achieved using currents that generate a strong, non-painful TENS sensation at the site of pain, and for most situations is the method of choice in the first instance. This is because most successful long-term users of TENS select conventional TENS and it is easier to administer the technique therefore promoting adherence to regular usage. Furthermore, patients taking opioids on a regular basis are more likely to respond to conventional TENS (see section on diet and concurrent medication, Chapter 4, 91). Pain relief from conventional TENS is generally rapid in onset and offset so long treatment sessions (e.g. >45 minutes) administered regularly throughout the day are necessary to manage persistent pain. Patients do not appear to become fatigued from prolonged delivery of continuous TENS. AL-TENS is used whenever patients are resistant to conventional TENS and it is claimed that AL-TENS may be more effective than conventional TENS for pains arising from deep-seated structures such as muscle and the visceral organs, and when pain is widespread, at multiple sites, or pain requires prolonged post-TENS pain relief (Johnson, 1998). Pain relief from AL-TENS is slower in onset and offset and may cause muscle fatigue and delayed onset muscle soreness and stiffness the following day. Individuals are advised to administer AL-TENS for approximately 20–40 minutes once or twice a day initially, progressing to three to four times per day once the technique has been mastered.

The physiological intention of using AL-TENS is to generate non-painful phasic muscle contractions (twitching) in myotomes segmentally related to the origin of the pain. This is achieved by stimulating large-diameter α motor neurones which generate muscle contractions that indirectly lead to small-diameter A-δ (Group III) afferent activity. When low-frequency single pulsed currents are used, smaller bundles of muscle fibres are activated and this results in small muscle 'twitches'. The electrical charge necessary to achieve this can cause discomfort at certain body sites so burst patterns are often used. When burst or amplitude-modulated pulse patterns are used the amplitude and surface area of the phasic muscle contraction is larger because of stimulation driven by high-frequency pulsed currents within the burst train, although this depends in part on the position of electrodes. In many circumstances it will not be possible to remain ambulatory in the presence of muscle twitching/contractions.

Safe and appropriate positioning of electrodes and appropriate choice of electrical characteristics used for stimulation are the critical factors in success for both TENS techniques. The principles for conventional TENS will be described first as many of these principles are also common to AL-TENS.

Principles of safe and appropriate electrode positioning for conventional TENS

Often it is possible to use similar electrode positions for conventional TENS and AL-TENS, although subtle differences exist in some circumstances. TENS electrodes must be positioned on healthy innervated skin where sensation is intact so checking skin sensation at electrode site is critical. In patients where skin sensation over the site of pain is normal then electrodes are positioned so that TENS sensation is perceived within the pain. In patients where skin sensation is not normal, conventional TENS can be delivered using electrodes positioned over nerve bundles so that TENS sensation is

In general, electrodes for conventional TENS are positioned on sensate skin on the outer margins of the pain, or:

- over main nerve bundles proximal to the site of pain
- paravertebrally in dermatomes related to the origin of pain
- on contralateral dermatomes at sites that mirror the pain
- on acupuncture points
- on trigger points

projected to the painful area, or by applying electrodes to generate TENS sensation at areas that are related to the dermatome associated with the origin of the pain.

Electrode placement on the outer margins of the pain

Commonly, two electrodes (single channel) are applied on opposite sides of the outer margins of the pain so that TENS sensation permeates the painful area (Figure 4.1). Thus, low-threshold cutaneous afferents (A-β) are stimulated generating nerve impulses that enter the same spinal segment as impulses conducted in nociceptive fibres associated with the origin of the pain (i.e. the same dermatome).

A dermatome is the area of skin innervated mainly by one spinal nerve root, although the borders of dermatomes partially overlap (Figure 4.2). There are 31 pairs of spinal nerves:

- Cervical (C1–C8) innervating the posterior head and neck and the upper limbs
- Thoracic (T1–T12) innervating the trunk
- Lumbar (L1–L5) innervating the lower abdomen and anterior lower limbs
- Sacral (S1–S4) innervating the buttocks and posterior lower limbs
- Coccygeal (Co) innervating the buttock

Dermatomal distributions can be seen in conditions that affect individual spinal roots. For example, infection with the herpes zoster virus which hibernates in spinal nerve ganglia and causes chickenpox and herpes zoster results in a rash and pain across the affected dermatome.

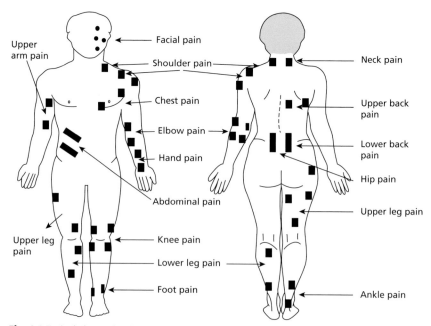

Fig. 4.1 Typical electrode placement sites on outer margins of pain when there is normal skin sensation.

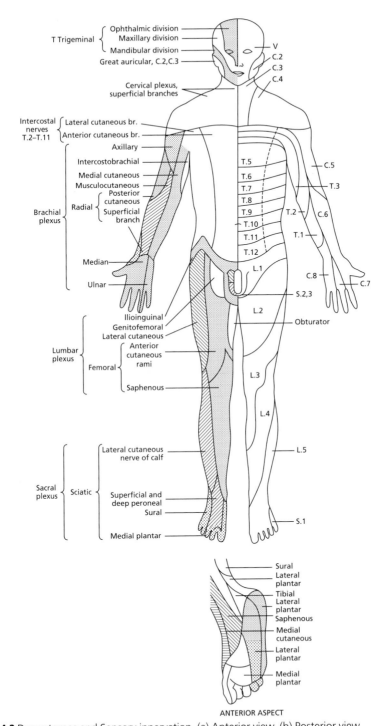

Fig. 4.2 Dermatomes and Sensory innervation. (a) Anterior view. (b) Posterior view.

Reproduced from Murray Longmore et al. (eds.), *Oxford Handbook of Clinical Medicine*, 6th edition, pp. 338–339, Copyright © 2004, by permission of Oxford University Press.

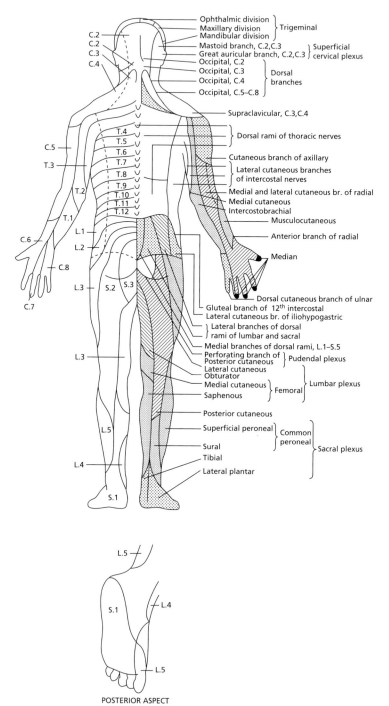

Fig. 4.2 (Continued)

Whether electrodes are aligned horizontally or vertically depends on the location of the pain with the key determinant being optimal coverage of pain with TENS sensation. It may be necessary to adjust the location of the electrodes through a systematic process of trial and error to achieve optimal positions.

It may be necessary to use dual-channel stimulation with double electrode pairs for pains that cover large areas. Currents from each channel may remain independent using parallel electrode positions or they may intersect using criss-cross electrode positions (see Figure 7.3, Chapter 7). Intersecting currents using criss-cross electrode positions are used during interferential current therapy where the intention is for two independent out-of-phase 'carrier currents' to intersect to generate a third amplitude-modulated interference current (see Chapter 10, 204–205). Interestingly, the interference pattern of two intersecting TENS currents of similar or different frequencies is not known. Field testing using healthy pain-free volunteers in our laboratory has found that TENS sensations are not affected by delivering the currents in parallel or intersecting electrode positions even when the two channels administer markedly different pulse frequencies or pulse patterns. Dual-channel devices are also used for pain at multiple sites such as low back pain with sciatica or for pains which change in their location and quality over a short time period, e.g. during childbirth. Conventional TENS may be combined with AL-TENS to maximize the effects of TENS. For example, conventional TENS may be delivered to the lower back and AL-TENS over the area of sciatic referred pain (see Figure 7.3, Chapter 7). Applying conventional TENS and AL-TENS at the same body site so that currents intersect is another means of trying to maximize sensory input during TENS. Most standard TENS devices do not provide independent control of output characteristics other than pulse amplitude. Consequently, it may be necessary to use two separate TENS devices to combine AL-TENS with conventional TENS.

The positing of the cathode (black lead) and anode (red lead) electrodes affects the intensity, distribution, and quality of TENS sensation. However, the outcome is rarely predictable and may vary according to device manufacturer. When using monophasic or asymmetric biphasic waveforms the cathode (black lead) is the active electrode and will excite neural tissue, so it should be positioned over the peripheral nerve to be stimulated. When both electrodes are aligned along a peripheral nerve the cathode is usually positioned proximal to the anode to prevent anodal block of the nerve impulse. Generally, a stronger TENS sensation in the distribution of the nerve is achieved when the cathode rather than the anode is placed over a peripheral nerve, and this seems to occur even when the anode is placed proximally. Some TENS instruction guides specify that the black lead should be placed on the peripheral nerve between the spine and the painful area, and the red lead alongside the vertebrae on the dermatome where the peripheral nerve enters the spinal cord, with the anode closest to the head (King, 1998). In this instance the cathode will stimulate the peripheral nerve proximal to the pain. If electrodes are straddling a painful area the cathode is normally placed proximal to the anode, unless one of the positions lies over a peripheral nerve, in which case the cathode should be positioned over the nerve. In practice, a systematic process of trial and error is used to find the most beneficial distribution, quality, and intensity of TENS sensation.

There are circumstances when a practitioner may decide not to apply electrodes on the outer margins of the pain, including:

- pains that cover a large area
- pains that are deep seated
- pains where it is difficult to place electrodes (hands, feet, body creases)
- altered skin sensation over the site of pain
- the absence of a body part (e.g. phantom limb pain)
- the presence of a skin lesion
- if there is a 'precaution' or local contraindication (see Chapter 5)

In these situations alternative electrode positions may be used as follows:

- over the main nerves proximal to the site of pain
- close to vertebrae of spinal segments
- over contralateral dermatomes

Electrode placement along the main nerves proximal to the site of pain

Placing electrodes over or around the pain sometimes fails to permeate TENS sensations within the pain especially for deep-seated pain. Delivering TENS directly over peripheral nerves may generate stronger TENS sensations that permeate deep tissue and cover larger areas (Hughes et al., 2013). Also it may not be possible to apply electrodes to skin with tactile allodynia and/or hyperalgesia (e.g. neuropathic pain), so electrodes can be positioned along peripheral nerves proximal to the site of pain to radiate TENS sensation into the painful area. This should be performed carefully because stimulation of low-threshold touch afferents (A-β) that contribute to allodynia may inadvertently worsen the pain. Paradoxically this is not always the case.

When it is not possible to place electrodes at or around the site of pain—e.g. radiating pain (sciatica), missing body parts (e.g. amputee pain) or on hands, feet, and body creases—it is possible to stimulate peripheral nerves to project TENS sensation into the painful area. For example, electrode positions over the median nerve can be used to project TENS sensation into painful fingers in rheumatoid arthritis, phantom pain, complex regional pain syndrome, or trigeminal or post-herpetic neuralgia. Conventional TENS over mixed peripheral nerves may inadvertently cause muscle contraction and users can tolerate a small amount of muscle contraction, but currents should be reduced if strong tetanic contraction is produced. Strong, non-painful sensations of conventional TENS without concurrent muscle contraction is easily achievable by stimulating mixed peripheral nerves innervating large muscle masses (e.g. legs, buttock, back, or shoulders) because of higher motor thresholds in these regions.

Often it is necessary to adjust electrode positions along the course of the main nerves using a trial-and-error approach before you hit the optimal distribution of TENS sensations for a region (Table 4.1). Often these sites correlate to where nerves or nerve plexi course run close to the surface of the skin so a working knowledge of anatomy aids optimal location (Figure 4.3). Positioning electrodes at sites where nerves or nerve plexi course run close to the surface of the skin will reduce the amount of current needed to activate the nerve and increase the likelihood of stimulation within the nerve territory. Practical

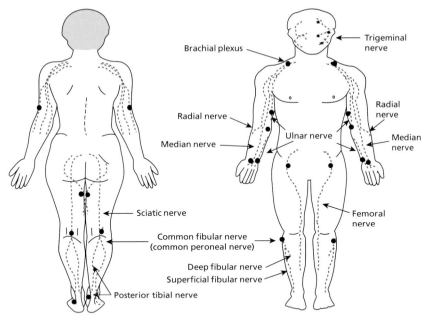

Fig. 4.3 Location of main peripheral nerves. Circles represent where nerves course close to the skin surface being ideal targets for placement of the (cathode) electrode.

Table 4.1 Peripheral nerve bundles and their branches commonly used as targets for peripheral electrical nerve stimulation techniques including TENS

Target	Clinical use
Radial, ulnar, median, and sciatic nerves	Upper and lower limb neuropathies, complex regional pain syndrome, and back pain
Hypoglossal nerve	To stimulate the genioglossus muscle for obstructive sleep apnoea
Occipital nerve	Severe migraine headache, occipital neuralgia, cluster headaches
Sacral nerve	Refractory overactive bladder syndrome, urge incontinence, non-obstructive urinary retention, interstitial cystitis, constipation, dysfunctional elimination syndrome in children, faecal incontinence, and chronic pelvic pain
Pudendal nerve	To stimulate pelvic floor musculature for dysfunctional bowel and bladder conditions and urogenic, iliac crest, and abdominal pain (similar to sacral nerve stimulation)
Trigeminal nerve	Cranial and facial pains including trigeminal neuralgia, post-herpetic neuralgia and supraorbital neuralgia, and also treatment-resistant seizures, depression, and attention hyperactive disorder
Vagus nerve	Which controls a wide range of motor and sensory functions of visceral organs and is used to manage seizures and depression

techniques to help locate optimal electrode sites to stimulate main superficial nerves to achieve TENS sensation within the appropriate painful (i.e. the 'sweet spot') are described in Chapter 6, 128–129.

Stimulation of peripheral nerves to project TENS sensation into areas of neuropathic pain may be inappropriate if the patient or the practitioner is concerned that TENS may exacerbate pain, or if it is impossible to find a large enough area of sensate skin to position electrodes (e.g. tactile allodynia covering one side of the face). In these circumstances, TENS sensations are generated at body parts where there is no pain by applying electrodes over contralateral dermatomes or on skin close to vertebrae of spinal segments related to origin of pain.

Electrode placement on contralateral dermatomes (mirror sites) or paravertebral

Electrode positions to generate TENS sensations within a non-painful contralateral dermatome ('mirror sites') have been reported to be successful for phantom pain, complex regional pain syndrome, or trigeminal or post-herpetic neuralgia. The rationale for using these sites is that afferents activated during TENS will conduct impulses into the central nervous system via the same segment as nociceptive afferents from a contralateral site with interaction between collaterals from each side of the body 'closing the pain gate'.

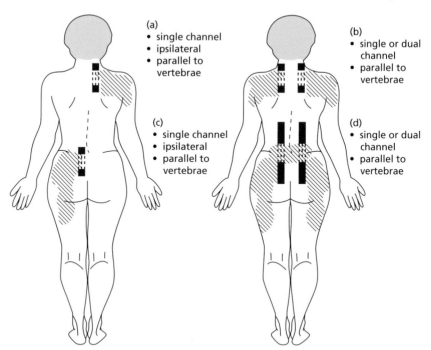

Fig. 4.4 Paravertebral electrode positions. (a) Unilateral upper-arm, shoulder, and neck pain, (b) unilateral upper leg and/or lower back pain, (c) bilateral neck, shoulder, and/or upper arm pain, and (d) bilateral upper leg, and/or low back pain. Diagonal shading area indicates pain. Dashed line indicates currents.

Electrodes can be positioned close to vertebrae of spinal segments that are related to the origin of pain. If the pain is located on one side of the body (unilateral pain) then electrodes are placed parallel to the vertebra on the ipsilateral dermatome (Figure 4.4a and 4.4c.). The skin from this region enters the spinal cord at the same segment as nociceptive information arising from the body part and therefore TENS-induced activity in A-β afferents will inhibit central transmission of nociceptive information (i.e. closing the pain gate at the same spinal segment). If the pain is located on both sides of the body (bilateral pain) then electrodes are placed to straddle vertebra so that dermatomes on both side of the body are stimulated (Figure 4.4b and 4.4d.). Input from TENS-induced activity in A-β afferents from either side of the skin overlying the vertebrae will be at the same segment as nociceptive information arising from areas from both sides of the body to inhibit central transmission of nociceptive information (i.e. closing the pain gate). Alternatively, two sets of electrodes could be positioned parallel to the vertebra on each side. This would be a more powerful way of generating input A-β afferents from either side of the skin overlying the vertebra but it requires a dual-channel stimulator.

Principles of safe and appropriate electrode positioning for AL-TENS

Electrode positioning for AL-TENS uses similar principles described for conventional TENS with electrodes positioned to activate myotomes rather than dermatomes. A myotome is group of skeletal muscles innervated mainly by one spinal root and is the muscle equivalent of a dermatome. Skin and muscle areas are innervated by the same spinal nerve root except in the limbs and head. For example, gluteal muscles are innervated from L4 to S1 whereas the overlying skin is innervated mainly from L1 to L3. The spinal nerve L4 innervates muscle of the medial and anterior thigh (vastus and adductor muscles), and skin from the lateral and anterior thigh, and down the medial aspect of the lower leg (Figure 4.5). When using TENS to manage pain arising from protective skeletal muscle contraction (i.e. reflex spasms) due to damage to cutaneous tissue it should be remembered that different myotomes and dermatomes may be affected. Also it is likely for most pains that more than one dermatome or myotome may be affected.

AL-TENS is used to activate large-diameter α motor neurones to create a muscle contraction/twitch. The cathode electrode is positioned over a motor point or a mixed nerve bundle that courses close to the skin surface (superficial) to reduce the amount of electrical current needed to elicit a strong, comfortable muscle contraction (Figure 3.13b). A motor point is the point at which a motor nerve enters a muscle and

In general, electrodes for AL-TENS are positioned on sensate skin over ipsilateral motor points of myotomes related to the pain, or:

♦ over main nerve bundles of innervating muscles related to the pain

♦ over contralateral motor points of myotomes that mirror the pain

♦ over trigger points

♦ over acupuncture points

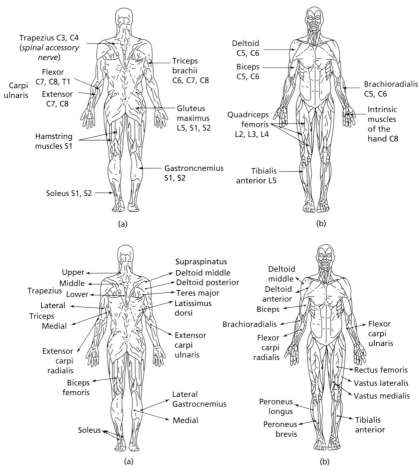

Fig. 4.5 (a) Myotomes and (b) motor points.

Reproduced with permission from Johnson, Mark I., 'Acupuncture-like transcutaneous electrical nerve stimulation (AL-TENS) in the management of pain', *Physical Therapy Reviews*, Volume 3, Number 2, pp. 73–93 (21), Figures 6 and 7, Copyright © 1998, available from www.maneypublishing.com/journals/ptr and www.ingentaconnect.com/content/maney/ptr.

is taken as a point on the skin over a muscle where electrical stimulation will cause contraction of the muscle. The cathode, which should be placed over the motor point, should be applied distally with respect to the anode because nerve impulses in a motor neurones will be travelling towards the periphery.

Instances where AL-TENS may be more beneficial than conventional TENS

Alterations in skin sensitivity

AL-TENS of ipsilateral myotomes may be effective in the presence of hypoaesthesia if it is not possible to achieve a strong, non-painful TENS sensation using conventional

TENS. AL-TENS of contralateral myotomes is preferable in the presence of hyperaesthesia although over time it may be possible to progress towards applying AL-TENS on the site of hyperaesthesia (i.e. ipsilateral) but this should be done with caution and only when the patient clearly understands that TENS may worsen the pain.

Radiating pain

Neuropathic pain that radiates in the limbs including lumbar and cervical rhizopathy can be managed using a dual-channel stimulator. One channel (electrode pair) is used to deliver conventional TENS over the origin of the pain (i.e. nerve root), and the other channel is used to generate muscle twitching via AL-TENS over the radiating pain.

Pain arising from deep structures

The afferent input from deeper-seated structures during AL-TENS may be more effective than conventional TENS at inhibiting onward transmission of nociceptive transmission of deep-seated skeletal muscle and visceral tissue (e.g. pelvic, abdominal, and myalgic pains), although contractions of already painful muscles may cause further discomfort. AL-TENS applied at contralateral myotomes or at trigger points may prove useful. Conventional TENS, AL-TENS, intense TENS, and interferential current therapy have all been reported to reduce pain associated with primary dysmenorrhoea suggesting that deep-seated afferent input during TENS is not a prerequisite for success (see Chapter 8, 158).

Widespread pain, multiple-site pain, and prolonged post-TENS pain relief

The more powerful, widespread, and prolonged pain relief associated with AL-TENS suggests that it may be more beneficial than conventional TENS for poorly localized pain (e.g. central pain), pains in multiple locations, or when prolonged post-stimulation pain relief is needed prior to activities such as driving, operating machinery, or exercise.

Electrode placement over acupuncture points

The delivery of TENS to acupuncture points (acu-TENS) requires no training in needling technique, although knowledge of appropriate acupuncture points to use for different painful conditions is necessary. Scepticism about the existence of acupuncture points remains in some quarters although systematic reviews and meta-analyses are positive for many conditions and acupuncture is recommended by the National Institute of Health and Clinical Excellence for non-specific low back pain in the UK (National Institute for Health and Clinical Excellence, 2009b).

Generally, acupuncturists use a combination of local points close to the site of pain and distant points that have analgesic properties. In general local points correspond to electrode positions used when TENS is delivered at the site of pain. Less precision is needed for the placement of TENS electrodes on acupuncture points compared with acupuncture needles because TENS electrodes are large (e.g. 5 cm × 5 cm) whereas acupuncture points and needles are small (e.g. 1 mm). Commercially available acupuncture point finders may be useful in locating acupuncture points with precision.

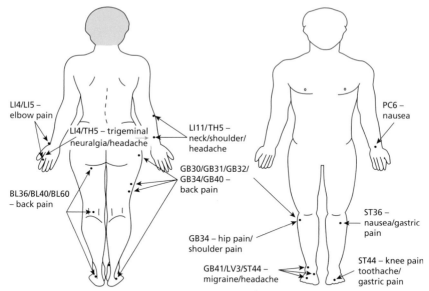

Fig. 4.6 Examples of some distant acupuncture points used to relieve various pains. TENS at these sites (acu-TENS) may be useful when local electrode placement is not possible.

Using TENS at distant points (Figure 4.6) may be useful when skin sensitivity close to the pain is heightened or diminished. Low-frequency, single pulsed high-intensity currents are often used to mimic the hyper-stimulation achieved during acupuncture, although some practitioners deliver conventional TENS on acupuncture points. The cathode should be placed directly over the acupuncture point as this is the active electrode, and small-diameter circular electrodes (1 cm diameter) may be used. Practitioners determine which acupuncture points based on point selection techniques used by acupuncturists as described in acupuncture literature (King, 1999; White et al., 2008b). Administering TENS to acupuncture points may be an efficient means of eliciting visible muscle contractions as some acupuncture points correspond to motor points and trigger points.

Electrode placement over trigger points

Trigger points are hyperirritable spots in skeletal muscle associated with nodules in taut bands of muscle fibres that are often tender on palpation causing patterns of referred pain and/or a local twitch response (Figure 4.7). Double-blind RCTs have found that TENS reduced trigger-point sensitivity and improved symptoms associated with myofascial pain syndrome. Gemmell and Hilland (2011) found that TENS delivered by an electric point stimulation device increased pressure-pain threshold at the trigger point and reduced pressure-evoked pain over the trigger point in 60 individuals with upper-trapezius trigger points. Rodriguez-Fernandez and colleagues (2011) found that low-frequency TENS (burst pattern 2 bps, internal frequency 100 pps, 200 μs) over the upper trapezius for 10 minutes increased referred pressure-pain threshold over trigger

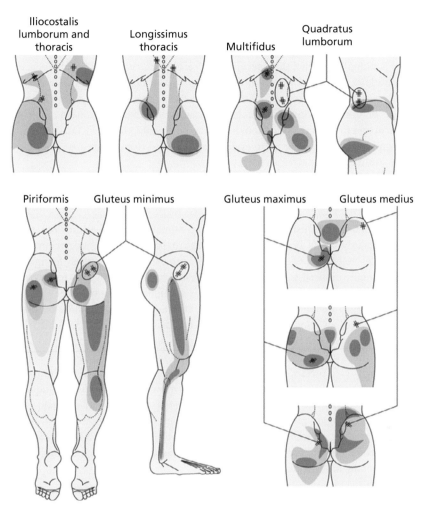

Fig. 4.7 Common trigger points (cross-hatch symbols) and pain referral patterns relevant to lower back and posterior hip-girdle pain created from a composite from multiple individuals. Darker areas represent common referral patterns and lighter areas represent less common referral patterns. The long axis of the trigger point is aligned with the direction of the muscle fibre for the relevant muscle.

Reproduced from Mike Cummings, Physical approaches to the management of back pain: III. Acupuncture, in Andrew Souter et al. (eds), *Oxford Pain Management Library Back Pain*, Figure 7.1, 72, Copyright © 2012, by permission of Oxford University Press.

points and cervical range of motion in rotation. Graff-Radford and colleagues (1989) found that 10 minutes of high-frequency, high-intensity TENS (100 pps, 250 μs) was more effective at reducing myofascial pain than high-frequency, low-intensity TENS (100 pps, 50 μs), or low-frequency, high-intensity TENS (2 Hz, 250 μs or control (n = 12 per group). Interestingly, TENS did not affect local trigger-point sensitivity.

Principles of safe and appropriate choice of electrical characteristics used for stimulation

There is a long-held belief that specific electrical characteristics of TENS influence the magnitude of pain relief. However, the number of possible combinations of electrical characteristics using a standard TENS device is vast. Experimental studies that expose animals or humans to noxious stimuli under controlled laboratory conditions are used as precursors to clinical studies looking at the relationship between TENS characteristics and hypoalgesia in order to evaluate efficacy and to establish dose and optimal technique, including electrical characteristics.

Studies using experimental pain to determine optimal settings

Experimental studies using healthy pain-free humans exposed to noxious stimuli are particularly useful because humans can verbalize and make judgements about experiences associated with exposure to the noxious stimuli. Methods for inducing experimentally induced pain are relatively safe and enable investigators to control the duration, intensity, and quality of the noxious stimulus and the treatment intervention including adherence (Staahl & Drewes, 2004). Various techniques are used to administer noxious stimuli to cutaneous, deep somatic (bone, muscle), and visceral (oesophagus, stomach, bladder) tissue without causing appreciable injury to the individual. These include blunt pressure algometry, sharp pressure algometry, contact thermal pain, cold pressor pain, electrical pain, and the submaximal effort tourniquet test for ischaemia pain. (Figure 4.8) (Staahl & Drewes, 2004). Some techniques are used to cause moderate injury to provide information about response to pain associated with pathological processes such as delayed onset muscle soreness (post-exercise muscle soreness), intramuscular injection of hypertonic saline, intradermal capsaicin, and experimentally induced wounds. Common measurements taken in studies using experimentally induced pain are:

- pain threshold, the point at which first sensation of pain is experienced
- pain tolerance, the point at which the pain is no longer bearable
- pain intensity, the strength/severity of the pain sensation
- pain unpleasantness, the 'bothersomeness' of the pain sensation

When compared with RCTs, studies using experimentally induced pain are less expensive, achieve statistical power using fewer participants, and enable fast and efficient evaluation of outcome. They should include comparison groups to determine which variables are contributing to any observable effect. Placebo controls are used to determine whether the active ingredient of a treatment is contributing to observed effects because non-specific effects associated with the act of receiving a treatment will contaminate observations.

Efficacy: TENS versus placebo

The most comprehensive systematic review of experimental studies to date included 43 studies that investigated the effects of parameter combinations of TENS on experimental

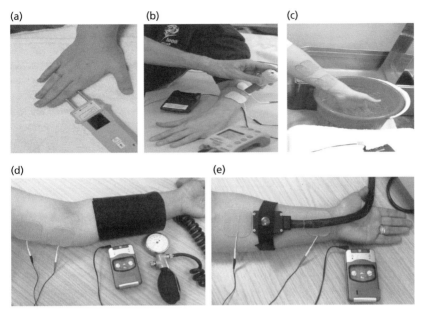

Fig. 4.8. Models of experimental pain. (a) Electrical pain, (b) blunt pressure pain (pressure algometry), (c) cold pressor pain, (d) ischaemic pain using the submaximal effort test, and (e) contact thermal pain using a contact thermode and a Thermal Sensory Analyser.

models in healthy humans and that were published up to December 2009 (Claydon et al., 2011). Overall, evidence was conflicting for the efficacy of TENS compared with placebo (no current) TENS, irrespective of the TENS parameters used, although findings from good quality studies consistently showed that conventional TENS was superior to placebo (no current) TENS for reducing pressure pain but not for reducing experimental pain induced by other pain models. Low-intensity, low-frequency, local TENS and 'barely perceptible' TENS were not efficacious, suggesting that current amplitude with sufficient strength to generate a strong TENS sensation was necessary to produce hypoalgesia. The reviewers concluded that the efficacy of TENS depended on combinations of parameters and on the experimental pain model used in the study but they were unable to recommend specific parameters for TENS. The possibility that strong, non-painful TENS sensations act as a general non-specific distraction was investigated by Marchand and colleagues (1991). If TENS acted by non-specific distraction, any distraction technique would produce similar effects. Marchand and colleagues (1991) found that TENS reduced the intensity of experimental pain in healthy participants but did not affect participants ratings of the intensity of visual stimuli, demonstrating that general distraction was not the major mechanism for TENS.

Optimal TENS amplitude (TENS intensity)

Increasing pulse amplitude activates cutaneous A-β fibres first to produce a non-painful TENS sensation and then cutaneous A-δ fibres to produce a pin-prick pain sensation followed by C-fibres to produce a burning pain sensation (Sang et al., 2003). Studies using

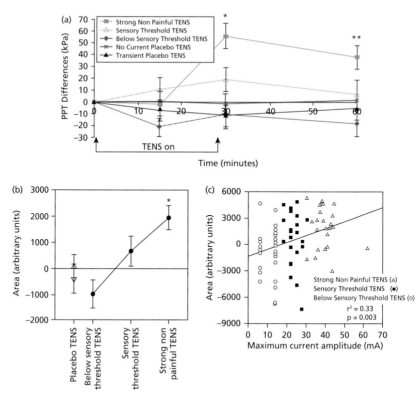

Fig. 4.9 Dose response for the intensity of TENS on experimentally induced pressure pain in healthy human volunteers ($n = 26$ per group). Strongest intensities show the greatest effect. TENS (80 pps, continuous pattern) was applied to the forearm for 30 minutes and pressure pain (PPT) recorded from the forearm before, during (at 15 minutes) and post-TENS (immediately and 30 minutes after switch off). (a) Differences in PPT from baseline (* = $P < 0.0001$ strong, non-painful TENS significantly different to below-sensory-threshold TENS, no current placebo TENS, and transient placebo TENS; ** = $P = 0.003$ strong, non-painful TENS significantly different to below-sensory-threshold TENS). (b) Mean area under the curve for the change in PPT. For comparison, areas for the two placebos (∇ = transient placebo; $\triangle$ = no current placebo; * = strong, non-painful TENS significantly different from below sensory-threshold and both placebo TENS groups). (c) Scatter plot of the maximum pulse amplitude (mA) used and the mean area under the curve for the change in PPT (kPa) for each participant ($n = 78$). A positive relationship was found (Pearson's correlation coefficient). Adapted from Moran et al., 2011.

Adapted from *The Journal of Pain*, Volume 12, Issue 8, Fidelma Moran et al, Hypoalgesia in Response to Transcutaneous Electrical Nerve, pp. 929–935, Copyright © 2011 by the American Pain Society, with permission from Elsevier, http://www.sciencedirect.com/science/journal/15265900

experimental pain have consistently found that strong, non-painful TENS is superior to TENS below or just at sensory-detection threshold in a dose-dependent fashion with stronger intensities producing stronger hypoalgesia (Aarskog et al., 2007; Lazarou et al., 2009; Claydon et al., 2011; Moran et al., 2011) (Figure 4.9). A meta-analysis of studies investigating TENS for the management of post-operative pain found larger reductions in post-operative analgesic consumption when TENS was applied at strong, non-painful intensities compared with application at weaker intensities (Bjordal et al., 2003). Thus, patients are instructed to titrate the amplitude of currents to achieve a strong, non-painful TENS sensation without muscle contraction for conventional TENS. For AL-TENS a strong but comfortable pulsate TENS sensation in the presence of muscle contractions is used. A strong, comfortable, non-painful intensity is easier to achieve when TENS is delivered to areas of muscle and soft tissue because of the larger current window (Hughes et al., 2013). The intensity of TENS fades (decreases) during treatment due to habituation so current amplitude needs to be adjusted to maintain a strong, comfortable, non-painful sensation and hypoalgesia (Pantaleao et al., 2011). Adjustments in amplitude have not been shown to affect hypoalgesia for interferential current therapy (Defrin et al., 2005).

Optimal pulse frequency

Different TENS frequencies elicit different neurophysiological mechanisms (DeSantana et al., 2008a). Studies of head-to-head comparisons of pulse frequency when the intensity of TENS is standardized are few because investigators often compare high-frequency, low-intensity TENS with low-frequency, high-intensity TENS. A systematic review of studies using healthy human participants found no difference in hypoalgesia between TENS frequencies during conventional TENS in ten out of 13 studies, although shortcomings in study methodologies compromised the finding (Chen et al., 2008). Since then, a series of methodologically stronger studies have found that strong, non-painful TENS at 80 pps was superior to 3 pps at reducing experimentally induced, blunt pressure mechanical pain (Chen & Johnson, 2010b), and ischaemic pain (Chen & Johnson, 2011), yet 3 pps was superior to 80 pps for cold pressor pain (Chen & Johnson, 2010a). This suggests that different frequencies may have different effects according to stimulus modality. Chen and Johnson (2009) also found no differences between constant-frequency TENS and frequency-modulated TENS on blunt pressure pain although both were superior to placebo TENS.

There is an absence of clinical research investigations into the relationship between frequency and diagnosis and pain relief when TENS intensity is standardized. A double-blind RCT found no differences in the relief of osteoarthritic knee pain between TENS at 2 pps, 100 pps, and alternating frequency between 2 pps and 100 pps, although all groups were superior to placebo TENS (Law & Cheing, 2004). An RCT using 163 chronic pain patients found that individuals with bone and soft tissue injuries were more satisfied with high-frequency TENS than individuals with osteoarthritis of the vertebral column or peripheral neuropathic pain, but there were no comparisons with low-frequency TENS so it was not possible to attribute the findings to high frequency per se (Oosterhof et al., 2008). An in-depth study that included 179 chronic pain patients using TENS successfully on a long-term basis failed to detect a relationship between patient, electrical characteristics of TENS, and outcome variables (Johnson et al., 1991c). Pulse frequencies between 1 pps and 70 pps were utilized by 75 per cent of patients although this may have been due in part to the logarithmic scaling of the frequency control dial on most devices. A small observational study that recorded pulse frequencies and patterns of TENS used by 13 chronic patients over a one-year period provided tentative evidence that long-term TENS users show individual preferences for TENS frequencies turning to similar pulse frequencies on subsequent treatment sessions (Johnson et al., 1991b). However, pulse frequency was not related to pain aetiology suggesting that patients prefer such frequencies and patterns for reasons of comfort rather than for more potent pain relief. It would be interesting to see whether preferences for different frequencies are related to the sensory quality of pain, e.g. a particular frequency may affect burning pain differently from aching pain. At present there is no clinical evidence to support this view.

As evidence is inconclusive individuals are advised to use frequencies that are comfortable for them at that moment in time for conventional TENS. For AL-TENS either low-frequency single pulsed currents or burst patterns are chosen to achieve a pulsate sensation with accompanying muscle contractions/twitching.

Optimal pulse pattern

A continuous pattern is often implied as a requirement for conventional TENS although activation of low-threshold afferents using any pattern is the important requirement from a physiological perspective. Thus, low-intensity burst-pattern TENS should be considered conventional TENS because it selectively activates low-threshold afferents. Few experimental studies have systematically investigated the effect of pulse patterns with other electrical characteristics held constant. Johnson and colleagues (1991a) found that strong, non-painful TENS without visible muscle contraction delivered using burst (2.3 bps, internal frequency 80 pps, 200 μs), amplitude modulation, random frequency, and continuous (80 pps, 200 μs) pulse patterns elevated cold pressor pain threshold and tolerance in healthy participants. However, there were no differences in the magnitude of hypoalgesia between the different pulse patterns. Burst pattern TENS increased pain threshold to a greater extent when delivered to produce forceful phasic muscle contractions of the brachioradialis muscle (2.3 bps, internal frequency 80 pps) compared with burst pattern TENS without muscle contractions (Johnson et al., 1992b). Conventional TENS (continuous pattern, 80 pps) and intense TENS (continuous pattern, 80 pps, fasciculatory muscle contractions) also increased pain threshold, with longer post-TENS hypoalgesia observed using AL-TENS compared with conventional TENS. An in-depth study of 128 patients successfully using TENS on a long-term basis found that 56 per cent preferred using a continuous pattern of stimulation, 23 per cent preferred burst, and 21 per cent alternated between the two (Johnson et al., 1991c).

In clinical practice patients are instructed to use conventional TENS with a continuous pattern in the first instance, but they are encouraged to experiment with other patterns to find what is comfortable for them at that moment in time. For AL-TENS burst and amplitude modulation patterns have been found to be most comfortable for forceful muscle contractions.

Optimal pulse duration

Strong TENS sensations are generated by increasing pulse duration, eventually causing pain according to strength–duration principles of fibre activation (Figure 3.12). It is suggested that AL-TENS should use longer pulse durations to generate hyperstimulation, and shorter pulse durations used to facilitate the passage of currents through the skin to stimulate deeper nerves. There is a lack of systematic research focusing on the influence of pulse duration on TENS outcome, although investigators have manipulated pulse duration simultaneously with other electrical characteristics within experimental studies. In clinical practice patients are encouraged to experiment with pulse durations to find what is comfortable for them at that moment in time.

Optimal pulse waveform

In most standard TENS devices pulse waveform cannot be adjusted by patients. There are very few studies that have investigated TENS waveforms on humans. Kantor and colleagues (1994) found that symmetrical biphasic waveforms required less pulse charge to excite peripheral nerves compared with amplitude-modulated sinusoidal waveforms or bursts of symmetrical pulses. In contrast, Petrofsky and colleagues (2009) investigated the effect of waveforms on muscle strength, pain, and current dispersion in 16 healthy volunteers and found that sine waves produced greater muscle strength and less pain than square, Russian, and interferential waveforms. Square wave stimulation was most painful. They suggested that the subcutaneous fat layer acted as a resistor-capacitor (RC) filter separating the conductive skin dermal and muscle layers which would form the plates of a capacitor allowing sine waves to pass to muscle more easily. Fary and Briffa (2011) found more adverse skin reactions occurred using monophasic waveforms than asymmetric biphasic waveforms, and concluded that monophasic electrical stimulation should be used with caution.

Optimal electrode positioning

There have been remarkably few experimental pain studies that have focused on the influence of different electrode sites without altering other parameters. Chesterton and colleagues (2002) conducted a double-blind, sham-controlled study measuring mechanical pain threshold from the first dorsal interosseous muscle in 240 participants randomized to receive TENS (200 µs) administered at ipsilateral segmental sites over the distribution of the radial nerve or, extrasegmental sites over the acupuncture point Gall bladder 34 (GB34), using different combinations of pulse frequency (4 pps or 110 pps) and intensity ('to tolerance' or 'strong but comfortable'). When compared with sham (no current) TENS, conventional TENS (high-frequency, 'strong but comfortable' intensity) at segmental sites elevated pain threshold during stimulation but not post-stimulation, whereas extrasegmental stimulation (low-frequency, high-intensity) produced an immediate elevation of pain threshold which remained elevated for 30 minutes post-stimulation. Stimulation at both sites simultaneously elevated thresholds to a greater extent than seen at each site on its own. A follow-up study by the same investigation team found that high-frequency, high-intensity segmental TENS, produced rapid onset hypoalgesia which was sustained for 20 minutes post-stimulation whereas other combinations of TENS frequencies (110 Hz or 4 Hz), intensities (strong but comfortable or highest tolerable) and sites (segmentally or extrasegmental) were no different to placebo (no current) TENS (Chesterton et al., 2003). Largest effects were seen when high-intensity stimulation at segmental and extrasegmental sites were used simultaneously, suggesting that the intensity of stimulation was a critical factor in effective technique (Claydon et al., 2008). Brown and colleagues (2007) found no differences in hypoalgesia in the arm exposed to experimental ischaemic pain induced by the submaximal effort tourniquet technique compared with TENS at the contralateral lower leg, which was at a site not related to pain. Cheing and Chan (2009) found no differences in the change in mechanical pain threshold when TENS was administered over acupuncture points versus peripheral nerve points, although there were no differences in the magnitude of response between the two active TENS interventions. Studies that investigate electrode placement on pain patients are even rarer. Rao and colleagues (1981) found no correlation between TENS electrode placement or stimulating parameters on pain relief in 114 chronic pain patients. Johnson and colleagues (1991c) found that successful long-term users of TENS place electrodes to generate strong non-painful electrical paraesthesiae at the site of their chronic pain.

Optimal dosage

There are many views about how often and for how long individuals should administer TENS, and whether dosing regimens should be prescriptive or open. For conventional TENS maximal pain relief occurs in the presence of a strong, non-painful TENS sensation so an open dosing regimen where individuals keep the TENS device switched on whenever the pain is present is likely to be optimal. Individuals should take regular, short breaks from stimulation by turning TENS off for ~10–15 minutes every 1–2 hours, although electrodes can remain in situ. Skin condition beneath the electrodes should be monitored as minor skin irritation may occur, and skin should be washed when electrodes are eventually removed. It is wise to apply electrodes to adjacent fresh skin on a regular basis. For AL-TENS, which is a stronger form of stimulation, muscle fatigue and delayed onset muscle soreness are a concern, especially if stimulation is prolonged and generating contractions of large muscle mass, so dosing regimens of 20–40 minutes a few times a day are advised.

Duration of onset and offset of TENS effects

Electrophysiological studies using animal models of nociception suggest that the onset and offset of inhibition of central nociceptive transmission is almost immediate for conventional TENS with short-lived post-stimulation effects, consistent with a simple neurosynaptic mechanism of action. For AL-TENS, the onset and offset of effects are more gradual, consistent with a more complex neurochemical mechanism of action utilizing supraspinal feedback loops and neuromodulators such as endogenous opioids.

Experimental pain studies using healthy human participants suggest that hypoalgesia for both conventional and AL-TENS occurs within minutes of the participant experiencing a strong, non-painful TENS sensation, although there is tentative evidence that the onset of hypoalgesia during AL-TENS is more gradual (Andersson et al., 1973; Andersson et al., 1976; Duranti et al., 1988; Johnson et al., 1992b). Many of these studies find that hypoalgesia following conventional TENS returns to baseline within 10–20 minutes post-TENS with tentative evidence that hypoalgesia post AL-TENS is more prolonged, lasting up to one hour, although head-to-head comparisons are few. Recently, Francis and colleagues (2011a) failed to detect differences in cold pressor pain threshold or pain intensity between conventional TENS and AL-TENS, but found that hypoalgesia persisted for 15 minutes after TENS was switched off for AL-TENS but not for conventional TENS (Francis et al., 2011b). Whether these differences are clinically meaningful is a matter for debate.

Post-stimulation pain relief has been reported to last anywhere between five minutes and 18 hours for patients in pain although systematic research is lacking. Cheing and colleagues (2003) measured the half-life of relief of osteoarthritic knee pain following strong but comfortable TENS of acupuncture points around the knee (continuous, 100 pps, 200 μs) for five days per week for two weeks. Similar magnitudes of pain reduction were seen immediately after 20, 40, or 60 minutes of TENS but more prolonged post-stimulation relief lasting up to 4.3 hours was found for longer durations of stimulation in a dose-dependent fashion. Moreover, the half-life of post-TENS increased between the first day and the tenth, suggesting a cumulative increase in post-TENS effects with repeated use. The authors suggested that 40 minutes of TENS each day would be an optimal dose to generate prolonged post-TENS effects.

Post-TENS effects are also influenced by a variety of other factors including natural fluctuations in pain over time, concurrent medication, and physical activity. For example, pain relief during TENS may be lower than expected if TENS was applied when pain intensity was on an upward trajectory. In such circumstance no alteration in pain intensity during TENS may reflect beneficial effects. It is important to synchronize concurrent medication so that the effects of medication do not decline at the same time as TENS is stopped as this may lead to rebound pain. Therefore, patients must be able to appropriately coordinate dosing of pro re nata (as needed) medication and TENS. Physical activity may exacerbate or improve pain which may affect pain relief during and post-TENS. Patients should be warned of the dangers of undertaking excessive physical activity whilst achieving pain relief from TENS as they may experience rebound pain the following day. A boom-and-bust approach to using TENS in order to undertake excessive physical activity should be discouraged. However, if physical activity is carefully managed it is possible that the additional low-threshold (A-β) input resulting from activity may prolong the duration of post-TENS pain relief.

Biological, psychological, and social factors influencing response to TENS

Response to TENS may be influenced by a vast array of biological, psychological, and social factors often unrelated to the pain (Mannheimer & Lampe, 1988). In general, attempts to determine the relationship between these factors and TENS success have failed and as a consequence, factors predicting treatment outcome have remained elusive. Nevertheless, awareness of these factors helps in troubleshooting non-response.

Biological factors

An individual's biological characteristics are likely to influence response to TENS although strong relationships between biological factors have not been found.

Type of pain

Robust studies on the relationship between type of pain and TENS outcome are few. Johansson and colleagues (1980) found that pains of neurogenic origin and pains located mainly in the extremities were predictors of a positive result with TENS in 72 chronic pain patients. Johnson and colleagues (1991c) failed to find a relationship between pain diagnosis and TENS outcome. Oosterhof and colleagues (2008) found that patients were more satisfied with TENS outcome if they had pain arising from bone and soft tissue injury (especially post-surgical pain) rather than pain from osteoarthritis (especially of the vertebral column) or peripheral neuropathy. The failure to find any reliable pathophysiology or aetiological variables predictive of treatment success means that any type of pain may respond to TENS. Interestingly, prolonged stress is known to deplete levels of endogenous opioids and TENS actions are mediated via the release of endogenous opioids. Consequently there is a possibility that the effects of TENS may be diminished in the presence of sustained intense pain, such as the later stages of childbirth.

Nervous system responsivity to electrical stimuli

It has been suggested that responders to TENS have nervous systems that amplify TENS input to a greater extent than non-responders, with a greater release of neurotransmitters and neuromodulators (Johnson et al., 1993). The amplitude and latency of waveform components of somatosensory evoked potentials reflect the sensitivity of the nervous system to various stimuli (Chapter 9, 182–184). Golding and colleagues (1986) found that healthy individuals with small baseline somatosensory evoked cortical potential amplitudes were less responsive to TENS reflected by small elevations in pain threshold and small reductions somatosensory evoked cortical potential amplitude. Johansson and colleagues (1981) found that chronic pain patients with large amplitude visual evoked cortical potentials were more likely to respond to TENS. Johnson and co-workers (1993) conducted a prospective study of 29 chronic pain patients given a trial of TENS and then categorized them into responders ($n = 22$) or non-responders based on pain scores at a one month follow-up. Non-responders had smaller baseline N1P1 and N1P2 amplitudes for somatosensory evoked potential elicited by electrical stimuli and auditory evoked potentials suggesting that individual variation in intrinsic cortical responsivity to electrical stimuli may influence response to TENS (Figure 4.10). Response was not related to baseline plasma concentrations of opioid peptides, the site, type, or severity of pain, electrical characteristics of TENS used, age, sex and gender, personality, or clinical ratings of anxiety or depression. Thus, there is tentative evidence that a relatively non-responsive nervous system to sensory stimuli maybe a characteristic of TENS non-responders.

Habituation and tolerance with repeated use of TENS

Habituation of response to TENS occurs whereby neurones and their sensory receptors require a stronger stimulus or a longer period of rest before they can generate another nerve impulse. This decreasing response to repeated and monotonous presentation of pulsed currents results in the intensity of TENS fading over time. In addition, tolerance, a physiological phenomenon whereby larger doses of a treatment are required to achieve the same therapeutic outcome, contributes to long-term decline in response to TENS. Healthy human and animal studies have found that tolerance to repeated daily application of high-frequency TENS resulting in opioid tolerance occurs by day four

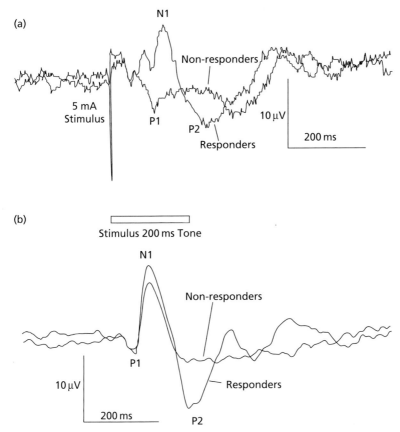

Fig. 4.10 Cortical recorded evoked potentials recorded at Cz reference to linked mastoids in chronic pain patients categorized as TENS responders (*n* = 22) and TENS non-responders (*n* = 7). (a) Somatosensory evoked potentials to 30 monophasic square wave electrical stimuli delivered at 5 mA (interstimulus interval random between 1 and 3 seconds). (b) Auditory evoked potentials to 30 tonnes delivered at 60 dB (1000 Hz, 200 ms, interstimulus interval random between 1 and 3 seconds).

Reproduced from Johnson, M.I., Ashton, C.H., and Thompson, J.W., A prospective investigation into factors related to patient response to TENS: The importance of cortical responsivity, *European Journal of Pain*, 14, pp. 1–9, Copyright © 1993, by permission of the author.

and by day five for low-frequency TENS (Chandran & Sluka, 2003; Liebano et al., 2011) with cholecystokinin (DeSantana et al., 2010) and NMDA receptors (Hingne & Sluka, 2008) being involved.

Providing the nervous system with a continuously changing (novel) input prevents habituation and tolerance. Sato and colleagues (2012) demonstrated in rats that increasing the intensity of TENS by 10 per cent per day delayed the development of analgesic tolerance to repeated use of TENS. Sandkühler (2000) suggested that delivering strong, non-painful conventional TENS punctuated with periods of high-intensity TENS using low-frequency (AL-TENS) or high-frequency (intense TENS) currents may reduce habituation and may be useful for background pain with incidents of breakthrough pain. They termed the technique 'sequential TENS'. Melzack and colleagues (1980) suggested that habituation to TENS can be reduced by swapping the type of afferent input using cold, heat, or massage. Codetron, a TENS-like device, was developed in the 1980s and was shown to reduce habituation by delivering acupuncture-like TENS to stimulation points on the body in a random order (Fargas-Babjak et al., 1992), although no additional benefits were observed when it was added to an active exercise regimen (Herman et al., 1994). Delivery of conventional TENS using random pulse frequencies has been attempted although users report that the irregular presentation of pulses is unpleasant and creates anxiety (Johnson et al., 1991a). More recently, alternating and modulating patterns of pulses have been developed to reduce habituation and tolerance. Desantana and colleagues (2008b) found that alternating (4 pps and 100 pps) or mixed frequency (4 pps on one day, 100 pps on the next day) TENS at sensory intensity (20 minutes per day for two weeks, 100 μs) delayed the onset of tolerance by approximately five days compared with low- or high-frequency TENS on its own. Tong and colleagues (2007) found that alternating or frequency modulated patterns produced greater hypoalgesia compared with constant frequency TENS whereas Chen and Johnson (2009) did not. Hamza and co-workers (1999) found that alternating or frequency modulated patterns produced greater pain relief in women undergoing major gynaecological procedures but Law and Cheing (2004) did not find the same for osteoarthritic knee pain. Thus, evidence suggests, but is not irrefutable, that techniques to reduce nervous system habituation and physiological tolerance may improve TENS.

Psychological factors

Psychological factors, including personality, fear avoidance, catastrophizing, and expectation of treatment outcome, play a major role in chronic pain and an individual's response to treatment. Bates and Nathan (1980) reported the results of seven years of experience in treating pain with TENS and found that individuals with psychological and social problems tend not to respond well to TENS. Nielzen and colleagues (1982) measured the incidence of psychiatric factors in 66 chronic patients using TENS under blind condition and found that patients with mental illness and pathological personality traits were less likely to respond to treatment. Johansson and co-workers (1981) found that high values of the Lie scale of the Eysenck Personality Inventory reflecting socially conforming behaviour were related to positive outcome with TENS. However, other studies have failed to find a relationship (Andersson et al., 1976; Johnson et al., 1991c). Oosterhof and colleagues (2008) analysed the findings from 163 chronic patients who were participants of an RCT and found that response to high-frequency conventional TENS was not related to pain catastrophizing or mechanisms of pain behaviour and perceived control of pain. A fear of electricity and of technology is likely to hinder success and may even prevent an individual from trying TENS in the first instance.

The situational context in which treatments are delivered influences expectation of response. TENS produces an unfamiliar sensation as part of the therapeutic effect, yet the research on expectancy of treatment outcome has largely been ignored. Lampl and colleagues (1998) found that many patients overestimated the potential benefit from TENS, which is similar to many pain-relieving treatments. Patients discontinued TENS use because it did not relieve pain, required too much effort to administer, or the pain condition had worsened. This demonstrates the need for careful patient evaluation and education, and the need for patients to commit to the necessary effort to achieve treatment success. Patients with an external locus of control, expecting health-care professionals to provide a cure for their pain, often fail to accept responsibility for self-administering TENS and are less likely to respond. It is important to assess patient expectations and establish a clear understanding from the patient that they need to engage fully with the search for a personalized, successful TENS-treatment strategy that fits into their activities of daily living. Sometimes patients are stubborn with their refusal to accept that TENS is not a cure for their pain and that their pain is likely to return after each treatment, and that they will probably need to use TENS regularly to manage their pain.

Whether treatment is perceived as logical is likely to affect outcome. Dementia or senility may compromise understanding of how to operate TENS although a caregiver may be able to administer TENS providing the caregiver is able to understand changes in the patients behaviours or facial expression that convey appropriate TENS sensation and pain relief. Similarly, patients with physical disability that prevents them from administering TENS themselves can have a caregiver administering TENS. Generally, however, patients that are dependent on a caregiver to administer TENS are less likely to continue with TENS in the long term. Thus, evidence suggests that psychological factors are important for TENS success, although relationships between specific factors and outcome are not known.

Sociocultural factors

Societal and individual attitudes and beliefs associated effect response to pain treatments and may present barriers to TENS as a viable treatment option.

TENS and gender

The prevalence of chronic pain and pain sensitivity response to experimental stimuli are higher in women than men with biological differences in reproductive physiology and psychosocial differences in gender role expectation playing a role (Fillingim et al., 2009; Alabas et al., 2012). There is only one experimental pain study with a primary focus to compare TENS responses between men and women. Lund and colleagues (2005) found increased pain thresholds to electrical stimuli for women but not men during 20 minutes of high-frequency TENS, but there were no differences in sensory-detection thresholds, suggesting sex differences in response to TENS. Investigators have failed to detect meaningful differences in response in patient populations. Johansson and colleagues (1980) found that sex had no predictive value on response to TENS in chronic pain patients, and Johnson and colleagues (1991c) failed to detect differences between men and women in the way that they used TENS to relieve pain or in the amount of pain relief achieved. Pragmatically, women may have difficulty attaching the TENS device to items of clothing that do not have a belt, although this will affect women and men equally in cultures where women and men do not wear trousers and skirts (e.g. South Asia and the Middle East).

TENS, ethnicity, and culture

It is plausible that genetic variation may influence nervous system responsivity to TENS. To date there have been no studies investigating the relationship between ethnicity and response to TENS. Cultural attitudes and beliefs may also influence acceptance of TENS as a viable treatment. In China and the Far East stimulation-produced analgesia has a long history and may be more culturally acceptable as a treatment modality than in other regions of the world such as Africa (Tashani & Johnson, 2009). It has been found that response to acu-TENS is culturally determined, with Chinese individuals reporting that they expected acu-TENS to be more beneficial than conventional TENS perhaps because acupuncture is a culturally accepted treatment (Brown et al., 2009). Likewise, response to placebo TENS is influenced by ethnicity. Johnson and Din (1997) found that first-generation, UK-born Asian participants had larger elevations in cold pressor pain threshold during placebo TENS than white Anglo-Saxon participants.

Research on TENS in culturally diverse and resource-limited countries tends to use sample populations from urban hospital settings reflecting modern biomedical models of practice. In India, the prevalence of chronic pain in the general population is 19 per cent and prevalence of musculoskeletal pain 25.9 per cent (Bihari et al., 2011), and attitudes towards the use of TENS in physiotherapy are positive (Babu et al., 2010). Case series in urban settings support acceptability of the treatment with patients (Mittal et al., 1998; Dhindsa et al., 2011), and RCTs conducted in urban physiotherapy and hospital settings are plentiful with the majority having positive outcomes (for example, Ratna & Rekha, 2004; Chandra et al., 2010; Rajpurohit et al., 2010; Prabhakar & Ramteke, 2011). However, research on the use of TENS in rural settings of India is limited to one study that found that TENS was used successfully for patients with trigeminal neuralgia in a rural outdoor patient department (Singla et al., 2011). Nevertheless, TENS appears to be a viable treatment option for culturally diverse and resource-limited populations, even in rural communities.

Adherence to TENS treatment regimen

Non-adherence to dosing regimens is common for pain treatments. The amount of effort to administer TENS and the ability to sustain motivation to use TENS influences long term response. Pallett and colleagues (2013) found that only one of 35 (3 per cent) patients fully adhered to a protocol for using TENS for chronic low back pain for one hour each day and reporting pain score four times throughout the day. The finding was surprising as patients were aware that the purpose of the study was to monitor TENS use and pain score reporting. Interestingly, some of the cases of non-adherence were due to patients using TENS for longer than prescribed. Some standard TENS devices record TENS usage, parameters, and electronic pain scores which may help to motivate patients to adhere and monitor treatment, but most do not include utilization monitoring technology because it increases the cost of the TENS device. Concern about the fidelity of research studies that require patients to self-administer TENS for multiple sessions has been revealed in an evaluation of Cochrane reviews that found that TENS treatments were too short, too infrequent, or with inadequate technique (Bennett et al., 2011). The use of electronic data monitoring is critical in future research to validate adherence to TENS protocols.

Diet and concurrent medication

Substances that affect the action of biochemicals including neurochemicals may interact with the physiological actions of TENS. The influence of diet on response to TENS has largely been neglected. Caffeine is a competitive, non-selective adenosine receptor antagonist at A1 and A2a spinal cord receptors that have been implicated in TENS actions. A placebo-controlled study found TENS did not reduce experimentally induced pain when combined with a 200 mg caffeine pill (Marchand et al., 1995) although a follow-up study failed to detect differences in pain threshold during TENS following an above-average strength of a cup of coffee (100 mg of caffeine) compared with decaffeinated coffee (Dickie et al., 2009). Thus, occasional ingestion of a normally caffeinated drink probably will not affect TENS hypoalgesia although more habitual caffeine intake may reduce TENS effectiveness. TENS hypoalgesia is also mediated via central serotonin (5-HT) systems and serotonin synthesis depends on the availability of its precursor tryptophan from eggs, meat, poultry, and dairy products. In principle the effect of TENS may be enhanced with a diet high in tryptophan, although to date there has been no empirical research on the topic.

The influence of concurrent medication in response to TENS has also been neglected. Habitual use of diazepam, a serotonin depleting agent, may reduce the effectiveness of TENS. However, diazepam also binds to a subunit on the GABA(A) receptor enhancing the effect of the neurotransmitter GABA which is a key neurotransmitter involved in TENS action. Therefore, diazepam might also act synergistically with TENS. The most important drug interaction is with habitual use of opioids. TENS actions are mediated via opioid receptors within the central nervous system and there is evidence that long-term use of opioid medication may impact negatively on response to TENS. Opioid medication (e.g. morphine) acts via μ-opioid receptors and habitual opioid use results in physiological tolerance. Low-frequency TENS also acts via μ-opioid receptors and Sluka and colleagues (2000) found that low-frequency TENS was ineffective in morphine-tolerant rodents. The effects of high-frequency TENS acting via δ-opioid receptors were preserved. Leonard and colleagues (2011) confirmed this finding in chronic pain patients by comparing the analgesic effect of conventional (high-frequency) and acupuncture-like (low-frequency) TENS in 12 opioid-treated chronic pain patients and 11 opioid-naive chronic pain patients. They found that conventional TENS reduced pain for both the opioid and non-opioid patients whereas AL-TENS only reduced pain in the non-opioid group. The investigators attributed the lack of pain relief during AL-TENS to the development of μ-opioid receptor tolerance. One clinical implication of this finding is that pain patients regularly taking opioids are more likely to benefit from conventional TENS.

Summary

1 In general, conventional TENS is the technique of choice and AL-TENS used if patients are resistant to conventional TENS.

2 Maximal pain relief occurs with electrodes positioned on sensate skin to generate a strong, non-painful TENS sensation within the site of pain. Alternative sites include nerve bundles, paravertebrally, and contralateral dermatomes.

3 Patients are advised to administer conventional TENS constantly whenever pain relief is required using pulse frequencies, durations, and patterns that are comfortable for them at that moment in time.

4 There are no reliable predictors of treatment success so any type of pain may respond to TENS.

5 Analgesic tolerance to TENS may develop from repeated daily use but can be overcome by increasing the intensity of TENS each day or by changing the electrical characteristics of stimulation. Patients taking opioids on a regular basis may respond less well to AL-TENS.

Further reading

- Claydon, L.S., Chesterton, L.S., Barlas, P., and Sim, J. (2011) Dose-specific effects of transcutaneous electrical nerve stimulation (TENS) on experimental pain: a systematic review. *Clin J Pain*, **27**, 635–47.

- Mannheimer, J., and Lampe, G. (1988) Factors that hinder enhance and restore the effectiveness of TENS: Physiological and theoretical considerations. In Mannheimer, J., Lampe, G. (eds) *Clinical Transcutaneous Electrical Nerve Stimulation*. FA Davis Company, Philadelphia, PA, 529–70.

- Moran, F., Leonard, T., Hawthorne, S., Hughes, C.M., McCrum-Gardner, E., Johnson, M.I., Rakel, B.A., Sluka, K.A., and Walsh, D.M. (2011) Hypoalgesia in response to transcutaneous electrical nerve stimulation (TENS) depends on stimulation intensity. *J Pain*, **12**, 929–935.

In Chapter 5 the hazards associated with TENS are reviewed.

Chapter 5

Contraindications, precautions, and adverse events

Introduction

Hazards associated with using TENS need to be assessed against risks of using other available treatments including drug medication, and patients need to be informed of these hazards to provide valid consent to treatment. In many instances TENS evaluates favourably. The decision to offer TENS to a patient is based on the professional judgement of the practitioner and it is always wise to seek the views of colleagues if uncertain. Not treating pain can involve risks to health and may even be fatal. For example, if an elderly person with fracture ribs remains in pain whilst breathing or coughing, it can lead cough suppression and an increased risk of pneumonia and under-ventilation affecting blood gases. The purpose of this chapter is to discuss contraindications, precautions, and adverse events associated with TENS by covering:

- National safety guidelines
- Contraindications to TENS, including device implants and pre-existing conditions
- Hazardous electrode sites
- Adverse reactions

National safety guidelines

Judgements about whether it is safe to use TENS are guided by whether TENS has the potential to increase the likelihood of an adverse event (Table 5.1). Practitioners should adhere to safety guidelines on the safe use of electrophysical techniques by professional bodies including the Australian Physiotherapy Association (Robertson et al., 2001), the Chartered Society of Physiotherapy in the United Kingdom (Chartered Society of Physiotherapy, 2006), and the Canadian Physiotherapy Association (Houghton et al., 2010). Guidelines from the Canadian Physiotherapy Association are comprehensive and supported by physiological rationale and research evidence.

As a rule of thumb, TENS can be used with little risk to manage pain in most patients. If there is concern that TENS may adversely affect the underlying medical condition then the situation must be discussed with the patient and their physician and all risks and consequences disclosed. Often it is possible to administer TENS at a body site away from the tissue of concern.

Table 5.1 Terminology

Term	Definition
Adverse event	Undesirable response that could harm the patient
Hazard	A situation that poses a threat resulting in a negative outcome (i.e. 'something' with the potential to cause harm)
Risk	The probability of threat being realized (hazard severity × likelihood of occurrence)
Contraindication	Situations where a treatment should not be used because it may do more harm to the patient than good
Absolute contraindication	No reasonable circumstances for giving the treatment
Relative contraindication	There are circumstances for giving the treatment despite there being risks of harm but these are outweighed by benefits
Local contraindication	Situations where the treatment should not be given to a specific body region
Precaution	When a treatment can be given but there is a moderate risk of an adverse event. The treatment should proceed but with caution and careful monitoring, and actions need to be put in place to reduce the risk of harm
Categories of adverse events	
Minor	Causing inconvenience which would resolve spontaneously and of limited consequence such as exacerbation of pain, mild erythema, and mild itchiness
Moderate	Temporary event that requires medical attention but will not seriously affect the patients overall health such as an electrical skin burn, infection, temporary paralysis, sensory loss, and tissue necrosis
Serious	Life-threatening events causing death or permanent disability or discomfort such as permanent paralysis or sensory loss, seizures, cardiac dysfunction and foetal abnormality

Judgements can be based on the following considerations (Houghton et al., 2010).

1 Is the patient competent to use TENS?

2 Does the patient have a pre-existing disease or illness and is there a potential for TENS to interfere with physiological functioning?

3 Does the patient have an implant or external attachment (e.g. drainage system)? If so, could the electrical currents from TENS

 • be electrically conducted by the implant and interfere with the normal operation of the implant or cause discomfort to the patient at the implant–tissue interface?

 • cause mechanical stresses in tissues which may interfere with the normal function of the implant, such as TENS-induced muscle contraction or blood vessel constriction or dilatation?

 • cause chemical reactions or iontophoresis?

Contraindications to TENS

A summary of contraindications form professional bodies is shown in Table 5.2. Manufacturers list cardiac pacemakers, pregnancy, and epilepsy as absolute contraindications because it may be difficult to exclude TENS as a potential cause of a problem in these patient groups from a legal perspective. Practitioners have used TENS for such individuals providing TENS is not applied over the area of concern and the patient's progress is carefully monitored throughout (i.e. local contraindication). TENS should not be applied over the chest in patients with cardiac failure, over areas where there is active malignancy for patients with 'treatable' tumours, or over areas where there has been recent haemorrhage.

Electrically active device implants

There is a risk of interference when TENS is applied close to an active electrical device implant because the implanted electrical device needs to discriminate between true electrical activity from biological tissue such as the heart and the electrical current generated by the TENS device. If TENS caused a malfunction of some of these devices it could be life-threatening or necessitate surgery to replace the device. Whether active implants are an absolute or relative (local) contraindication has been a matter for debate. The general consensus is that TENS is contraindicated for cardiac pacemakers, implantable cardioverter defibrillators, bone-growth stimulators, and neural stimulators such as spinal cord and brain stimulators, unless there are exceptional reasons following evaluation by a medical specialist from a pain clinic or cardiology clinic. If TENS is to be used on a patient with an active implant, the supervised trial should be performed under medical supervision where resuscitation facilities are available. Prior to implantation of an active device it is necessary to establish whether or not patients have been using TENS for a pre-existing pain condition.

Cardiac pacemakers and implantable cardioverter defibrillators

TENS is used to manage refractory angina and coronary artery disease and some of these patients may have been implanted with a cardiac pacemaker to correct bradycardia. Pulsed currents during TENS may be interpreted by the cardiac pacemaker as electrical signals from the heart resulting in inhibition of the intrinsic heart rhythm, pausing between heart beats, and bradycardia. Under-sensing may cause the pacemaker to operate at its basal rate resulting in suboptimal atrioventricular synchrony and pacemaker syndrome, with decreased cardiac output, decreased atrial contribution to ventricular filling, and reductions in total peripheral resistance response. There is a greater risk of TENS affecting demand-type pacemakers which adjust pacemaker rate according to the individual's heart rate than TENS affecting fixed-rate pacemakers. The potentially serious hazardous effects are most likely if TENS electrodes are placed over the pacemaker, i.e. on the chest. Filters can be used to reduce electromagnetic interference by electronic devices. It is likely that adverse symptoms would abate when the TENS device was switched off.

Research suggests that most patients with permanent cardiac pacemakers could safely use TENS providing it is not applied over the chest. There were no episodes of TENS

Table 5.2 TENS contraindications and precautions

Condition	Synthesis of recommendations	Canadian Physiotherapy Association Guidelines	UK Chartered Society of Physiotherapy Guidelines	Australian Physiotherapy Association Guidelines	Adverse reaction	Quality of research evidence
Implants						
Electronic (e.g. pacemakers or cardioverter defibrillators)	C-L following consultation with cardiologist	C-L	C	C-L	Serious	Moderate
Metal	P monitor skin condition	S	S	?	Minor	Low
Non-metallic e.g. plastic, cement	S	S	?	?	Minor	Absent
Conditions						
Impaired cognition or communication	C	C for TENS; P for NMES/HVPC	C	P	Minor	Moderate
Deep-vein thrombosis	C for active or suspected DVT; P for conventional TENS but only for individuals with history of DVT after successful management with anticoagulant therapy	C	P	?	Serious	Moderate
Impaired circulation	C for AL-TENS in severe arterial disease and C-L for moderate arterial disease; P for conventional TENS	P but C for severe arterial disease	P	P	Minor	Low

Table 5.2 (continued) TENS contraindications and precautions

Condition	Synthesis of recommendations	Canadian Physiotherapy Association Guidelines	UK Chartered Society of Physiotherapy Guidelines	Australian Physiotherapy Association Guidelines	Adverse reaction	Quality of research evidence
Infection/Tuberculosis/Osteomyelitis	C in the presence of underlying osteomyelitis C-L over infected region	C-L	?	P	Moderate	Low
Pregnancy	C-L over abdomen, pelvis, or acupuncture points associated with uterine contraction. Also C-L for AL-TENS/NMES over lower back	C-L	C-L	C-L	Serious	Moderate
Malignancy	C-L regions of suspected malignancy in oncology; P for individuals close to the end of life	C-L	C-L	P	Serious	Low
Seizure/Epilepsy	C-L over neck or head	C	C	?	Moderate	Moderate
Cardiac failure/Dysrhythmia	C-L over chest	C-L	C-L	C-L	Serious	Low
Haemorrhagic conditions/Bleeding disorders (haemophilia)	C-L in regions of uncontrolled bleeding; P in bleeding disorders after successful management of coagulopathy	C	C	P	Serious	Moderate
Skin damage and/or disease	C-L on damaged tissue	C-L	P	P	Minor	High
Recently radiated tissue	C-L over affected tissue	C-L	P	P	Serious	Moderate

Table 5.2 (continued) TENS contraindications and precautions

Condition	Synthesis of recommendations	Canadian Physiotherapy Association Guidelines	UK Chartered Society of Physiotherapy Guidelines	Australian Physiotherapy Association Guidelines	Adverse reaction	Quality of research evidence
Recent fracture or suture/Osteoporosis	C-L for AL-TENS; S for conventional TENS	S for TENS; C for NMES/HVPC	?	?	Moderate	Moderate
Impaired sensation	C-L over non-sensate skin	C-L for TENS; P for NMES/HVPC	P	P	Minor	Moderate
Chronic wound	P infection control measures needed and monitor bleeding	S	?	?	Moderate	Low
Skin disease (e.g. eczema)	P monitor skin condition	P	?	?	Minor	Low
Active epiphysis in children	P	P	?	?	Moderate	Absent
Hypertension	S	S	?	?	Minor	Low
Inflammation/Acute injury	S	S	?	?	Moderate	Low
Photosensitivity or systemic lupus erythematosis	S	S	?	?	Moderate	Absent
Electrode sites						
Anterior neck/Carotid sinus region	C	C	C	?	Serious	Low
Chest/Intercostal muscles/Heart	C for AL-TENS; S for conventional TENS	P for TENS/HVPC; C for NMES	P	C	Minor	Moderate

Table 5.2 (continued) TENS contraindications and precautions

Condition	Synthesis of recommendations	Canadian Physiotherapy Association Guidelines	UK Chartered Society of Physiotherapy Guidelines	Australian Physiotherapy Association Guidelines	Adverse reaction	Quality of research evidence
Transcranially	C	C	C	S	Serious	Moderate
Reproductive organs	C	C	C	S	Moderate	Absent
Eyes (transorbital)	C transorbital; P other positions	C	C	S	Serious	Absent
Lower abdomen	C for AL-TENS; S for conventional TENS	P for TENS/HVPC; C for NMES	?	?	Moderate	Moderate

Key: C = contraindication; C-L = local contraindication; P = precaution; S = safe; ? = not addressed; HVPC = high-voltage pulsed current; NMES = neuromuscular electrical stimulation

Source: Data adapted from Electrophysical Agents: Contraindications and Precautions: An Evidence-Based Approach to Clinical Decision Making in Physical Therapy, *Physiotherapy Canada*, **62**, 5, Special Issue 2010, 1–80, Copyright © Canadian Physiotherapy Association, 2010. All rights reserved. DOI: 10.3138/ptc.62.5.

interfering with the performance of 20 different models of pacemakers in 51 patients when TENS was applied to the lumbar area, cervical spine, left leg, and lower arm area ipsilateral to the pacemaker (Rasmussen et al., 1988). Investigators did not evaluate the effects of electrodes placed parallel to the pacemaker electrode vector. Unusual electrocardiogram (ECG) artefact misinterpreted as runaway pacemaker activity has been reported for TENS delivered via parasternal electrodes. Carlson and colleagues (2009) assessed the effects of TENS at 2 pps and 80 pps applied above each mamilla on permanent pacemaker function in 27 patients. TENS intensity was increased to the maximum level tolerated for 30 seconds or until there were signs of interference on the ECG, and it was found to inhibit one or more pacemaker stimuli in 22 (81 per cent) cases. The incidence of interference was reported to be higher during TENS at 2 pps than 80 pps although differences were not statistically significant. There was no evidence of under-sensing by the pacemaker. Carlson and colleagues (2009) recommend that ECG monitoring should take place during the first application of TENS, especially if TENS is going to be applied over the chest, and they have developed a testing procedure to be performed at the pacemaker outpatient clinic (Box 5.1). TENS should be withdrawn if any pacemaker interference occurs and alternative treatments should be considered. If there is no interference during TENS and the patient has an intrinsic rhythm during ventricular inhibited (VVI) pacing at 40 beats per minute, then they suggest that TENS could be used safely at the intensities of TENS used during the test. They recommend that the lowest acceptable sensitivity of the pacemaker should be used.

Implantable cardioverter defibrillators (ICDs, internal cardiac defibrillators), are used to correct sudden onset ventricular fibrillation and ventricular tachycardia which may result in sudden cardiac death. They monitor the rate and rhythm of the heart and deliver electrical shocks when heart rate exceeds a preset value in order to restore heart rate to that required. They also perform biventricular pacing in patients with congestive heart failure or bradycardia. If currents from TENS were interpreted as generated by the heart, the implantable cardioverter defibrillator may falsely diagnose this as ventricular fibrillation and produce defibrillator shocks to restore heart rate to normal.

There is strong evidence that TENS triggers inadvertent electrical shocks by implantable cardioverter defibrillators. Holmgren and colleagues (2008) found that TENS interfered with implantable cardioverter defibrillator operation in 16 out of a total of 30 patients. Ventricular premature extra beats were common and the investigators recommended that TENS should not be used by patients with implantable cardioverter defibrillators. If, under exceptional circumstances, a medical team decides to use TENS for such patients it is imperative that testing of TENS and implantable cardioverter defibrillator interaction should be undertaken immediately post-implant and at regular follow-ups.

Implanted neurostimulator devices

TENS should not be used on patients with implanted (permanent) peripheral nerve stimulators, spinal cord stimulators, and brain stimulators unless there is a clear rationale and the case has been discussed with the medical specialist. TENS has been used in combination with non-implanted stimulators such as electroacupuncture to augment pain relief at multiple body sites. However, applying TENS at the same site as another neural stimulator to maximize pain relief is not recommended because of hazards from

Box 5.1 Testing procedure for TENS and pacemaker treatment as suggested by Carlson et al. (2009).

Testing procedure

- Connect continuous ECG and apply permanent pacemaker programmer
- Apply TENS electrodes to treatment area
- Set permanent pacemaker to VVI mode
- Obtain continuous pacing (by increasing ventricular rate of permanent pacemaker)
- Lower ventricular sensing level to maximal sensing level (usually 1 mV)
- Increase TENS amplitude until inhibition of ventricular pacing or to maximum level tolerated by patient for at least 30 seconds
- Explore ECG for inhibition whilst TENS on
- Re-perform whole test for 2 pps and 80 pps
- Re-programme permanent pacemaker to clinical setting
- Conduct new test whenever any future permanent pacemaker reprogramming

Text extracts reproduced from Carlson et al., Interference of transcutaneous electrical nerve stimulation with permanent ventricular stimulation: a new clinical problem?, *Europace*, Volume 11, Issue 3, pp. 364–369, published on behalf of the European Society of Cardiology. All rights reserved. Copyright © The Authors 2008, by permission of Oxford University Press.

electrical signals of multiple devices interfering with each other resulting in device failure or additive effects.

Bone-growth stimulators (electrical osteogenesis stimulators)

Non-invasive techniques to enhance bone repair include ultrasonic fracture-healing devices (e.g. ultrasonic osteogenesis stimulators) and direct low-intensity electrical current bone-growth stimulator devices that use a coil or electrodes placed on the skin or on a cast or brace over a fracture. Implanted devices (e.g. for spinal fusion) deliver direct current to stimulate osteogenesis with electrodes implanted at the fusion site and the battery pack just beneath the dorsal fascia and an external device using pulsating electromagnetic energy to generate electrical currents in the tissue. TENS is a local contraindication because of the risk of an interaction with the bone-growth stimulator. Careful monitoring should take place if TENS were to be used at a site distant to the location of the bone-growth stimulator.

Mechanically active implants

Mechanically active implants include artificial hearts, ventricular assist devices, and robotic prosthetic limbs. Potential hazards include interference with conductivity of electrical components of the implanted device, TENS-induced muscle contractions creating mechanical stresses, or TENS altering physiological variables such as venous return that are then detected by the implanted device. For artificial hearts and ventricular assist devices a worst-case scenario could be serious so TENS is a local contraindication, although no adverse events have been reported in the literature. Decisions on whether to administer TENS in close proximity of other mechanically active implants is at the discretion of the practitioner. Careful monitoring is advisable if TENS were to be used at a site distant to the location of mechanically active implants, especially if they involve cardiac function.

Non-active implants

Non-active implants include any material that has been introduced in the body but is not powered by an external source including artificial joints, stents, prosthetic limbs, and intravenous and central lines. Non-metal implants used, for example, to fix structures in artificial joints are considered safe. A potential hazard of administering TENS over a metal implant is the metal conducting TENS currents producing thermal effects (unlikely) or electrical conductance at the metal–neural interface. How close metal must be to the skin to influence current flow during TENS is not known although most metal components of surgical implants are unlikely to conduct electrical current to any appreciable amount. Therefore, metal implants are generally considered safe although a skin burn resulting from stimulation over a metal implant has been reported (Ford et al., 2005). TENS should not be delivered over skin staples or tissues treated with dressings or topical agents containing metal ions (silver, zinc).

Artificial joints

TENS may be used as part of rehabilitation after joint replacement surgery. Prosthetic hip implants are usually made of a titanium hip prosthesis, with a ceramic head and polyethylene acetabular cup. Prosthetic knee implants are made of a flat metal plate and stem implanted in the tibia, a polyethylene bearing surface, and a contoured metal implant fitted around the end of the femur. Nowadays metals are cobalt–chromium alloy, titanium, and titanium alloy, tantalum, and zirconium alloy. Stainless steel was used in the past but not often used nowadays. Individuals have used neuromuscular electrical stimulation devices over knee joint replacements without adverse reactions (Avramidis et al., 2003). However, Ford and colleagues (2005) reported that a patient experienced a full-thickness skin burn over a metal implant following unicompartmental knee arthroplasty after 'electrical stimulation' for oedema control, quadriceps activation and strengthening, and interferential current therapy for pain control. Interferential current therapy rather than 'electrical stimulation' appeared to be the cause of the burn although it was not possible to assess the direct influence of the metal implant. Skin burns have been reported using interferential current therapy in individuals without metal implants.

Stents, percutaneous drainage systems, and central venous catheters

Stents are used to hold physiological passageways open such as the coronary arteries, ureter, urethra, and oesophagus, and may be made of a metal mesh with a special fabric covering. Hazards associated with electrical conductivity seem minimal because TENS currents remain superficial. TENS has been used to manage pain associated with percutaneous drainage systems that aid removal of fluid from an area of the body such as the chest, abdomen, or pelvis. Central venous catheters (central lines) are made of flexible synthetic tubing placed into large veins in the neck, chest, or groin to administer fluids and medication, and to obtain measurements of blood and cardiovascular status. Mechanical stresses to surrounding tissue induced by higher intensity TENS may pull on catheters so AL-TENS is contraindicated close to the site of the catheter. It should be safe to use low-intensity conventional TENS with careful monitoring to ensure the absence of TENS-induced muscle contractions.

Pre-existing conditions

Compromised consciousness, cognition, or communication including non-adherent patients

Individuals who refuse TENS treatment, do not cooperate with instructions, or do not comprehend instructions should not be given TENS, including individuals with learning difficulties, mental illness, or phobias to electricity. Used inappropriately TENS can cause physical harm and it could be used in subverted acts such as connecting electrode lead pins to metal objects to produce inadvertent shocks. Therefore, individuals must understand that they are responsible for using and storing TENS safely and are competent at administering TENS safely to themselves.

TENS has been used to arouse persons with reduced levels of consciousness and acute coma under supervision by health-care professionals (Chapter 10, 198). However, TENS should not be administered to relieve pain when an individual is experiencing an altered state of consciousness because the individual's ability to provide reliable feedback about the intensity of stimulation will be compromised. TENS can be used on children providing they understand what to expect during TENS and can provide reliable feedback. Caregivers can help the patient in the operation of TENS.

Pregnancy

Practitioners have been fearful of administering any electrophysical agent to patients who are pregnant as it may be difficult to exclude these agents as a potential cause of a pregnancy-related problem. There has been much debate about whether TENS should be contraindicated in pregnancy. There is one review of evidence which concluded that there were no published reports of deleterious effects of TENS on pregnancy (Crothers, 2003, update available from: <http://acpwh.csp.org.uk/publications/acpwh-guidance-safe-use-transcutaneous-electrical-nerve-stimulation-tens-musculo>; accessed 29 November 2013). TENS compares favourably when balancing risks against the use of analgesic medication that could cross the placental barrier and affect the foetus.

Potential hazards when using TENS are the induction of uterine contractions with the potential of premature labour or even causing a miscarriage. This risk seems more likely in the first and third trimesters of pregnancy. Opinion leaders recommend that it is safe to apply TENS providing it is not in the vicinity of the abdomen. The Canadian

Physiotherapy Association recommends that TENS should not be administered over the lower back. However, currents generated for conventional TENS remain superficial and are unlikely to penetrate to a sufficient depth to stimulate uterine muscle so it seems reasonable that strong, non-painful TENS without muscle contractions could be administered over the lower back.

TENS could stimulate uterine nerves that may facilitate contractions. There are reports of TENS affecting uterine function when applied at acupuncture points distant to the uterus. For example, Dunn and colleagues (1989) reported that TENS administered at a 30 pps over acupuncture points—Spleen 6 (SP6, lower leg) and Liver 3 (L3, foot)—increased the frequency and intensity of uterine contractions when compared with placebo (no current) TENS. Other relevant acupuncture points include the dorsal aspect thumb web (LI4), lower-half of the leg and ankle (SP6; BL60 and BL67), middle of trapezius (GB21), head of fibula (LI4; ST36), head of fibula (GB34), ankle (BL60), and top of head (GV20). Therefore, TENS over specific acupuncture points may have physiological effects at other body sites so some electrode positions may inadvertently stimulate acupuncture points. Nevertheless, hazards when using TENS distant from the abdomen seem minimal, although it would be wise to monitor progress regularly.

There are no reports of effects of TENS on foetal development and the potential for teratogenicity or effects on foetal heart conduction and other aspects of physiology seem small because currents would not permeate to such a depth. Literature suggests that there are no adverse effects on the newborn when TENS has been used to treat low back pain and no foetal abnormalities have been reported in cases where TENS has been used by mothers for musculoskeletal pain or placental insufficiency. As the risk of teratogenicity is higher during the first trimester then careful consideration should be given before TENS is prescribed as a method of pain relief during this time, especially if electrodes are to be applied close to the abdomen.

There are no reports in the literature of TENS affecting foetal heart function when TENS is applied posteriorly over lumbosacral nerve roots on the lower back during childbirth. TENS does generate artefact on foetal monitoring equipment, and Bundsen and Ericson (1982) suggest that TENS current density should not be greater than 0.5 µA per square millimetre (mA/surface area electrode pad). Even higher output capacity TENS devices are unlikely to achieve this as the current density at the skin surface markedly diminishes by the time that it reaches the uterus due to dispersal within conducting tissues.

Thus, TENS is a local contraindication over the abdomen or pelvis or on acupuncture points that have an effect on uterine contractions, and AL-TENS (and neuromuscular electrical nerve stimulation) with phasic muscle twitching is contraindicated over the lower back. It seems wise to exert extreme caution if the woman has a history of early miscarriage.

Epilepsy

Seizures result from excessive hypersynchronous neuronal activity in the brain and in people with epilepsy they may be triggered by various stimuli including light, emotional, and/or physical stress, and sleep deprivation. High-amplitude electrical currents delivered to the head are used during electroconvulsive therapy (ECT) to produce seizures in people without epilepsy. Currents used during TENS are insufficient to trigger a seizure in people without epilepsy, even when applied across the temples (which is not recommended). There have been fears that low-frequency TENS (i.e. <10 pps) may trigger epileptic seizures in people with pre-existing epilepsy. For this reason, people with epilepsy, or those who are susceptible to epileptic seizures, need to use TENS with caution. Practitioners need to be vigilant when giving TENS to people with epilepsy as it may be difficult to exclude TENS as a potential trigger of a seizure. Interestingly, focal TENS, peripheral (vagal and trigeminal) nerve stimulation, spinal cord stimulation, and electroacupuncture have all shown promise for controlling seizures (Besio et al., 2007). Harreby and colleagues (2011) found that spinal cord stimulation at 4 Hz increased seizure susceptibility whereas 5 Hz produced a trend, although not statistically significant, towards decreased seizure susceptibility in rats.

Rosted (2001) reported a single case of repetitive tonic–clonic seizures in a post-stroke patient during TENS administered to the paralysed arm for 30 minutes three times a day. Initially, AL-TENS (two bursts per second of 100 pps) generating muscle contractions produced no improvement. When TENS intensity was increased and dosage progressed to four one-hour treatments per day, the patient developed a typical tonic–clonic seizure. The dosage of sodium valproate was increased and the patient continued to administer TENS but developed two further seizures in subsequent days and TENS treatment was withdrawn. No additional seizures occurred over the following three months. Some patients are prone to epileptic seizures following a stroke and in these cases it is advised that TENS should only be used in exceptional circumstances and with careful monitoring. TENS is commonly used for post-stroke pain with no reports of seizures.

Scherder and colleagues (1999) reported increased frequency of seizures when TENS was used to improve memory and behaviour for a girl who suffered from probable herpes simplex encephalitis two years earlier, and a boy with severe psychomotor problems and epilepsy due to meningoencephalitis, six years earlier. There were no beneficial effects of TENS on cognition and behaviour yet parent diaries suggested that during TENS treatment days the number of absence seizures was higher. Seizures persisted for two days after discontinuation of TENS. There are unpublished anecdotes that TENS may also trigger episodes of migraine in individuals with pre-existing migraine, so patients need to be made aware of this potential adverse event. Interestingly, TENS is used by some individuals to manage pain during migraine attacks usually by placing electrodes on the posterior neck or on the shoulder or both. At present, guidelines recommend that TENS should not be administered on the neck or head, including transcranially in patients with epilepsy, and that administering TENS elsewhere on the body should be performed with caution.

Malignancy

Electrical currents are known to stimulate DNA synthesis, cell growth, and cell replication in vitro and also the formation of new blood vessels to cancerous tissues and this has generated debate about the risk of TENS increasing tumour growth. Direct currents have been found to reduce tumour growth by interfering with mitotic spindle formation during cell division by Schaefer and colleagues (2008). To date, there are no studies that have assessed the effect of TENS on tumour growth and no known reports of TENS causing detrimental effects in patients. Clinical evidence suggests that TENS may alleviate pain and improve function and quality of life in individuals with cancer so the general consensus is that these benefits outweigh risks in people with advanced cancer (Searle et al., 2008; Hurlow et al., 2012). Published guidelines for providing acupuncture treatment for cancer patients are a useful resource for TENS and recommend that needling should be avoided in areas of spinal instability due to potential risk of cord compression due to muscle-relaxing properties and in lymphoedematous limbs because of a risk of swelling (Filshie & Hester, 2006). AL-TENS may relax skeletal muscle and increase blood flow so it would be wise to assume that AL-TENS is a local contraindication.

It is recommended that TENS should not be administered over confirmed or suspected malignancy in acute oncology settings. There needs to be caution when considering TENS in patients with undiagnosed pain and a history of cancer within the preceding five years. In the palliative setting TENS may be used with electrodes positioned on areas where there is known disease under the supervision of a palliative care specialist. TENS should not be used on irradiated skin in the immediate weeks after radiotherapy.

Cardiac disturbances

TENS is routinely administered over the anterior chest to relieve a variety of painful conditions including post-herpetic neuralgia and post-operative thoracotomy pain. It is safe to use TENS over the anterior chest to manage angina at intensities below motor threshold (i.e. conventional TENS). High-intensity TENS above motor threshold should not be applied using transthoracic electrode positions where electrodes are positioned antero-posterior thorax. Mann (1996) reported a case where a patient with unstable angina had administered TENS at a very high intensity through the chest using transthoracic electrode positions. This compromised pulmonary ventilation due to excessive stimulation of the intercostal muscles. It is recommended that TENS should not be applied over the chest in patients with cardiac failure or patients with cardiac disease including arrhythmias, although it should be safe to use TENS to manage other pain conditions in patients with arrhythmias, providing electrodes are applied away from the chest area and under the supervision of a cardiology specialist.

Circulatory conditions

Thrombophlebitis and deep-vein thrombosis Thrombophlebitis (White Leg) is related to a blood clot (thrombus) in a vein. A thrombus that has recently formed in a deep vein, usually in the legs, is at risk of being dislodged causing an embolism, which could be life-threatening if it affects a vital organ such as the lungs (i.e. pulmonary embolism). There is a risk that TENS at, or close to, the site of the thrombus could cause muscle contractions or increased blood flow that might dislodge the thrombus. TENS on a limb contralateral to the site of a thrombus may induce reflex vasodilatation in the opposite limb which could potentially dislodge a thrombus. TENS on certain acupuncture points may increase blood flow in other parts of the body, including the feet (see Brown et al., 2009, for review).

All published guidelines recommend that TENS should never be placed on a limb affected by a deep-vein thrombosis (DVT) or thrombophlebitis which is related to a thrombus in the vein (i.e. local contraindication). Inappropriately strong muscle contractions induced by a neuromuscular electrical stimulation device resulted in ischaemic colitis from colonic or vascular spasm and/or dislodging thrombi associated with atherosclerosis in an elderly male adult (Tsujimoto et al., 2004). The risk of low-intensity conventional TENS dislodging a thrombus is likely to be low but the worst case outcome could be death. Some published guidelines also emphasize the need to be cautious when applying TENS on other body sites because TENS on contralateral limbs or acupuncture points may cause reflex vasodilation at the site of a thrombus. The Canadian Physiotherapy Association recommends that TENS should be contraindicated at all sites, both locally and remote, when an individual has thrombophlebitis and deep-vein thrombosis (Houghton et al., 2010). If an individual has been successfully treated with anticoagulation therapy and the thrombosis has dissolved and been reabsorbed then TENS can be used with caution.

Haemorrhagic conditions TENS is known to increase regional and systemic blood flow and promote the release of vasoactive substances and pro-inflammatory mediators, and known to reduce platelet aggregation. TENS should not be applied over areas where there is haemorrhage, uncontrolled bleeding, or recent injury (including surgery) that had significant blood loss because TENS may cause further bleeding. Roche and co-workers (1985) have used TENS successfully to reduce pain without increased bleeding in individuals with haemophilia, so it is recommended that TENS can be used on individuals who have a bleeding disorder such as haemophilia providing coagulopathy has resolved following replacement factor treatment.

Impaired circulation When circulation to tissue is impaired, oxygen demand can exceed supply causing pain, ischaemia, and necrosis. In the skin, impairment of arterial or venous circulation can lead to oedema and deterioration of skin condition. TENS may increase the metabolic demands of tissue and therefore there is a risk of worsening the situation in severe arterial disease. Furthermore, if TENS is administered across frail or damaged skin there may be uneven distribution of currents. This may cause further damage resulting in a wound or skin burn. TENS has been found to increase regional blood flow leading to improvements in oxygenation of tissue in a variety of conditions including peripheral obstructive arterial disease of the lower limbs (Forst et al., 1997). AL-TENS and neuromuscular electrical stimulation have been used successfully to treat arterial insufficiency and claudication due to advanced arterial disease (Anderson et al., 2004).

It should be safe to use conventional TENS in individuals to improve wound healing and reduce claudication with arterial disease. However, the Canadian Physiotherapy Association recommends that neuromuscular electrical stimulation is contraindicated in the presence of severe arterial disease and therefore AL-TENS with muscle contractions should be too. It is safe to use TENS in individuals with hypertension and cold hypersensitivity resulting from Raynaud's, cryoglobulinaemia, or haemoglobulinaemia.

Osteoporosis, unstable bones, and recent surgery

There is a risk that forceful muscle contraction could cause further damage to bone fractures and tendon and ligament repairs, and could also cause unstable vertebrae in individuals with cancer. At post-operative incision sites it can disrupt skin sutures or staples. Hartkopp and colleagues (1998) reported a fracture of the lateral femoral condyle of a paraplegic subject with severe osteoporosis by transcutaneous electrical stimulation used to measure maximal isometric torque of the quadriceps with the knee flexed at an angle of 90 degrees. Ansari and colleagues (2006) reported that an electronic muscle stimulator caused rupture of a flexor pollicis longus repair in a body builder. Thus, AL-TENS is contraindicated at the site of recent bone fractures, ligament or tendon repairs, joint replacements, and post-operative incision sites. AL-TENS is also contraindicated in individuals with severe osteoporosis and in individuals with unstable vertebrae from metastases. It should be safe to use TENS below motor threshold locally in these situations but attention should be given to ensuring that no muscle contractions occur beneath the electrodes.

Infectious conditions including tuberculosis and osteomyelitis

Electrical currents have been shown to inhibit bacterial growth and therefore have been used to treat infected open wounds (Szuminsky et al., 1994). Surface electrodes used during treatment with electrophysical techniques including TENS have the potential for cross-contamination although Cottell and colleagues (2011) assessed skin microflora and found no serious hazards associated with bacterial contamination from reusable self-adhering TENS electrodes over a four-week period, provided that pads were handled and stored in accordance with manufacturers' instructions. Nevertheless, there is a risk that TENS could spread bacteria in localized infections such as abscess formations and chronic wounds. It should be safe to use TENS with antimicrobial therapy to open wounds that are only superficially infected using techniques to reduce cross-contamination from contact with electrodes and practitioner. There is a risk of TENS and other electrotherapies activating or spreading tuberculosis lesions, although the effect of TENS on latent or active tuberculosis is not known. Therefore, TENS is contraindicated in individuals with tuberculosis. Osteomyelitis is an infection of bone or bone marrow. TENS is contraindicated at the site of localized abscess formations and open chronic wounds when an individual has underlying osteomyelitis because an exit site is required for drainage.

Skin conditions

Delivering TENS over frail and damaged skin may create uneven current flow through the skin with a risk of further damage from a skin burn. This is because there is lower skin impedance in thin, broken skin than in intact skin. TENS electrodes may cause contact dermatitis and may cause skin damage due to mechanical stresses on removal of electrodes from the skin resulting in further skin loss. The most common adverse effect of TENS is skin irritation and therefore TENS electrodes should only be applied on healthy skin. Extreme care needs to be taken when applying TENS electrodes to individuals with frail, damaged, or diseased skin including systemic lupus erythematosis or eczema. TENS can be placed over healthy skin around or proximal to an area of damage and has been used successfully in this way for pruritus (Tinegate & McLelland, 2002; Hettrick et al., 2004). However, the situation needs to be monitored as electrical currents may increase regional blood flow and stimulate release of pro-inflammatory substances which may exacerbate inflammation caused by an underlying skin condition such as eczema or dermatitis.

TENS is contraindicated on tissues that have been radiated within the previous six months because the effect of TENS on changes to cellular or circulatory activities resulting from radiation treatment is not known. There is a risk that TENS may promote growth of malignant cells remaining after radiation therapy because electrical currents have been shown to stimulate cell growth and replication angiogenesis. TENS is also contraindicated over open wounds, and if applying TENS electrodes close to an open wound, careful monitoring of exudate should take place in case of excessive bleeding or fluid loss. Practitioners should be especially cautious if positioning electrodes close to inflamed tissue resulting from burn or physical trauma. Likewise, TENS electrodes should not be applied directly on inflamed tissue and if TENS is to be used close to lymphedemas tissue the situation needs to be monitored because TENS may increase swelling.

Altered skin sensation

Heightened sensation—allodynia and hyperalgesia TENS of skin with heightened sensation such as allodynia and/or hyperalgesia may exacerbate pain. Allodynia is believed to be mediated in part via amplification of low-threshold afferent activity and as TENS activates low-threshold afferents it would be expected that TENS would worsen pain, although paradoxically, this is not always the case. TENS electrodes should not be positioned on skin with altered sensation but instead positioned on sensate skin adjacent to the site of allodynia. Hence, skin sensitivity should be mapped prior to determining electrode positions. It may be possible to generate TENS sensation within the painful area by delivering TENS at sensory-detection threshold (barely perceptible) in an adjacent area of healthy skin for at least five minutes and then increasing intensity so that a stronger TENS sensation begins to permeate the painful area. AL-TENS applied over healthy skin to activate muscles in contralateral myotomes may be more appropriate.

Diminished skin sensation—hypoaesthesia TENS of skin that has diminished sensation, numbness, or insensitivity to touch is likely to be less effective because it will be difficult to achieve TENS sensation due to nerve damage. There is also a risk that unduly high-amplitude currents will be used to achieve a strong, non-painful TENS sensation and this could cause skin damage or burns. Electrodes can be positioned along the main nerves proximal to the site of pain to see if it is possible to project TENS sensation within or close to the site of pain. Alternatively, applying electrodes to sensate tissue on the margins of the numb area to achieve TENS sensation close to the site of pain may prove beneficial. AL-TENS, interferential current therapy, high-voltage pulsed currents, and neuromuscular electrical nerve stimulation over intact motor nerves to induce muscle contractions may be beneficial in conditions which produce lack sensory awareness such as spinal cord injury. The Canadian Physiotherapy

Association recommends that this should only be attempted by experienced practitioners using device settings that have been tested on a body part with intact sensation and with careful monitoring for adverse reactions. Direct current should never be applied to hypaesthesic skin as it is associated with a greater risk of skin burn.

Other

Using TENS with transdermal patches

TENS should not be delivered close to transdermal drug delivery systems such as fentanyl or buprenorphine patches because there is a risk that electric fields generated during TENS may cause electro-migration and electro-osmosis of drugs across the surface of the skin leading to drug toxicity. Positively charged chemicals will be repelled across the skin at the anode and negatively charged chemicals will be repelled at the cathode. The risks of this happening seem low using biphasic waveforms that result in zero net current flow beneath electrodes, but may be higher in monophasic waveform devices. As there are no known reports of adverse events in the literature and no systematic experimental investigation of the hazard in the literature it seems wise to classify TENS as a local contraindication.

Operating hazardous equipment

TENS should not be used while operating vehicles or potentially hazardous equipment as a sudden surge of current may cause an accident. From a legal perspective it would be wise for TENS users to place their TENS device in a glove compartment whenever driving as the cause of an accident may be attributed to TENS if it were attached to a drivers belt (even if it was switched off). TENS does not transmit electromagnetic waves so it will not interfere with aeroplane instruments. However, TENS may be considered a dangerous item to carry in hand-luggage so it would be advisable to check prior to travel and to have a signed letter from a health-care practitioner describing what TENS is, and why it is important for the individual to travel with it.

Hazardous electrode sites

There are several electrode positions that have the potential for harm (Figure 5.1).

Anterior neck

TENS should not be delivered over the anterior neck because there is a risk that currents may stimulate the carotid sinus which may cause a vasovagal reflex with a rapid fall in blood pressure and possibly syncope. TENS on the anterior neck may also stimulate laryngeal tissue leading to laryngeal spasm compromising ventilation.

Transthoracic using high-intensity TENS

High-intensity TENS should not be delivered through the chest using transthoracic electrode positions using anterior and posterior electrode positions because it can cause intercostal muscle spasm and compromise breathing (Mann, 1996). There is also a risk that high-intensity transthoracic TENS may drive currents into deeper tissues

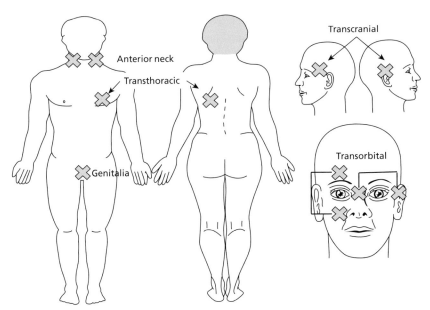

Fig. 5.1 Hazardous electrode sites.

within the chest which may interfere with electrical conductivity and mechanical actions of the heart and associated blood vessels. It has been suggested that electrodes should not be positioned arm to arm or leg to arm as currents may take a path through deeper tissue, including the chest. There are no known reports of adverse events in the literature and no systematic experimental investigation of these hazards. Furthermore, the characteristics of currents used during TENS are designed to target superficial tissue and skin even at higher intensities so it seems unlikely that currents would be able to penetrate to depths that would affect the heart.

Transcranial and transorbital

It is unwise to administer conventional or AL-TENS using electrodes on each side of the forehead because skin is thin and there is a lack of underlying soft tissue to conduct currents. Therefore, it is difficult to titrate current to achieve a strong, comfortable TENS sensation without causing overt pain. Transcranial TENS-like devices are commercially available and utilize microampere currents that are 1000 amperes lower than currents used in a standard TENS device (Chapter 10, 207–208). In theory, delivering TENS across the eye socket may increase intraocular pressure of the eye by exciting extraocular musculature, and this may be particularly hazardous in individuals with glaucoma. TENS can be used to manage facial pains and headaches using electrode positions on the face, but if TENS sensations are experienced in the eyelids or within the eyes the electrodes should be repositioned.

Internally and on reproductive organs

TENS should only be administered internally in the mouth, rectum, or vagina using TENS devices designed for dental, vaginal, and rectal stimulation respectively. TENS and neuromuscular electrical stimulation have been used with success to stimulate pelvic floor muscles to manage urinary and faecal incontinence using specialized rectal and vaginal electrode probes. Electrical stimulation using a rectal probe has also been used for electroejaculation for sperm retrieval in spinal-cord-injured men (Engin-Uml Stun et al., 2006). In these instances, electrical currents were used to induce muscle contractions and advanced expertise was needed to use the technique. Electrode positions that cause TENS currents to permeate reproductive organs or genitalia may be hazardous because the effects of currents on gametogenesis are not known.

Adverse reactions

In general, adverse reactions to TENS are rare and are often due to inappropriate technique. TENS worsens pain in some individuals and may produce a vasovagal response leading to nausea, dizziness, and even syncope although the proportion of patients in which this occurs is unknown. This can often be detected in the initial supervised trial of TENS and subsequent follow-up (Chapter 6).

TENS exacerbating pain

Some patients experience increased pain when using TENS for the first time and this may persist after stimulation has ceased. Reports of elevations in pain during and after TENS may be due to:

- reporting artefacts such as exaggerating the account of pain following a period of pain relief from TENS
- the after-effects of increased physical activity during TENS
- TENS being stopped when pain intensity is naturally fluctuating on an upward trajectory, or when the effects of concurrent medication are wearing off
- TENS aggravating already sensitive peripheral and central nervous system neurones
- TENS causing the release of histamine and other neurochemicals at the site of the electrodes, or at distal terminals of peripheral fibres (e.g. via axon reflexes)
- TENS being used excessively at a high intensity resulting in delayed onset muscle soreness in following days

Careful assessment of the cause is necessary to ensure that TENS is not incorrectly dismissed as unsuitable.

Autonomic reactions to TENS

Some patients may be very anxious and fearful when trying TENS for the first time. Neurological reactions to TENS, termed a vasovagal response, may manifest as a drop in blood pressure, profuse sweating, general uneasiness and discomfort, nausea, lightheadedness, and even syncope (fainting). The incidence of such events is not known although clinical experience suggests that they are rare. Caution should be taken when TENS is being given to individuals with a history of autonomic reactions, and especially syncope, to medical procedures. The risk of sustaining a fall injury associated with fainting should be controlled by making sure the patient is sitting or lying during the first treatment session. Some patients do not like the sensation created during TENS but do not have an autonomic reaction. Very occasionally individuals react to TENS with emotional responses such as sadness, happiness, crying, or giggling, although these effects are usually transient.

Skin reactions

An in-depth study of successful long-term users of TENS found that 31 per cent encountered skin reactions to the tape, gel, or electrodes, which presented as redness, irritation, or a rash (Johnson et al., 1991c).

Contact dermatitis

Dermatitis is inflammation of the skin due to an allergic response usually triggered by exposure to chemicals but also by cold or hot temperatures and sunlight. Dermatitis at the site of contact with the electrodes results from the constituents of electrodes, electrode gel, or adhesive tape causing redness of the skin (erythema), itchiness, and occasionally a rash (Corazza et al., 1999). Constituents associated with skin reactions include various polyacrylates in TENS conductive gels, karaya gum used in electrodes, and nickel in TENS electrode plates. The development of self-adhering hypoallergenic electrodes has reduced the incidence of contact dermatitis. Washing skin and electrodes when indicated by the manufacturer and applying electrodes to fresh skin on a daily basis reduces dermatitis. There are unpublished anecdotes of cases where TENS has caused an allergic response with severe redness, blotching, and irritation at local and distant sites to TENS. It is difficult to confirm the validity of such reports and whether symptoms are a direct result of TENS.

Shearing stresses of removing electrodes

A common cause of erythema and itchiness is shearing stresses during the removal of electrodes from the skin. The severity depends on the stickiness of the adhesive gel or tape, and the condition of the skin. Frail skin is particularly prone to damage when removing electrodes.

Electrical currents

There are no known published reports of allergic reactions resulting from exposure of the electrical currents of TENS, although there are unpublished anecdotes of individuals experiencing erythema, swelling, and itchiness only when currents during TENS are being delivered. Such cases need to be published to determine the extent of the problem. There is a debate about whether some people have an idiopathic environmental intolerance to electromagnetic fields (electrosensitivity) resulting in chronic headaches, depression, and insomnia. It seems reasonable to assume that some individuals may be sensitive to currents used during TENS resulting in amplified autonomic and neurological responses such as dizziness, nausea, headache, and even syncope.

Erythema and itchiness is more likely to occur at higher current densities due to the use of higher pulse amplitudes and/or electrodes with small surface areas. Fary and Briffa (2011) investigated the rate of adverse skin reactions in 25 healthy participants exposed to 10 minutes of pulsed electrical stimulation of the knee. They found that 52 per cent of participants experienced adverse skin reactions with a monophasic waveform compared with 4 per cent ($n = 1$) with asymmetrically biphasic waveforms. They recommended caution is needed if using monophasic waveforms.

TENS-induced vasodilatation and the axon reflex

Currents during TENS may stimulate excitable tissue controlling the flow of blood through capillary beds causing vasodilation and erythema at the site of electrodes. At high intensities TENS may initiate an axon reflex. An axon reflex occurs when peripheral nerve activation results in impulses travelling in afferent neurones towards the periphery. TENS of afferent axons creates impulses that travel towards the central nervous system (orthodromic) and also towards the periphery (antidromic). Antidromic impulses in high-threshold afferents that travel distally towards the periphery initiate the release of chemicals from the distal terminals of free nerve endings including substance P, and this triggers a local inflammatory response including vasodilation and erythema. TENS-induced activity in autonomic efferents may affect smooth muscle control of blood vessels and TENS-induced skeletal muscle pumping may also affect blood flow contributing to regional erythema.

Electrical burns

The likelihood of an electrical burn during TENS is low and is likely to be due to negligent technique.

Reports of skin burns during electrical stimulation of the skin are rare and are usually related to the use of TENS-like devices. Nadler and colleagues (2003) claimed that burns were responsible for 40 per cent of complications caused by functional electrical stimulation seen by athletic trainers. Satter (2008) described a patient who experienced a third-degree burn in an area treated with interferential current therapy, and Ford and colleagues (2005) reported that a patient who experienced a full-thickness skin burn over a metal implant following unicompartmental knee arthroplasty after using interferential current therapy for pain control. Barkana and colleagues (2010) reported a case of a woman attending a health spa who received massage administered using a neuromuscular electrical stimulator for 10 minutes using eight pairs of electrodes. It appeared that several electrodes became partially unstuck from the skin resulting in current distributed over a smaller area and a third-degree burn to a depth of 2 mm to 5 mm. This demonstrates the importance of maintaining the integrity of reusable electrodes. Actions to reduce the incidence of skin burns include using large surface electrodes with good conducting material and uniform contact between the electrode and the skin, and ensuring that there is not wire insulation damage or sharply cut electrode corners.

The likelihood of experiencing a burn during conventional TENS and AL-TENS using a standard TENS device is low compared to using some TENS-like devices. Micropunctate burns during TENS were more common in the past when carbon–rubber electrodes and conductive wet electrolyte gel were used because gel dried out or electrodes were inflexible and did not follow the contours of the skin, resulting in current 'hot spots'. The use of self-adhesive electrodes with more even current distribution has reduced the potential for micropunctate burns. Patriciu and colleagues (2005) found that regions of increased current density were correlated with tissue burns induced by electrical currents delivered as monophasic square waveforms at 20–35 mA and 200 pps for 30–135 minutes. Their experimental study using a porcine-skin-gel model suggested that the burns resulted from electrochemical mechanisms rather than thermal mechanisms. Many standard TENS devices use biphasic rather than monophasic waveforms resulting in zero net current to reduce electrochemical changes beneath electrodes because DC may cause an alkaline environment beneath electrodes from electrolysis of surface moisture leading to epidermal damage.

Summary

1 The safety profile of TENS compares very favourably against other available treatments including medication.

2 Judgements about whether it is safe to use TENS are informed by safety guidelines published by professional bodies.

3 Absolute contradictions include patients who have electronic implants such as cardiac pacemakers and implantable cardioverter defibrillators or who do not understand TENS.

4 Local contraindications and precautions include pregnancy, epilepsy, active malignancy, deep-vein thrombosis, and frail or damaged skin. Hazardous electrode sites include transorbital, transthoracic, transcranial and the anterior neck.

5 Adverse reactions include aggravating pain, autonomic reactions, and minor skin reactions.

Further reading

- **Carlson, T., Andrell, P., Ekre, O., Edvardsson, N., Holmgren, C., Jacobsson, F., and Mannheimer, C.** (2009) Interference of transcutaneous electrical nerve stimulation with permanent ventricular stimulation: a new clinical problem? *Europace*, **11**, 364–9.
- **Chartered Society of Physiotherapy.** (2006) *Guidance for the clinical use of Electrophysical agents*. Chartered Society of Physiotherapy, London.
- **Houghton, P., Nussbaum, E., and Hoens, A.** (2010) Electrophysical agents. Contraindications and Precautions: An Evidence-Based Approach to Clinical Decision Making in Physical Therapy. *Physiother Can*, **62**, 5–80.
- **Robertson, V., Chipchase, L., and Laakso, E.** (2001) *Guidelines for the clinical use of electrophysical agents*. Australian Physiotherapy Association, Melbourne.

Chapter 6 will explore the practicalities of using TENS on a new patient by discussing the procedures for undertaking a supervised trial of TENS.

Chapter 6

Evaluating TENS on a new patient—the supervised trial

Introduction

The principles and practicalities of using TENS described in previous chapters provide the foundation for good clinical practice based on physiological rationale. In principle, conventional TENS should be efficacious for pains arising from somatic 'superficial' structures rather than visceral 'deep-seated' structures. Potentially, AL-TENS may be more useful for deep-seated pain and neuropathic pain where hyperaesthesia and/or dysaesthesia are prominent features. There are no robust indicators to identify whether a new patient will respond to TENS so the only way to determine which type of TENS is best for each patient is by a process of systematic trial and error. Lampl and colleagues (1998) investigated factors that predict response to TENS in 482 patients with various types of chronic pain over a 48-month follow-up period and found that patients who understood the principles of TENS and were competent in TENS technique were more likely to have treatment success. Patients need to be able to self-administer TENS. In in-patient settings, health-care professionals are readily available to provide advice when patients self-administer TENS. When TENS is used in out-patient settings, patients need to self-administer TENS without direct support from a health-care professional. Therefore, new patients not only need to be assessed for their suitability for TENS but they also require a period of TENS training and learning with appropriate follow-up. The most efficient means of achieving this for in-patients (e.g. within a ward for post-operative pain) and out-patients (e.g. chronic pain patient at home) is to provide a trial of TENS under the supervision of a health-care professional. The purpose of this chapter is to provide a framework for undertaking a supervised TENS trial by covering:

- Screening for suitability
- Trying TENS on the patient and troubleshooting issues
- Evaluating the patient's initial response to TENS and their ability to self-administer TENS
- Setting treatment goals
- Instigating and evaluating an extended TENS trial
- Strategies to improve treatment effect

Practicalities of a supervised TENS trial

The aim of the supervised trial is to assess the patient's suitability for TENS and to train the patient how to self-administer TENS. This can be achieved by using a systematic approach (Box 6.1).

Too often practitioners rush patients through their first experience of TENS leaving them confused, uncertain of technique, and with unrealistic expectations of TENS outcome. The patient achieves limited pain relief, dismissing TENS as a non-effective treatment and returning to clinic dissatisfied and requesting another treatment, adding further pressure to service provision. Ideally, a supervised trial of TENS should last at least 30 minutes as it may take this length of time for a patient to respond. In out-patient settings a dedicated TENS clinic is a good way of making this process cost-effective so that a group of new patients can be assessed over a morning or afternoon. The health-care practitioner can assess and train one patient whilst other newly trained patients can try TENS in a waiting room. Expert patient volunteers who are experienced TENS users are a valuable asset to facilitate TENS training for new patients. The supervised trial can be structured into a series of stages (Box 6.2).

Orientation to TENS and the trial process

New patients should be asked not to take medication in the preceding 4–8 hours before the trial. The key to success when assessing an individual in pain is to connect with the patient through an alliance between practitioner and patient. Fishman (2012) offers excellent advice on how to communicate effectively with pain patients, including the following pointers:

1 Slow down and take time when communicating with patients.

2 Focus on the whole patient not just the pain.

3 Use reflective skills to listen carefully and non-judgementally to what the patient says.

Box 6.1 Objectives of a supervised TENS trial

- Check contraindications and precautions
- Test skin sensation
- Make sure that TENS does not aggravate pain
- Help to determine whether the patient is likely to respond
- Troubleshoot problems arising from poor response
- Provide instruction on equipment use and expected therapeutic outcome
- Familiarize the patient with TENS sensations
- Train the patient on how to apply TENS
- Check that the patient can apply TENS appropriately and safely on their own

> ## Box 6.2 Stages of a supervised trial of TENS on a new patient
>
> - Orientation to TENS and the trial process
> - Screening for suitability for TENS and taking consent
> - Trying TENS on the patient and troubleshooting issues
> - Evaluating patient ability to self-administer TENS
> - Evaluating initial response to TENS
> - Setting treatment goals
> - Instigating and evaluating an extended TENS trial

Establish the patient's prior knowledge of their pain and its prognosis to help manage the patient's expectation of what TENS can do for them. At this stage a simple explanation of what pain is and why TENS has been suggested as a treatment is useful, perhaps using a short video such as 'Understanding Pain: What to do about it in less than five minutes?'; available at: <http://www.youtube.com/watch?v=4b8oB757DKc>.

As the patient has not been screened for their suitability for TENS as yet it is wise to leave the practicalities of applying TENS and how it works until later in the supervised trial. At this stage a prompt such as '*TENS acts by electrically rubbing pain away*' may be useful to explain to patients how TENS mimics the act of rubbing for pain relief. The patient is likely to experience information overload during the TENS trial so explanatory handouts are encouraged.

Screening for suitability for TENS and taking consent

Patients need to be carefully assessed for suitable for TENS. Sometimes it is not possible to make a precise pain diagnosis but it is critical that a medical history and physical examination has been taken to make sure that there are no 'red flags' requiring further investigation or immediate treatment. The health-care professional supervising the TENS trial should assess the appropriateness of the patient, including contraindications and precautions, and a simple screening proforma can be useful to record decisions and any control measures put in place. Document the location, character, and time course of the pain; exacerbating and relieving factors; sleep and mood disturbances; ongoing medical concerns; and how pain affects daily function and quality of life. A body chart should be used to record the location of pain and electrode sites used in the trial.

The patient must be fully informed of risks, adverse events, precautions, and practicalities of self-administering TENS before consenting to trying it. A simple handout for the patient can be used to list common adverse events and control measures. Managing the expectations of pain patients can be challenging so practitioners should try to negotiate goals for TENS treatment to help the patient develop realistic expectations of treatment outcome. It is important that the patient understands that he or she takes responsibility to self-administer TENS-treatment as advised by the practitioner, and that it is important that he or she carefully follows instructions on how to use TENS. Identifying the support provided by the clinic including patient–clinic interface and procedures for loaning, buying, or renting-to-buy TENS devices and accessories is worthwhile at this stage.

Trying TENS on the patient, and troubleshooting issues

A process of systematic trial and error is used to determine electrode positions and electrical characteristics for TENS. It is advisable to use conventional TENS with a continuous pulse pattern when the patient uses TENS for the first time because a continuous pattern is chosen by most successful long-term users of TENS, and it is easier to demonstrate how TENS sensations vary with alterations of pulse amplitude, frequency, and duration. Once patients have mastered conventional TENS it will be possible to demonstrate how to apply AL-TENS. Explaining the principles and practice for both conventional TENS and AL-TENS, and checking patient competence to self-administer TENS within the first supervised trial is likely to lead to information overload for the patient. Therefore, it may be wise to demonstrate only one technique, usually conventional TENS, in the first supervised session. If AL-TENS is the first line of treatment the first supervised trial should focus on skills associated with mastering this technique. If the patient does not respond then the other TENS technique can be tried during the extended trial phase.

Demonstrating safe clinical technique

It is critical that the practitioner demonstrates safe clinical technique to the patient, including:

1 Testing skin sensitivity

2 Preparing the skin for electrodes

3 Placing the electrodes on the skin and delivering currents

4 Experimenting with stimulator settings

5 Removing electrodes from the skin and storage

Testing skin sensitivity It is important to check that the skin is sensate using a simple 'blunt' and 'sharp' test where the individual closes his or her eyes and the practitioner presses a blunt (e.g. end of a pencil) and a sharp (e.g. cocktail stick) object against the skin, and the individual identifies which is which. Comparisons with adjacent and contralateral areas can be used for comparison. Do not place electrodes on skin with altered skin sensitivity.

Preparing the skin for electrodes Soapy water is used to remove oil, lotions, and make-up from the skin surface as chemicals may react with electrodes and/or reduce conductivity. Pre-treatment skin preparations to improve adhesion and electrode conductivity can be useful but not essential for most patients. It may be necessary to trim areas of skin with a lot of body hair using scissors. Shaving or waxing is not recommended because it may lead to 'hot spots' where current follows the path of least resistance down exposed hair follicles. Soft-gel electrodes for sensitive skin have a thicker layer of hypoallergenic gel and can be useful for people with excessive perspiration, body hair, or sensitivity to ordinary electrodes (for example, see: <http://www.physiomedical.co.uk/tens-electrodes/best-tens-electrodes/pals-blue-sensitive>).

Placing electrodes on the skin and delivering currents It is important to verbalize each step of the technique used when applying TENS for the first time to help patient understanding (Box 6.3). When applying self-adhesive electrodes to skin it is important to press firmly and smooth down all edges, and to check that electrodes are not peeling away from the skin at the sides. Adhesion increases the closer that the temperature of the electrode is to the temperature of the skin. Sometimes the adhesive is too sticky and strong especially with new electrodes, and this stickiness can be reduced by moistening the surface of the gel by spreading a few drops of tap water across the surface of the gel. It may be necessary to add adhesive tape around the edges of the electrode to prevent clothes lifting the edge of the electrode due to abrasion. It may also be necessary to tape sections of the electrode lead to anchor it to the skin, especially if it is going to be left in place for long periods of time, but it is important that the lead remains relatively loose. Do not loop the lead wire back on itself close to the pin as this will weaken the pin connector.

Box 6.3 Safe technique for administering TENS

1 Make sure:
- the stimulator is switched OFF with no flashing lights 'on'
- amplitude dials are set to zero
- electrode lead wires are not attached to the stimulator

2 Adjust TENS device settings to:
- Pattern = continuous (C) or Normal (N)
- Frequency = 40–80 pps (mid-range)
- Duration (width) = 150–200 µs
- Timer = continuous (C)

3 Attach electrode lead wire pins to electrodes.

4 Attach the electrodes to the skin at chosen site.

5 Attach jack plug of electrode lead wire to one channel on TENS device and ensure it snaps into place.

6 Switch the stimulator ON but DO NOT increase amplitude. Ask the patient whether they feel anything.

7 Explain that you are about to slowly increase the amplitude dial and you would like them to tell you when they feel the very first 'tingling' sensation from TENS.

8 Increase the amplitude dial very slowly. The patient may be anxious so do not lose their confidence by a sudden appearance of a strong TENS sensation.

Box 6.3 Safe technique for administering TENS (continued)

9 When the patient experiences the very first tingling sensation immediately stop increasing amplitude. Assess the patient's experience, being attentive to autonomic reactions or unpleasant feelings.

10 If appropriate, explain to the patient that you will slowly increase amplitude again. They should tell you when they feel a 'strong, non-painful tingling sensation'. This intensity should not be painful or cause muscle contraction.

11 Assess the patient's experience of strong, non-painful TENS for a few minutes.

12 Slowly turn the amplitude setting back to zero whilst checking that TENS intensity is diminishing as you do so.

13 Switch the device off.

14 Ask the patient to switch the stimulator on themselves without increasing the amplitude.

15 Ask the patient to follow steps 1–13 to achieve a 'strong, non-painful tingling sensation' and assess their ability to do this.

16 Ask the patient to increase amplitude so that the intensity of TENS is slightly too high and then ask them to return to a 'strong, non-painful tingling sensation'. This helps the patient to internalize the therapeutic level of stimulation and to gain confidence of using high intensities of stimulation.

If TENS worsens the pain at any step the practitioner needs to review the situation. Alternative electrode positions or different TENS settings could be tried. Sometimes the patient will refuse to continue with the TENS trial.

Experimenting with stimulator settings Once the patient is confident that they can titrate the intensity of TENS themselves then it is possible to demonstrate how to alter frequency and duration (Box 6.4). In the first instance, the practitioner should take control of the TENS device and talk through each step to aid patient understanding. A set of audio speakers (or headphones) can be plugged into the output sockets of some TENS devices to demonstrate the sound of pulses and improve patient understanding of TENS output characteristics (Figure 6.1a).

To demonstrate pulse pattern it is important to switch the device off before switching pattern from continuous to another setting (e.g. burst). Pulse frequency and pulse duration should remain mid-range. The TENS device can be switched on and pulse amplitude increased until the patient experiences a strong, non-painful TENS sensation. Emphasize that

♦ stimulator settings should not be altered without turning down amplitude first otherwise it is possible that an unpleasant intensity surge may occur

♦ whenever other stimulator settings have been altered it is necessary to titrate pulse amplitude back to achieve a 'strong, non-painful TENS sensation'

Box 6.4 Protocol for demonstrating the electrical characteristics available in a standard TENS device

1 Set pattern to continuous, duration to 150–200 µs and frequency to mid-range (40-80pps).

2 Increase amplitude until the patient experiences a strong, non-painful TENS sensation.

3 Slowly decrease frequency—intensity should start to diminish.

4 Increase amplitude to maintain a strong, non-painful TENS sensation as frequency is decreased until the lowest possible frequency setting is reached.

5 Slowly increase frequency—intensity should start to increase.

6 Decrease amplitude to maintain a strong, non-painful TENS sensation as frequency is increased until the highest possible frequency setting is reached.

7 Allow the patient to experiment with pulse frequency settings whilst they also titrate amplitude to maintain a strong, non-painful TENS sensation.

8 Repeat steps 1–2 for pulse duration. Intensity will decrease as pulse duration increases.

(a)

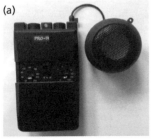

(b)   (c)

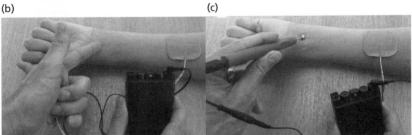

Fig. 6.1 (a) Audio speakers (or headphones) plugged into TENS device. Technique for locating optimal electrode position using (b) finger, or (c) metal probe as a pointer.

Box 6.5 Safe procedure for removing electrodes from the skin

1 Turn the TENS device off.
2 Remove the electrode lead wire from the TENS device.
3 Remove the electrodes from the skin.
4 Place the electrodes on the plastic sheet.
5 Remove the electrode lead-wire pins.
6 Check the condition of the skin.

Removing electrodes from the skin and storage At the end of the demonstration switch off the device and disconnect the electrode leads from the TENS device before removing electrodes from skin (Box 6.5). Peel off the electrode by gripping the leading edge of the electrodes and pull off in the direction of the hairs of the skin. Never pull electrodes off using the lead wires as this will damage them.

This is a good opportunity to advise patients about electrode care. Reusable self-adhesive electrodes are estimated to achieve 15–100 uses before they deteriorate significantly, although many patients use electrodes more than 100 times. Electrodes should be replaced onto the plastic carrier sheet supplied with the electrodes and stored at room temperature in the reusable plastic bag. Do not store in the fridge or freezer unless instructions accompanying the electrodes say so. Electrodes can be disposed of in household waste and should not be incinerated or flushed down the toilet. If the gel becomes contaminated with dirt, hair, or skin, a moist sponge can be used to wipe and clean the electrode surface. Too much water applied to the gel surface may damage the electrode and the gel will begin to break down. Patients should not use other people's electrodes as this may cause cross-contamination.

Monitoring the condition of skin

Mild erythema (redness of the skin) and itchiness beneath the electrodes is common but extensive reddening, irritation, a rash, or soreness is more serious. If this happens the skin should be washed and aloe vera and vitamin E cream applied. It may be necessary to discontinue TENS for a few days to allow the skin to recover. It is important to find out the reason for and alleviate the cause of extensive reddening, which may be contact dermatitis from constituents of electrodes, electrode gel, or adhesive tape, deterioration or dryness of electrodes, or increased skin sensitivity resulting from steroid use or pre-existing inflammation. It may be necessary to move electrodes to a different area of skin, replace electrodes, or change the type of electrodes.

Evaluating patient ability to self-administer TENS

It is important to check that the patient is able to self-administer TENS using safe technique. A simple tick-box checklist can be used to test competence. Encourage the patient to set the mode/pattern to continuous, and the frequency and duration to mid-range during each TENS application, and then to search for the optimal setting for his or her pain at that moment in time. Uncertainties and queries can be resolved whilst watching the patient self-administering TENS. Patients should use TENS on their own in the clinic for a further 15–30 minutes so that an initial evaluation of outcome can be made.

Evaluating initial response to TENS

An individual can be considered not suitable for TENS when:

◆ they refuse to use TENS in the future

◆ a serious adverse event occurs

◆ they do not understand the principles of using TENS

◆ they are unable to self-administer TENS (unless a caregiver takes on the responsibility to do so)

◆ TENS worsens the pain and it was not possible to resolve the cause of the worsening pain during the supervised trial

Failure of TENS to relieve pain during the initial trial should not be taken as non-response. Even with systematic positioning of electrodes and electrical characteristics few patients achieve their *best* result during the TENS trial.

Setting treatment goals

It is important to negotiate the objectives of TENS treatment and to manage the patient's expectation of TENS outcome. Treatment with TENS requires commitment from the patient to self-administer treatment regularly. A treatment agreement, formalized in writing, can be useful to prevent misunderstanding and to engage the patient in collaborative decision-making and treatment delivery. It can also serve as a motivational reminder to the patient about the treatment regimen. It is important to document the patient's expectations about pain prognosis, medication, and TENS treatment outcome including factors that may hinder success such as how TENS might interfere with daily functions.

Setting a goal of achieving zero pain is often unrealistic unless there are strong reasons to believe that pain pathology will resolve. Reducing pain by 20 per cent may be significant with respect to regaining function. Resist the urge to frame the *main* outcome of TENS as reductions in pain sensation or 'feeling better' as these are amorphous and akin to 'hitting a moving target'. Objectives framed as measureable functional goals that can monitor progress and can be verified with quantifiable changes in behaviour and quality of life are more effective (Table 6.1, see also Fishman, 2012). Patients should have a sense of ownership of treatment objectives generated through a process of negotiation that encourages honesty, transparency, and realism. A verification protocol to monitor progress of treatment objectives shows the patient the seriousness of agreement of functional goals. Photographs taken on a mobile phone is a simple way to show evidence of the achievement of goals, and these may be communicated to friends and family using social media to sustain motivation to self-manage the painful condition.

Table 6.1 Examples of specific measureable functional goals and verification evidence

Goal	Evidence
Walking around the block	Pedometer recording
Walking without crutches	Report by spouse/friend
Taking bus to the shops	Bus ticket
Performing daily exercise, playing sport	Gym membership, photograph
Returning to work	Letter from employer
Sleeping throughout the night without awakenings	Confirmation by spouse
Beginning physiotherapy or participation in pain support group	Letter from physiotherapist or physical group leader
Resume sexual relations	Confirmation by partner

Instigating and evaluating an extended TENS trial

At the end of the initial supervised trial out-patients should be given an extended trial of TENS of one month to determine whether TENS will produce effective pain relief under the normal everyday conditions of their lives. Some clinics and manufacturers allow patients to borrow TENS devices for a limited period with a view to purchasing the device. During this extended trial period patients should be instructed to self-administer TENS using the principle 'start low and go slow' in order to ensure that there are no adverse events associated with prolonged use (Box 6.6).

For out-patients a point of contact is critical and follow-up contact (via telephone or email) should be made after one week, after one month, and after six months. A follow-up via telephone instigated by the clinic should occur within a week to troubleshoot issues and provide further instruction (Box 6.7). The longer a patient has to wait for advice when a problem arises the less likely he or she will remain positive about TENS treatment. Do not assume that a patient who does not contact the clinic is satisfied and responding to treatment. It should be possible to terminate TENS for non-responders within three months of the initial TENS trial.

Adherence to TENS treatment instructions

Most patients have difficulty trying to integrate TENS treatment into daily life. They may report that TENS is not beneficial for a variety of reasons including:

- the presence of adverse effects
- uncertainty about the treatment regimen
- they are unable to achieve any beneficial effect (i.e. not responding)
- they are unable to improve the amount of existing treatment effect
- they are unable to sustain motivation to continue with treatment because they perceive that the amount of effort required to self-administer TENS is disproportionate to the amount of benefit achieved

Sometimes patients are uncertain about the treatment regimen. Being told to administer conventional TENS for as long as is needed may be counterintuitive, causing uncertainty

Box 6.6 Advice during the extended trial period

Conventional TENS

- ◆ 'For the first few days use TENS for a minimum of one hour no more than three times a day'
- ◆ 'Then adjust your usage of TENS according to your specific needs'
- ◆ 'Use as much as you like, but remember to turn TENS off for "rest periods" throughout the day'
- ◆ 'Try comparing the pain-relieving effect of different settings such as continuous and burst TENS, and then use which is best for you'
- ◆ 'Remember that the intensity of TENS must remain at a strong, non-painful level and you might have to adjust the intensity dial to maintain this level if TENS sensation fades away'
- ◆ 'You may get a bonus of pain relief after the stimulator has been switched off, but don't be disappointed if relief is limited to the time that the TENS device is switched on'
- ◆ 'If you have any problems with the treatment, for example with the stimulator or the electrodes, contact the clinic immediately for advice'

Acupuncture-like TENS

- ◆ 'For the first few days use TENS for 20–30 minute sessions once a day'
- ◆ 'Then increase usage but not more than three to four times a day with individual treatments no longer than ~ 30 minutes because excessive use may result in post-treatment muscle soreness'
- ◆ 'Compare AL-TENS using single pulses and burst patterns and also try conventional TENS'
- ◆ 'Then use whichever is best'

and misunderstanding. A DVD of existing patients talking about their experiences in using TENS can be invaluable. Also a simple advice sheet or a 'prescription' label attached to the front of the TENS device is useful, such as the following:

> Use conventional TENS whenever in pain with ten minute rests every hour. TENS sensation should be strong, comfortable, and not painful.

The follow-up period should be used to evaluate whether the patient is following instructions about how to use TENS. Obtaining reliable data about how frequently and for how long patients use TENS at home during and after the extended TENS trial is difficult. Self-reported usage from either patient interviews or patient diaries tends to overestimate usage so the patient needs to be able to solicit truthful self-reports of TENS usage without reprimand. One way to internalize the practical difficulties of using TENS regularly is for practitioners to follow a TENS treatment regime for themselves over a period of a week.

Box 6.7 The purpose of follow-up contact

- To evaluate TENS effectiveness over the longer term
- To evaluate declining response and offer suggestions for improving effectiveness
- To evaluate adherence to instructions of TENS use
- To address compatibility of TENS with lifestyle, adverse effects, forgetfulness, confusion about regimen, and motivation to tolerate effort and side effects
- To sustain the patient's motivation and maintain realistic expectations
- To recall TENS devices that have been borrowed from the clinic and are no longer required
- To monitor pain progression, especially if the individual has ongoing disease where new symptoms are likely to evolve following diagnosis

There has been little objective utilization and adherence monitoring in TENS research and most conducted to date has measured cumulative duration totals of individual treatment sessions rather than patterns of use, making it impossible to differentiate between one ten-hour TENS session and ten one-hour TENS sessions. Oosterhof and colleagues (2006) found that generally chronic pain patients complied with instructions about regular daily TENS treatment using their device on average 9.8–11.6 hours per day. This finding is consistent with other investigations (Johnson et al., 1991c; Fishbain et al., 1996). Some TENS devices have incorporated data capture software into their design although these devices are more costly. In the future it is hoped that relatively inexpensive TENS devices that log usage, electrical characteristics, and pain scores with the capability of downloading into electronic diary software will become available at a reasonable cost.

Strategies to try to improve treatment effect

It is important to make a detailed assessment of what patients mean if they claim they are 'not responding' (Table 6.2). Establish whether they have previously experienced a 'beneficial response' to TENS. TENS may be reducing pain intensity but this lower intensity has now become bothersome or the patient's pain condition may have worsened. Temporarily withdrawing TENS treatment for a week or two can help a patient evaluate whether TENS was improving pain and function. Declining response may be due to physiological tolerance. Tolerance may be overcome by providing the nervous system with a continuously changing (novel) input to prevent habituation. Tolerance may also be overcome using a stronger peripheral input by simultaneously delivering conventional TENS and AL-TENS or intense TENS via a dual-channel stimulator (2 × 2 electrode pairs), or by combining TENS with different types of afferent input such as cold, heat, massage, or acupuncture (Chapter 4, 86–88). Sometimes, initial enthusiasm for the new treatment wanes so the practitioner will need to revisit patient

Table 6.2 Potential reasons for non-response

Potential reasons for non-response	Action
Unrealistic expectations of outcome	Revisit and modify treatment goals
Equipment failure	Establish that a strong TENS sensation is possible (check device produces an output by checking batteries, condition of electrodes, and that plugs and pins have 'snapped' into sockets
Inappropriate technique	Establish that a strong TENS sensation is being used rather than barely perceptible current
Inappropriate electrode positions	Establish that a strong TENS sensation is being achieved and explore techniques to improve hitting the 'sweet spot' if necessary
Inappropriate dosage	Establish the regimen being used and recalibrate expectations of effects (e.g. TENS for a few minutes at a time will not produce pain relief)
Lifestyle factors that hinder or mask potential improvements	Activities, diet, concurrent medication
Development of tolerance	Regularly change TENS settings including using alternating or modulating patterns of pulse delivery to provide a novel sensory input to the nervous system
Change in pain condition	Re-evaluate the use of TENS within the overall treatment strategy
Disproportionate effort needed to apply TENS for amount of relief obtained	Discuss expectations

expectation of outcome. If the patient is genuinely experiencing no physiological, psychological, or social benefit from using TENS a different treatment approach may be necessary.

Practical techniques to help locate the electrode 'sweet spot'

It is relatively easy to position electrodes so that TENS sensation permeates superficial pain, yet many pains are deeper and patients become frustrated because TENS sensation does not quite 'hit the spot', i.e. insufficient coverage and/or insufficient depth. Stimulating over nerve bundles that run superficially generates stronger and deeper TENS sensations distributed throughout the receptive field of the nerve. Making small adjustments to electrode positions during a treatment session can be cumbersome as the user needs to switch the TENS device off, peel one or both of the electrodes off the skin, perhaps rehydrate the electrodes with drops of water, and reposition them back on the skin. A convenient approach to locate superficial nerve bundles was described by Berlant (1984). One TENS electrode is positioned at a potentially useful site on the body and the second electrode is held in the hand of the patient, health-care professional, or caregiver. With the TENS device switched on, the index finger of the hand with the electrode probes the skin to locate the best site to place the second electrode (Figure 6.1b). The patient and/or therapist will feel TENS sensation when the circuit is completed by touching the patient's skin. Whilst probing the patient's skin with the index finger the intensity of TENS sensation will increase whenever it crosses a superficial nerve bundle and this will help to target an effective electrode site. It is important to use low current amplitudes to avoid discomfort. It is possible to use a metal probe instead of an index finger to achieve the same effect (Figure 6.1c).

Summary

1 There are no robust indicators to predict whether a new patient will respond to TENS so new patients need to be given a supervised trial of TENS.

2 The supervised trial should screen for suitability, familiarize the patient with TENS, and evaluate competence to self-administer, evaluate initial response, set treatment goals, and instigate an extended TENS trial.

3 Treatment goals should be framed as measureable functional outcomes that can monitor progress and can be verified with quantifiable changes in behaviour and quality of life.

4 A dedicated TENS clinic can be cost-effective and provide patients with access to various TENS devices and accessories and educational materials.

5 The use of long-term TENS users as 'expert patients' to help with the clinical rota and support new patients can be valuable.

Further reading

◆ Fishman, S.M. (2012) *Listening to pain. A clinician's guide to improving pain management through better communication.* Oxford University Press, Oxford.

◆ Fox, J., and Sharp, T. (2007) *Practical Electrotherapy. A guide to safe application.* Churchill Livingstone Elsevier, Edinburgh.

◆ The Pain Toolkit website; available at: <http://www.paintoolkit.org>.

Chapter 7 will discuss how general principles and practicalities of good practice are adapted in specific clinical conditions.

Chapter 7

Practicalities of using TENS for specific conditions and situations

Introduction

Mainstream treatment for most acute and chronic pain is pharmacological with non-pharmacological techniques used as adjuncts. Research studies have failed to find superiority of different TENS techniques for specific conditions. When TENS is used to manage pain for specific conditions the principles described in previous chapters inform operational procedures. Usually, conventional TENS delivered at a strong, non-painful intensity at the site of pain is used in the first instance with patients selecting pulse pattern, frequency, and duration for reasons of comfort. The purpose of this chapter is to demonstrate how the general principles of good practice are applied when managing various painful conditions by covering:

◆ Acute pain including post-operative pain and labour pain
◆ Chronic musculoskeletal pain, including back pain and osteoarthritis
◆ Chronic neuropathic pain, including peripheral and central neuropathic pain
◆ Cancer pain
◆ TENS for children and the elderly

Acute pain

Post-operative pain

Post-operative pain is often severe and localized around the incision but may also spread because of soft-tissue injury from surgical trauma and retraction and may include neuropathic elements with hyperalgesia and tactile allodynia. Local policy and practice dictates whether TENS is offered. In 1997, a survey of pain management after thoracotomy in 24 Australian hospitals found that TENS was used infrequently, which may be a reflection of concern about effectiveness at that time (Cook & Riley, 1997). Evidence suggests that TENS can reduce post-operative pain at rest and movement from major thoracic, abdominal, and orthopaedic surgery including thoracotomy, post-open-heart surgery, coronary artery bypass graft (CABG) surgery, cholecystectomy, appendectomy, myomectomy, haemorrhoidectomy, tonsillectomy, hernia, surgery for retroperitoneal lymph node dissection, gynaecological surgery, post-caesarean pain, and pain associated with dental procedures (Chapter 8, 157). Studies have also shown that TENS reduces analgesic consumption, ileus, nausea and vomiting, and pulmonary atelectasis, and length of stay in the recovery room.

Conventional TENS is often used at the site of incision pain. TENS intensity should be below motor threshold to reduce risks associated with mechanical stress causing additional trauma to the site of surgery. Electrodes should be placed at least 5 cm from the scar to prevent mechanical damage of the incision site when removing electrodes. Sterile 'strip-like' electrodes are used for large areas of pain following major thoracic, abdominal, or spinal surgery (Figure 7.1). Alternatively, dual-channel TENS devices with four electrodes can be used with one channel at the site of pain and the other channel over proximal nerves or paravertebrally at the relevant spinal segment. Examples include:

◆ Coronary artery bypass surgery (CABG) surgery—either side of the incision scar and parallel to the spinous processes at T1–T5 on the affected side

◆ Cholecystectomy—either side of the incision scar and parallel to the spinous processes at T7–T10 on the affected side

◆ Knee surgery—medial and lateral to knee around scar and parallel to the spinous processes at L3–L4 on the affected side

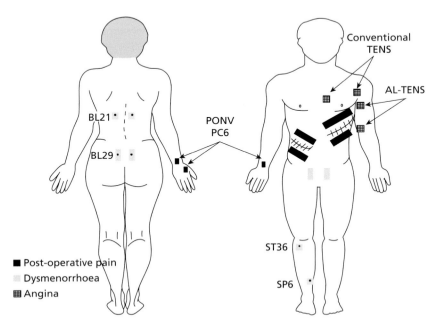

Fig. 7.1 Electrode positions when using TENS for post-operative pain (black), dysmenorrhoea including over acupuncture points (grey shading) and angina (grid). PONV = post-operative nausea and vomiting.

In certain circumstances it is advisable to place electrodes along the main nerves proximal to pain, rather than the incision site itself, including:

◆ when TENS sensations cannot be produced close to the scar

◆ when dysaesthesia and/or tactile allodynia is present

◆ when a body part is absent following amputation (e.g. limb or breast)

◆ when tissue is fragile (e.g. hand or foot reconstructive surgery where electrodes can be positioned over major nerve bundles to project TENS sensation into the distal limb)

◆ when there is an open wound

Dual-channel stimulation is also useful when managing pain and ileus or nausea simultaneously (Chapter 10, 198–201).

If possible a pre-operative TENS trial should be conducted to prepare the patient for using TENS following surgery (see Johnson & Bagley, 2009, for review). Ideally, TENS should be tried at the site to be used post-operatively. The forearm is a practical alternative when this is not possible. Record settings preferred during the pre-operative TENS trial and use these settings in early post-operative stages, although settings preferred during a pre-operative trial in the absence of pain may differ from those preferred in the presence of post-surgical pain. Patients should be warned that a successful pre-operative trial does not necessitate success post-operatively and that there is a possibility that TENS may worsen pain following surgery. It should be emphasized that there should be no muscle twitching near the incision site because it may hinder healing and cause further damage in underlying tissue. If the surgical procedure requires a dressing then TENS electrodes need to be applied in the operating room (Box 7.1). If it does not then electrodes can be applied in the recovery room or ward. It is critical that infection-control processes are carefully adhered to. If appropriate, remind patients that electrodes will be applied whilst they are under general anaesthesia.

Labour pain

During stage 1 of labour the cervix dilates causing backache and abdominal pain. During contractions there are strong, menstrual-cramp-like sensations distributing into the suprapubic regions. During stage 2, the baby is pushed down the vagina and pain becomes stretching-like, progressing to burning and stinging during crowning. Augustinsson and colleagues (1977) pioneered the use of TENS for childbirth pain when they reported that 88 per cent of 147 women obtained pain relief during TENS. A larger survey of 10 077 women found that 71 per cent reported 'excellent' or 'good' relief of pain using TENS and 91 per cent would use TENS again in the future suggesting satisfaction with the use of TENS (Johnson, 1997). TENS is often used in the early stages of labour as a stand-alone treatment for backache either at home, during the journey to the hospital, or in the labour suite. TENS is less effective for the second stage of labour when pain becomes more intense and distributed into the suprapubic region.

Obstetric TENS devices are specially designed to be dual-channel, and include a 'boost' control button to produce a stepwise increase in current amplitude to relieve more intense contraction pain. They are a little more expensive than a standard TENS

Box 7.1 TENS procedures in the operating room, hospital ward, and recovery room

TENS procedures in the operating room

- Check the condition of the patient's skin prior to applying electrodes
- Sterile electrodes and aseptic procedures should be used when placing electrodes along the incision site in the operating theatre
- Skin should be rinsed and dried before electrodes are applied if an iodine-based surgical preparation has been used
- The scrub nurse removes electrodes once packaging is open and applies electrodes to patient skin parallel at least 5 cm away from any sutures.
- Ensure all parts of the electrodes adhere to the skin
- Apply wound dressing and remember to protrude the electrode's lead-wire connection from under the dressing so that it can be connected to electrode leads and TENS device at a later time

TENS procedures in the hospital ward or recovery room

- Start TENS once patient is sufficiently alert and able to provide verbal feedback—the patient needs to be fully conscious to control the TENS device
- Attach TENS device to electrode lead wires with settings preset to those preferred in the pre-operative TENS trial
- Nurse or patient, if able, switches TENS on and increases TENS intensity to the first TENS sensation and then slowly to a strong, non-painful level
- Patient takes control of TENS and is encouraged to keep TENS on as long as needed—devices with timers that automatically switch TENS off after 30–60 minutes can be useful
- Check patient frequently in early stages of TENS treatment to ensure no adverse effects
- Discontinue TENS if post-operative complications occur or pain worsens
- If possible monitor skin under the electrodes and close to the incision by lifting the corner of electrode
- Itchiness may indicate that electrodes need to be replaced
- All incidents related to TENS should be recorded

device (e.g. approximately GB£40.00). One pair of electrodes are positioned paravertebrally at T10–L1 to target low-threshold afferents from segments associated dilation of the cervix and contraction of the uterus,and the other pair of electrodes is positioned at S2–S4 to target low-threshold afferents from segments associated with distension

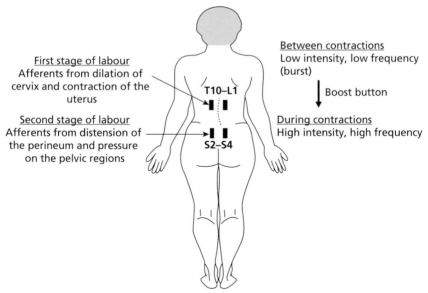

Fig. 7.2 TENS for labour pain.

of the perineum and pressure on the pelvic regions (Figure 7.2). TENS sensations are distributed on the thoracic and sacral regions which are prominent during the first stage of labour but not the second stage of labour when pain distribution progresses to the lower abdomen and suprapubic region. Women and their partners should practise using TENS in advance (e.g. as part of antenatal class education) so that they are famil- iar with how to use TENS.

Dysmenorrhoea

Dysmenorrhoea is excessive lower abdominal menstrual pain in the umbilical or su- prapubic region of the right or left abdomen radiating to thighs and lower back with sharp, throbbing, dull, nauseating, burning, or shooting qualities. Primary dysmenor- rhoea occurs in the absence of an underlying cause although inflammatory mediators such as prostaglandins have been implicated. Secondary dysmenorrhoea is associated with underlying pathology. TENS may be used as a stand-alone treatment or in combi- nation with any of the other treatments using electrode positions (Figure 7.1):

- over the abdomen, medial to the anterior superior iliac spine just below the um- bilicus, so that TENS sensation covers the painful area
- paravertebrally at nerves corresponding to afferent innervation from uterus (i.e. T10, T11, T12)
- over the abdomen (one channel) and lower back (one channel) using two pairs of electrodes
- over acupuncture points used for abdominal problems including BL21, BL29, SP6, SP10, and ST36

Conventional TENS is commonly employed when abdominal and lower back electrode positions are used and AL-TENS when acupuncture points are used. Examples of TENS parameters used in studies are 100 pps, 95 μs; 125 pps, 30 μs; 70–100 pps, 200 μs for conventional TENS, and 1 Hz, 40 μs; 2 Hz, 250 μs for AL-TENS with stimulation duration varying from 30 minutes to 8 hours. No approach has shown superiority. Examples of TENS devices specifically marketed for dysmenorrhoea include OVA Period Pain Reliever (GB£28.00) and Digital TENS—Period Pain Reliever (Kinetick, GB£20.00).

Angina

Angina pectoris is chest pain presenting as pressure, heaviness, tightness, squeezing, or burning, and referred pain in the inner left arm, shoulders, epigastrium (upper central abdomen), back, shoulders, neck, and jaws. Stable angina is precipitated by activity and managed with glyceryl trinitrate, beta-blockers, or calcium channel blockers to reduce the frequency of attacks. Unstable angina occurs at rest and may be treatment-resistant so coronary artery bypass graft or coronary angioplasty is used. TENS is used for chronic angina and the general consensus is that is TENS is unlikely to mask pain of a potential myocardial infarction. However, apprehension remains, so many practitioners consult a physician or cardiologist to confirm that is TENS is appropriate.

Mannheimer and co-workers pioneered TENS for chronic angina pectoris that was refractory to other treatment demonstrating that TENS improved microcirculation and coronary artery insufficiency, raised the ischaemic threshold of cardiac muscle, increased working capacity, and decreased ST-depression of the electrocardiograph (for reviews, see Borjesson, 1999; Moore & Chester, 2001). Recently it was found that TENS provided long-term benefit for angina pectoris-like chest pains in individuals refractory to medication (de Vries et al., 2007). TENS generated vasodilation in the forearm of healthy participants but not in individuals with refractory angina suggesting that systemic vascular responses may differ (Hallen et al., 2010).

TENS can be administered using conventional TENS over the chest and AL-TENS over muscles of the left arm to manage referred pain (Figure 7.1). Electrodes are placed over the painful area on the anterior aspect of chest wall so that TENS sensation covers the painful area. Electrodes can also be placed over referred painful areas of the left arm and on spinal nerve roots related to the heart, i.e. T1–T3. TENS has been used both to suppress pain during an attack and also as a prophylactic. During an angina attack TENS is administered using the principles of conventional TENS by increasing intensity so that it covers the pain. Some commentators suggest that stimulation should be delivered using high-frequency, high-intensity pulses of short duration lasting 30–60 seconds until the pain is gone, repeating two to three times if necessary. Others suggest that TENS should be delivered at the site of chest pain at a strong, non-painful level for the entire duration of the attack. TENS appears to alter pain sensation so that it is less bothersome and distressing and reduces the duration of the angina attack. When TENS is used as a prophylactic it is administered on the anterior aspect of the chest wall prior to physical activity using treatment sessions lasting approximately one hour for two to three times a day. AngioTENS was developed as a specific TENS device for angina and neuropathic chest wall pain, although it may no longer be commercially available. See <http://217.33.237.40/document_uploads/Case_Studies/David%20Trenbath%20Case%20Study%20(Sharing)_05d3d.pdf>.

Chronic pain

Musculoskeletal pain

Musculoskeletal pain affects muscles, ligaments, tendons, and bones, and has a wide variety of causes. Musculoskeletal pain presents as aching pain occasionally with burning sensations and twitching in muscles, and is often associated with fatigue and sleep disturbances. Treatment depends on the condition with electrophysical techniques popular as adjuncts or stand-alone treatments. TENS may not be practical for minor musculoskeletal injuries or multiple severe injuries where appropriate analgesics should be prescribed. In sports settings TENS may be used to manage localized, short-lived pains resulting from strains or tears of ligaments or muscles. Combining conventional and AL-TENS is recommended for musculoskeletal pain that is referred from sciatica, arthritis, and central pain states.

Back, neck, and shoulder pain

There are a variety of possible causes for back, neck, and shoulder pain including muscle or soft-tissue sprain or strain, torticollis, degeneration of vertebrae and discs (spondylosis), ankylosing spondylitis, herniated vertebral disc(s), inflamed, compressed, or ischaemic nerves (radiculopathy), whiplash, and adhesive capsulitis (frozen shoulder) to name but a few! Pain is characterized by aching soreness, tension, or stiffness in the lower back and also in the neck and shoulders. Pain may radiate into the buttocks and limbs with pins-and-needles and numbness in the presence of radiculopathy. A sensation of stiffness is common with decreased movement and postural difficulties. Non-specific back, neck, or shoulder pain is not caused by a recognizable primary disease and is managed with simple analgesics, exercise, and various physical therapies and acupuncture. TENS is often used either as an adjunct or a stand-alone treatment. Evidence of effectiveness is inconclusive with few good-quality RCTs, and therefore best-practice guidelines are contradictory.

In general, conventional TENS is used in the first instance with electrodes positioned around the painful area and unilateral electrode positions used if the pain is located on one side of the body. AL-TENS can be used to generate phasic muscle contractions of large muscle masses using burst patterns of stimulation, or more discrete muscle groups perhaps at trigger points using single pulses and this may be useful to release muscle spasm. In the presence of sciatica conventional TENS can be administered to the spine and AL-TENS over the muscles innervated by the same spinal segment as radiating pain (Figure 7.3). TENS belts with Velcro fastening to aid body fit and good electrode–skin contact may be useful. An RCT found that TENS administered via a lumbosacral orthosis was superior to conventional TENS delivered using normal electrodes for pain associated with degenerative disc disease in the lumbosacral spine (Pop et al., 2010).

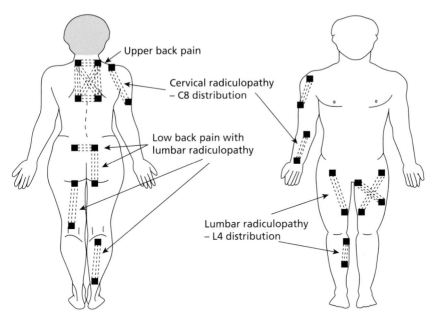

Fig. 7.3 TENS for low back pain with lumbar radiculopathy and for upper back pain with cervical radiculopathy.

Non-inflammatory rheumatic diseases

Osteoarthritis and related conditions

Osteoarthritis is a degenerative disease of joints, articular cartilage, and subchondral bone of the knees, hips, and hands causing pain and tenderness in joints and associated tissue, decreased movement, stiffness, and muscle atrophy. Exercise is used to improve local muscle strengthening and general aerobic fitness in association with simple analgesics. TENS is used as an adjunct to core treatment for short-term benefit.

Conventional TENS using electrode positions to permeate TENS sensations into the site of pain has been used extensively for osteoarthritis. Care needs to be taken not to deliver excessive pulse amplitudes resulting in contractures of the painful joints of the fingers and toes which can exacerbate pain. Some patients use mild AL-TENS using burst patterns of stimulation to generate mild twitching of the fingers to relieve pain and promote movement but this should be undertaken with care. Glove and sock electrodes are available for painful osteoarthritic hands and feet, and a placebo-controlled study on healthy participants demonstrated that conventional TENS delivered using a glove electrode had similar hypoalgesic effects as normal electrodes projecting sensation into the hand (Cowan et al., 2009). Glove electrodes have an advantage that they also keep the hand warm, yet a stronger TENS sensation within the hand is generated using normal electrodes over proximal nerves to the hands (Chapter 3, Figure 3.12).

Conventional TENS delivered using a dual-channel stimulator and two pairs of electrodes can be used to give full coverage of pain within osteoarthritic knees. It is possible to walk whilst delivering conventional TENS providing intensity is kept below motor threshold, although patients need to extremely careful because TENS will affect proprioceptive sense with a risk of an accidental fall. Conductive knee braces with electrodes integrated into the brace using conductive fabric strips are also available which will provide additional knee support.

Bone fractures and osteoporosis

Bone fractures may occur from a variety of causes including impact, stress, or weakened bones from bone metastases or osteoporosis. Fractures cause pain due to activation of nociceptors because of damage to the periosteum or endosteum, and oedema and protective muscle spasms with reduced in mobility. Fractures of vertebrae may lead to sudden onset back and radicular pain due to nerve root compression. Conventional TENS either side of the fracture may reduce pain and improve function. For example, Oncel and colleagues (2002) found that 30 minutes of conventional TENS (80 pps, 50 µs), twice a day was more effective than non-steroidal anti-inflammatory drugs (NSAIDs) in controlling pain when two pairs of electrodes were placed on either side of the fracture along the lines of intercostal nerves. It is important that the intensity is below motor threshold in order to reduce hazards associated with muscle contractions causing mechanical stress at the site of the fracture. AL-TENS with forceful muscle contractions should be avoided at osteoporotic sites because there is a risk of further damage to bone fractures (Hartkopp et al., 1998).

Fibromyalgia syndrome and myofascial pain syndrome

Fibromyalgia is a chronic widespread pain accompanied by allodynia, stiffness, fatigue, and sleep disturbances. Fibromyalgia may be idiopathic, perhaps with a genetic component, or associated with other conditions such as rheumatoid arthritis and systemic lupus erythematosus. Myofascial pain syndrome shares common symptoms with fibromyalgia but is characterized by chronic pain with multiple trigger points with tenderness, muscle hardening at the trigger point on palpation, and reproduction and referral pain on trigger point palpation. Stretching and trigger-point release techniques using manipulation, massage, acupuncture, electroacupuncture, or TENS are often used in combination.

Conventional TENS over painful sites is used for fibromyalgia or myofascial pain syndrome and has been show to produce comparable pain relief as superficial warmth therapy (Lofgren & Norrbrink, 2009). Dual-channel stimulation can be used to get sufficient coverage of TENS sensation when pain is widespread. TENS over acupuncture points segmentally related to the distribution of pain may also be used. AL-TENS over trigger points may be beneficial for trigger point release.

Inflammatory rheumatic diseases including rheumatoid arthritis and ankylosing spondylitis

Rheumatoid arthritis is a systemic inflammatory disorder affecting tissues, organs, and especially synovial joints causing pain in joints accompanied by swelling, stiffness, and general tiredness. Symptoms may worsen during 'flare-ups' which are unpredictable. Treatment includes disease-modifying antirheumatic drugs, physical therapy and exercise to maintain strength and joint mobility, although exercise in an active inflammatory state may make pain worse. TENS is recommended as an adjunct to core treatment for short-term benefit. Ankylosing spondylitis is a chronic inflammatory disease of the axial skeleton affecting the spine and sacroiliac joint presenting as chronic back pain and stiffness with pain from the sacroiliac joint referred to the buttock or back of thigh. Treatment is similar to that described for rheumatoid arthritis.

TENS is administered for rheumatoid arthritis and ankylosing spondylitis using similar techniques described for osteoarthritis. Careful monitoring of pain and swelling is necessary as there may be a risk of exacerbating an active inflammatory state due to TENS increasing blood flow. TENS may be useful for patients with ankylosing spondylitis who find it difficult to sit or stand for prolonged periods of time (e.g. <20 minutes).

Soft-tissue periarticular disorders

Soft-tissue periarticular disorders encompass a range of painful conditions of tendons and associated tissue including lateral and medial epicondylitis, Achilles tendonitis, plantar fasciitis (Policeman's heel), rotator-cuff injuries, and bursitis. There is no universally accepted treatment for most of these conditions, although the principles of management of these conditions are similar to that described previously for musculoskeletal conditions using a combination of medication and physical therapy, and surgery when appropriate. Conventional TENS is administered for soft-tissue periarticular disorders using similar techniques as described for myofascial pain syndrome. Care must be taken not to generate muscle contractions that could cause additional strain on injured tendons and surrounding tissue. TENS elbow and ankle sleeves, and hand and sock electrodes may be beneficial.

Neuropathic pain

Neuropathic pain is caused by a lesion or disease of the peripheral or central components of the somatosensory system and presents as spontaneous and/or evoked pain with allodynia, hyperalgesia, and hyperpathia. Pain is characterized in the skin as burning, stabbing, or pricking, and in muscle and bone as aching, cramping, or throbbing. Electrical paraesthesiae and shock-like shooting pains are common. Pharmacological management includes tricyclic antidepressants (e.g. amitriptyline), membrane stabilizing drugs (e.g. gabapentin, carbamazepine), and topical preparations (e.g. capsaicin). TENS has been used with success for post-herpetic and trigeminal neuralgias, phantom limb and stump pain, radiculopathies (cervical, thoracic, and lumbar), diabetes, HIV-associated neuropathy, complex regional pain syndromes, entrapment neuropathies (carpal tunnel syndrome), cancer pain (neoplasm nerve compression, infiltration by tumour, cancer treatment), post-surgical neuropathic pain, central post-stroke pain, spinal-cord-injury pain, spinal surgery, and multiple sclerosis (Barlas & Lundeberg, 2006; Johnson & Bjordal, 2011). Peripheral neuropathic pain may respond better than central neuropathic pain. There is one case report of long-term remission of neuropathic pain following TENS (Thorsen & Lumsden, 1997).

Peripheral neuropathic pain

Diabetic peripheral neuropathy

Up to half of all patients with diabetes present with neuropathy and a quarter of these have neuropathic pain. Research using models of diabetes in rats suggests that electrical stimulation can normalize nerve-conduction velocities and improve endoneurial blood flow (Cameron et al., 1993). Conventional and AL-TENS have been used for diabetic neuropathy delivered around the site of pain. The presence of hypoaesthesia and altered sensation at the site of pain needs to be considered and this may result in electrodes being placed proximal to the pain over the main nerve distributions. Dual-channel TENS using four electrodes may be beneficial. Sock electrodes have been used.

Post-herpetic and trigeminal neuralgias

Neuralgia describes pain in the distribution of a nerve or nerves. Post-herpetic neuralgia is caused by the varicella zoster virus following infection from herpes zoster (i.e. shingles) with burning pain, allodynia, and paraesthesia presenting in the dermatome of the affective nerve when herpes zoster vesicles begin to heal. Trigeminal neuralgia may be caused by compression of the nerve with demyelination of axons from a wide variety of aetiologies. Trigeminal neuralgia presents as superficial burning-like pain and a dull aching pain with episodes of intense, sharp, shooting pain following the distribution of the three branches of the trigeminal nerve, resulting in pain on the side of the face including an ear, eye, lips, nose, scalp, forehead, cheeks, teeth, or jaw. Mild stimuli such as touch or wind may evoke an attack of the pain.

Conventional TENS over the distribution of the relevant peripheral nerve is often used in the first instance. Hyperaesthesia may prevent electrodes from being placed directly over the site of pain so nerve bundles proximal to the site of pain or contralateral mirror sites can be used (Figure 7.4). AL-TENS may also be used. Extreme care needs to be taken when using TENS on the face for trigeminal and facial pains, as accidental provocation of an attack will cause much suffering for the individual. Titrating currents to generate TENS sensations or mild muscle twitching of intercostal or facial muscles can be challenging. The size of electrodes used on the face may need to be smaller than those commonly used.

Amputation pain

Following amputation of a body part, individuals may experience pain in the residual body part (limb), sometimes termed 'stump pain', presenting as sharp, dull, burning, squeezing, cramping, shooting, and shock-like electrical sensations. The residual body part may be sensitive to touch because of the presence of neuroma. Pain in the location of the missing (amputated) body part, termed 'phantom (limb) pain', presents as tingling, itching, burning, and aching. Non-painful sensations of tingling, movement,

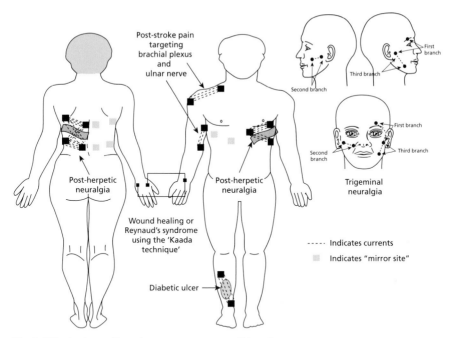

Fig. 7.4 Electrode positions for common neuropathic pains.

and distortion of size and shape of the absent body part may also be present. Electrical stimulation of afferents proximal to the stump may generate sensations of touch, joint movement, and position in phantom limbs. An open-label study found that projecting conventional TENS into a painful phantom limb reduced pain on movement and at rest when electrodes were placed over peripheral nerves in the residual limb (Mulvey et al., 2012). Furthermore, some participants reported that TENS sensations arose from the prosthetic limb, suggesting that TENS may facilitate perceptual embodiment of the prosthetic limb (Mulvey et al., 2009). Improvements in phantom limb pain and sensations have also been reported following TENS delivered to the contralateral limb (Giuffrida et al., 2010).

Conventional TENS is used in the first instance, progressing to AL-TENS if patients do not respond. The choice of whether to use an ipsilateral or contralateral site for stimulation is made on a patient to patient basis taking account of the sensitivity of the residual body part and the wishes of the patient. Some patients may express concern at TENS 'reawakening the phantom'. It is possible to apply TENS electrodes to the residual limb and project TENS sensation into an allodynic stump or painful phantom, but this needs to be performed with care (Figure 7.5). Electrodes should be placed on skin with normal sensation and proximal to or either side of areas of tactile allodynia. In some but not all people it is possible to apply electrodes to project TENS into the phantom through a process of trial and error. Participants can wear their prosthesis with TENS electrodes in situ and they may be able to stand and walk with lower-limb prosthesis, but careful monitoring of skin condition is needed. Electrodes should not be positioned at sites prone to excessive

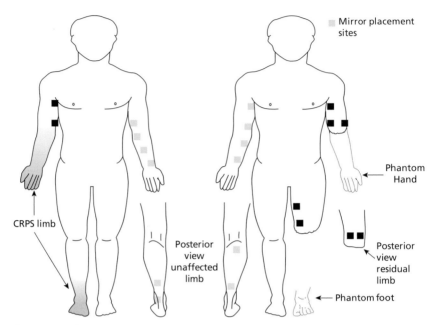

Fig. 7.5 TENS for amputation pain and complex regional pain syndrome.

pressure from the prosthesis such as on the stump of a lower limb because this may lead to skin abrasion.

Complex regional pain syndrome

Complex regional pain syndrome (CRPS) type I occurs in the absence of nerve damage (reflex sympathetic dystrophy), and CRPS type II occurs following nerve damage (causalgia). CRPS usually affects an arm or a leg, although it can spread to other parts of the body, and presents as changes in skin appearance and temperature, and swelling with burning, stabbing and paraesthesiae. Moving or touching the limb is often intolerable. Spinal cord stimulation is used for severe cases for CRPS type I (Cruccu et al., 2007). No studies have specifically focused on the efficacy of TENS, although TENS is often listed as a useful treatment. The findings of a study using an animal model of CRPS type II found that high-frequency TENS reduced the development of tactile allodynia when delivered to the contralateral limb, and contralateral low-frequency TENS reduced the development of thermal allodynia (Somers & Clemente, 2006a).

Many patients with CRPS are unable to tolerate stimulation of the skin of the affected limb by touch or TENS until a programme of desensitisation has taken place close to the area of allodynia. TENS can be applied to the contralateral limb in the first instance and then moved to skin with normal sensation proximal to the affected area eventually projecting TENS sensations into the affected area (Figure 7.5). Barely perceptible TENS sensations should be used first and intensity slowly increased to a strong, non-painful TENS sensation. It may be possible for glove or sock electrodes to be used for patients with less sensitive limbs.

Central neuropathic pain including post-stroke and spinal cord injuries

Post-stroke pain

Post-stroke pain may present months to years after the cerebrovascular event. Individuals experience local pain in joints especially in the shoulder and central pain (thalamic pain syndrome) characterized by constant, moderate, or severe pain on part or all of the affected side. Pain is often cramping, burning, crushing, shooting, and in combination with dysaesthesia, hyperpathia, and mechanical and thermal allodynia. Pain may be dynamic in characteristics and location. Conventional TENS at the site of pain, often at the shoulder, is used providing a strong, comfortable sensation can be experienced by the patient (Figure 7.4). Proximal sites over main nerve bundles are used in the presence of hyperpathia and mechanical and thermal allodynia. If strong, comfortable TENS sensations are not possible then AL-TENS may be used. Practitioners should be attentive to the possibility of discomfort, increased pain, and local muscle spasms during TENS treatment. Caution is needed if TENS is used for individuals who are seizure-sensitive after stroke.

Multiple sclerosis

Multiple sclerosis is an inflammatory disease resulting in loss of myelin from axons of the central nervous system resulting in muscle weakness and spasms with difficulties in movement, coordination, balance, speech and swallowing, and altered sensory physiology. Pain presents as neuropathic in origin including trigeminal neuralgia, Lhermitte's sign (a brief, electric-shock-like sensation running from the back of the head down the spine), and burning, aching, or dysaesthetic neuropathic pain 'girdling' around the body. Pain may also present as secondary musculoskeletal pain in the form of aches, and cramps resulting from spasticity. TENS is used to manage neuropathic and musculoskeletal pain as previously described.

Spinal cord injury

Spinal cord injury denotes any type of trauma of the spinal cord, as opposed to disease, resulting in 'partial' or 'complete' loss of function below the injury (e.g. paralysis and incontinence) with associated pain, numbness, or a loss of sensation in relevant dermatomes. As early as 1974, TENS was identified as being useful for patients with spinal cord injury and more efficacious for pains at the site of injury rather than radiating or central pain. Conventional TENS is used over areas with intact or diminished but preserved sensation at, or directly above, the level of the lesion. A dual-channel stimulator with four electrodes positioned paravertebrally may also be useful. If it is not possible to achieve a strong, comfortable TENS sensation then AL-TENS can be used in a similar manner to central post-stroke pain. Discomfort, increased pain, and muscle spasms are possible during TENS.

Cancer pain

Cancer-related pain may be associated with the disease, the cancer treatments, and/or associated co-morbid conditions. Cancer pain may be of musculoskeletal, neuropathic, or nociceptive origin. Bone metastases causing pain on rest and on movement are a common cause of cancer-related pain. The WHO analgesic ladder is used in combination with non-pharmacological approaches. Surveys in anaesthetics-based palliative care programmes in Germany found that TENS was only indicated for 1–3 per cent of individuals over a ten-year period (Grond et al., 1999). Evidence from case series suggest TENS may be of benefit for pain from bony metastases, nerve compression and infiltration, and cancer treatment including chemotherapy-induced neuropathy, and post-surgery (see Johnson et al., 2008. for review).

Conventional TENS at the site of pain is the primary approach providing skin sensitivity is normal. Published case series have found that conventional TENS was acceptable at the site of cancer bone pain and that it may be useful for rest and movement pain with the rapid onset of analgesia associated with conventional TENS potentially useful for cancer breakthrough pain. However, because of the frailty of some of these individuals, especially towards the end of life, practitioners should be vigilant to the possibility of adverse events during TENS including increased pain and discomfort during and following TENS. TENS over the acupuncture point Pericardium 6 (PC6, Neiguan) may be beneficial for nausea and vomiting in these patients (Chapter 10, 201). Higher intensities of TENS generating muscle contractions should not be administered over unstable vertebrae and some practitioners may feel that the hazards associated with using even low-intensity TENS in these situations are too great. TENS has also been used for the management of lymphoedema by placing electrodes proximal to the lymphoedematous limb, although hazards associated with increasing lymphoedema may outweigh the potential benefit (Waller & Bercovitch, 2000).

Miscellaneous

Visceral pain

Visceral pain encompasses a wide variety of conditions and is usually considered to be nociceptive in origin, arising in thoracic, pelvic, or abdominal organs. Pain arising directly from visceral tissue is characterized as being diffuse and difficult to localize and often referred to somatic areas. Often the referred pain is more localized and sharper in quality than the pain in the visceral tissue itself. The use of TENS to manage pain arising from visceral tissue including labour pain, dysmenorrhoea, and angina has been dealt with previously. Currents used during TENS do not permeate to the depth necessary to stimulate visceral organs, and even if TENS excites visceral tissue, the resultant sensation is not as strong or clear as that obtained from somatic cutaneous structures. However, TENS can be useful for pain referred to somatic structures.

Wound pain

Conventional TENS on healthy skin around wounds or at low frequencies on auricular acupuncture points has been used successfully to relieve pain from dressing changes and debridement and the relief of burn pruritus in areas of severe itching once the area had healed (Ordog, 1987).

Headache and orofacial pain

There are over 100 categories of headache and orofacial pain and treatment depends on cause. It is difficult to permeate TENS sensations into deep-seated headache pain. It is possible to create a low-intensity TENS sensation across the forehead and scalp using electrodes above the eyes but this should be performed as a last resort because of the sensitivity of the skin. Applying TENS to the scalp can create unpleasant sensations because of the lack of underlying soft tissue and the difficulty of attaching electrodes because of hair. Conventional TENS is useful for tension headache when applied over musculature of the posterior neck. Transorbital and transcranial electrode positions are not advised because of the danger of increasing intraocular pressure (Chapter 5, 111).

Conventional TENS and AL-TENS have been used for orofascial pain using similar techniques to those described for trigeminal neuralgia. When TENS is administered on the face unilateral electrode placements are used. Two pairs of electrodes with each channel positioned unilaterally are used for bilateral facial pain. Electrodes can be positioned on either side of the midline of the upper face (e.g. bilateral cheek) so that currents permeate the nose, although extreme care needs to be taken as the skin and underlying tissue of the face is sensitive and the dense neural innervation of the face means that currents often permeate other structures. Generally, conventional TENS is used first. AL-TENS has been be used for atypical facial pain presenting as continuous burning and aching pain sensations in combination with numbness or dysaesthesia.

TENS for children and the elderly

TENS has been successfully used for children with complex regional pain syndrome, dental pain, and minor procedures including venepuncture and wound-dressing changes for open perineal wounds following burn trauma (Lander & Fowler-Kerry, 1993; Merkel et al., 1999). Children as young as four years are able to tolerate TENS providing the child is able to understand in simple terms what is happening. A caregiver or practitioner should be present to supervise treatment at all times. A trial of conventional TENS on an area of non-painful skin before trying TENS at the painful site usually reveals whether the child finds TENS sensation acceptable. Practitioners and/or caregivers need to monitor behavioural cues from the child about their experience with TENS and whether it is helping their pain.

Summary

1 A flexible approach should be taken when using TENS in clinical practice.

2 Infection-control processes should be followed when TENS is used in perioperative settings with electrodes applied in the operating room if a dressing is required.

3 Consider specialist equipment such as glove, sock, sleeve, brace, and belt electrodes, and obstetric TENS devices with 'boost' control for labour pain.

4   Consider dual-channel TENS for widespread and/or multiple pains including referred pain where conventional TENS can be administered to the source of the pain and AL-TENS over the referred pain.

5   Electrodes should be positioned on sensate skin and over main nerves or contralaterally when hypoaesthesia, allodynia, or hyperalgesia is present. Projecting TENS sensation into the painful area may be possible.

Further reading

◆ Johnson, M.I., Oxberry, S., and Robb, K. (2008) Stimulation-induced analgesia. In Sykes, N., Bennett, M., and Yuan, C.-S. (eds) *Cancer Pain. Clinical Pain Management Second Edition*. Hodder Arnold, London, 235–50.

◆ Johnson, M.I., Oxberry, S., and Simpson, K. (2008) Transcutaneous Electrical Nerve Stimulation (TENS) and acupuncture for acute pain. In Macintyre, P., Walker, S., and Rowbotham, D. (eds) *Acute Pain. Clinical Pain Management Second Edition*. Hodder Arnold, London, 271–90.

◆ Johnson, M.I., and Bagley, J. (2009) Transcutaneous electrical nerve stimulation in perioperative settings. In Cox, F. (ed.) *Perioperative pain management*. Wiley-Blackwell, Chichester, 248–76.

◆ Johnson, M.I., and Bjordal, J.M. (2011) Transcutaneous electrical nerve stimulation for the management of painful conditions: focus on neuropathic pain. *Expert Rev Neurother*, **11**, 735–53.

Chapter 8 will review clinical research evidence to determine the efficacy and effectiveness of TENS for pain management.

Chapter 8

Clinical research on the efficacy of TENS

Introduction

The acceptance of a treatment into mainstream medicine is influenced by a wide variety of factors including the patient and practitioner circumstances and preferences, and the context in which the treatment is being used, including political, philosophical, ethical, economic, and aesthetic values of society. Traditionally, practitioners relied on information gathered from personal experience although this can be misleading so emphasis is now given to experience coupled with the findings of clinical research. The purpose of this chapter is to present an overview of the evidence from clinical research on the clinical efficacy of TENS for the management of pain by covering:

- Evidence-based practice
- Clinical research on TENS for:
  - acute pain including post-operative pain and labour pain
  - chronic musculoskeletal pain, including back pain and osteoarthritis
  - chronic neuropathic pain, including peripheral and central neuropathic pain
  - cancer pain
- Challenges in TENS research

Evidence-based practice

Evidence-based practice integrates clinical experience with clinical research to inform effectiveness of treatments. Clinical observation on its own cannot determine whether an active ingredient of a treatment produces beneficial effects because non-specific effects associated with receiving a treatment, including practitioner–patient interaction, contaminate observations. Randomized controlled clinical trials (RCTs) are considered to be the gold standard of clinical research to determine efficacy because they attempt to remove biases that confound clinical observation (Table 8.1). Clinical effectiveness is investigated using pragmatic trials. The majority of clinical research on TENS has used RCTs and therefore has tested efficacy. Often the terms 'efficacy' and 'effectiveness' are used interchangeably.

Table 8.1 Terminology

Term	Definition
Evidence-based medicine	The use of current evidence to make medical decisions about the care of individuals
Clinical experience	Knowledge and judgement that clinicians acquire through clinical practice that relies on clinical observation to gather wisdom about the effectiveness of treatments
Clinical research	Any research on humans that produces knowledge for the understanding of human disease, preventing and treating illness, and promoting health
Efficacy	How well a treatment works in a controlled situation (e.g. experiment)
Effectiveness	How well the treatment works in 'real-world' situations, such as clinical practice, including potential side effects
Randomized controlled clinical trial	A scientific experiment used to test the efficacy of an intervention within a human population, usually patients, that compares a treatment under study with a comparison (control) intervention
Placebo control	A fake or dummy treatment without an active ingredient that has no specific biological activity on the illness or complaint under study
Blinding	Concealing knowledge about whether an intervention is a treatment control from study participants and/or investigators and/or therapists
Systematic review	A review that identifies, appraises, and synthesizes all research evidence that meets pre-specified eligibility criteria to answer a given research question
Meta-analysis	A statistical technique that combines (pools) the data from independent studies to estimate treatment effect taking into account the sample sizes of the different studies (weighted)
Cochrane review	A systematic review published in the Cochrane Database of Systematic Reviews (<http://www.cochrane.org/cochrane-reviews>) on treatment interventions, diagnostic test accuracy, or research methodology, and prepared and supervised by a Cochrane Review Group according to methodology published in the Cochrane Handbook for Systematic Reviews (<http://www.cochrane.org/training/cochrane-handbook>)

Randomized controlled trials (RCTs)

Randomized controlled clinical trials (RCTs) investigate the effects of a treatment with a comparison intervention which may be:

+ a no treatment control
+ a placebo control
+ another treatment

Patients have an equal chance (randomized) of receiving the treatment or comparison (control) intervention. Placebo controls are used to isolate effects caused by the active ingredient of the treatment from the act of receiving a treatment. Placebos used in RCTs of medications contain inert substances that have no known specific physiological effects. They are identical to the active (real) medication to enable investigators to conceal (blind) which intervention is the placebo and which intervention is 'real' from trial participants and assessors. The validity and reliability of RCT findings depend on the methodological quality of the study (Box 8.1). Methodologically weak RCTs tend to overestimate treatment effects resulting in the reporting of false positive findings or underestimate treatment effects resulting in false negative findings. Furthermore, RCT findings should not be taken in isolation because apparently similar RCTs may produce different results. When extrapolating RCT findings into a wider clinical context the following should be considered:

- Findings are generalized to populations and do not account for individuality in treatment response
- RCTs are conducted in an 'artificial environment' that does not reflect true treatment situations
- Similar outcomes measured in an RCT often produce inconsistent results
- RCTs are expensive which can bias research topics under study
- RCTs under-research certain groups such as ethnic minorities

Box 8.1 Attributes of good RCTs

Attributes of good RCTs

- Sufficient numbers of participants to ensure statistical power to detect any differences between treatment and comparison groups
- Clearly defined eligibility criteria so that the generizability of the findings to a patient population is known
- Sample selected randomly from the population under study
- Randomization of participants into active treatment and control groups
- Concealment of treatment allocation to participants, practitioners, and outcome assessors
- Use of an authentic placebo
- Use of treatment with adequate dosing and technque
- Blinding of participants, practitioners, and outcome assessors to intervention groups
- Sufficient time for any treatment effects to take place
- Minimal missing data

Systematic reviews, meta-analyses, and levels of evidence

Systematic reviews and meta-analyses of RCTs use explicit methods and attempt to minimize bias to produce reliable findings by:

◆ comprehensive searching for relevant studies from a number of different sources
◆ using predefined criteria for selection and evaluation of studies
◆ systematically collecting data
◆ synthesizing data for analysis

High methodological quality scores are given to RCTs with appropriate randomization and blinding although this is a challenge for TENS because of difficulties in designing and blinding authentic placebos. Furthermore, a methodological review of 38 RCTs included in Cochrane reviews on TENS for acute, chronic, and cancer pain revealed that inadequate TENS technique and infrequent treatments of insufficient duration in the treatment intervention (i.e. low implementation fidelity) contributed to negative outcomes and underestimation of TENS effects (Bennett et al., 2011). These methodological issues contaminate published clinical research on TENS.

Systems to rank evidence according to quality are used to aid development of health policy and clinical practice guidelines (Table 8.2). When assessing clinical efficacy and effectiveness systematic reviews and meta-analyses are at the top of the hierarchy of research evidence. Therefore the discussion of TENS efficacy will focus on this type of clinical research evidence.

Clinical research on TENS

Research literature on TENS is vast and has been increasing year-on-year (Figure 8.1). An unfiltered search on PubMed using the medical subject heading (MeSH) term 'transcutaneous electric nerve stimulation' on 4 October 2013 yielded 6025 hits, which reduced to 1367 hits when the limits 'clinical trials' was applied, 998 hits when the limit 'randomized controlled clinical trial' was applied, and 45 hits when the limit 'meta-analyses' was applied. The hits would need to be carefully screened to reveal studies specifically focused on TENS but the search demonstrates the large volume of available research literature.

Table 8.2 UK National Health Service levels of evidence

Level	Evidence
A	Consistent findings in RCTs or prospective cohort studies with the clinical decision rule validated in different populations
B	Consistent findings in retrospective, exploratory, or ecological cohort studies, outcomes research, case-control studies. Extrapolations from level A studies may be used
C	Case series or extrapolations from level B studies
D	Expert opinion without explicit critical appraisal, or based on physiology, bench research, or first principles

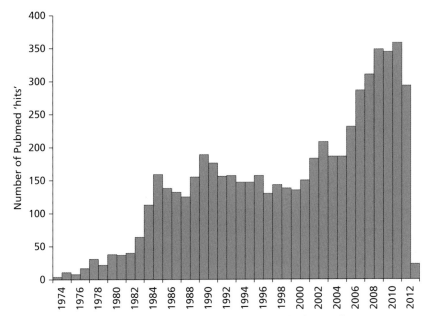

Fig. 8.1 Number of 'hits' by year for a PubMed search using the keyword 'transcutaneous electric nerve stimulation' on 24 May 2013; (search string: 'transcutaneous electric nerve stimulation'[MeSH Terms] OR ('transcutaneous'[All Fields] AND 'electric'[All Fields] AND 'nerve'[All Fields] AND 'stimulation'[All Fields]) OR 'transcutaneous electric nerve stimulation'[All Fields]).

The majority of patient-centred studies on TENS are cohort studies and case series and lack control groups but are a rich source of documented clinical experience about the usefulness of the overall TENS treatment package. However, randomized placebo controlled clinical trials would be necessary to isolate the effects of electrical currents on pain to answer the question 'Do you need to put batteries in the TENS device to get effects?' The first systematic review on TENS was published in 1996 and there have been many since (Table 8.3). In 2008, Claydon and Chesterton attempted to synthesize the findings of six systematic reviews on TENS for chronic pain including chronic low back pain, osteoarthritis of the knee, rheumatoid arthritis of the hand and chronic musculoskeletal pain (Claydon & Chesterton, 2008). They found evidence from three systematic reviews that TENS was superior to placebo. Higher intensity TENS produced optimal effects, although any inferences of dose-related responses were undermined because of inadequate study design, low statistical power, and variability in TENS protocols. A similar picture emerges for acute pain.

Acute pain

A Cochrane review on TENS as a sole treatment for adults with acute pain (<12 weeks) identified 1775 studies and excluded 145 because TENS was given in combination with

Table 8.3 Summary of systematic reviews on TENS

Reference	Condition	Data set and analysis	Reviewers' conclusion	Comment
Acute pain				
Walsh et al., (2009) Cochrane review	Acute pain	12 RCTs (919 patients) Descriptive analysis	Evidence inconclusive	Low-quality studies with small sample sizes
Carroll et al., (1996)	Post-operative pain	17 RCTs (786 patients) Descriptive analysis	Evidence of no effect	Comparison groups consisted of active and inactive interventions. Patients allowed free access to analgesic medication in some RCTs
Bjordal et al., (2003)	Post-operative analgesic consumption	21 RCTs (964 patients) Meta-analysis	Evidence of effect	Demonstrated that adequate TENS technique critical for effect
Freynet & Falcoz (2010)	Post-thoracotomy pain	Nine RCTs (645 patients) Descriptive analysis	Evidence of no effect as stand-alone treatment Evidence of effect as adjuvant	Most studies low-quality studies with small sample sizes
Sbruzzi et al., (2012)	Post-thoracic surgery pain	11 studies	Evidence of effect	TENS with pharmacological analgesia > placebo TENS with pharmacological analgesia at reducing pain for thoracotomy and sternotomy. TENS with pharmacological analgesia = placebo TENS with pharmacological analgesia for improvement in forced vital capacity
Carroll et al., (1997a)	Labour pain	Ten RCTs (877 patients) Descriptive analysis	Evidence of no effect	Comparison groups consisted of active and inactive interventions. Patients allowed free access to analgesic medication in some RCTs

Table 8.3 (continued) Summary of systematic reviews on TENS

Reference	Condition	Data set and analysis	Reviewers' conclusion	Comment
Dowswell et al., (2009) Cochrane review	Labour pain	19 RCTs (1671 patients) Descriptive analysis	Evidence inconclusive	Low-quality studies
Bedwell et al., (2011) Update of (Dowswell et al., 2009)	Labour pain TENS for pain relief in labour vs. routine care or placebo devices	14 studies (1256 women) [11 studies on TENS of the back, two studies on TENS of acupuncture points and one study using a cranial TENS-like device]	Evidence inconclusive	Women receiving TENS to acupuncture points were less likely to report severe pain. Women using TENS would use it again in a future labour. Use of TENS at home in early labour was not evaluated
Mello et al., (2011)	Labour pain	Nine studies (1076 women)	Evidence of no effect	TENS = placebo for pain relief during labour and for the need for additional analgesia Women desire to use TENS in future deliveries
Proctor et al., (2003) Cochrane review	Primary dysmenorrhoea	Seven RCTs (213 patients) Descriptive analysis	Evidence of effect-pain relief for HF TENS only	Low-quality studies with small sample sizes
McIntosh & Hall (2011)	Acute low back pain	One systematic review (Machado et al., 2009)	Insufficient evidence to judge	Evidence low quality
Chronic pain				
Nnoaham & Kumbang (2008) Cochrane review	Chronic pain	25 RCTs (1281) Descriptive analysis	Evidence inconclusive	Low-quality studies with small sample sizes and possibility of underdosing TENS
Johnson & Martinson (2007)	Musculoskeletal pain	32 RCTs on TENS, six RCTs on PENS (1227 patients) Meta analysis	Evidence of effect	Criticized for using multiple diseases creating heterogeneity

Table 8.3 (continued) Summary of systematic reviews on TENS

Reference	Condition	Data set and analysis	Reviewers' conclusion	Comment
Khadilkar et al., (2008) Cochrane review	Low back pain	Three RCTs (197 patients) Descriptive analysis	Evidence inconclusive Insufficient evidence to judge	Low-quality studies with small sample sizes and possibility of underdosing TENS
Poitras & Brosseau (2008)	Low back pain	Six RCTs (375 patients) Descriptive analysis	Evidence of effect	Low-quality studies with small sample sizes
Machado et al., (2009)	Non-specific low back pain (acute and chronic)	76 trials reporting on 34 treatments. Four RCTs (178 patients) were on TENS, (two acute, two chronic)	Evidence of effect	Low-quality studies with small sample sizes. Insufficient evidence to judge
Chou (2010)	Chronic low back pain	One systematic review (Khadilkar et al., 2008) and one additional RCT	Evidence inconclusive	Available evidence very low quality. RCTs heterogeneous in design and TENS technique
Dubinsky & Miyasaki (2010)	Painful neurological conditions Low back pain	Two RCTs (201 patients) Descriptive analysis	Evidence of no effect	Small sample sizes and possibility of under-dosing of TENS. Insufficient evidence to judge
Rutjes et al., (2009) Cochrane review	Knee osteoarthritis	18 RCTs (275 patients) Descriptive analysis	Evidence inconclusive	Low-quality studies with small sample sizes with some RCTs not using standard TENS device
Bjordal et al., (2007)	Knee osteoarthritis	Seven RCTs (414 patients) Meta-analysis	TENS effective in short term	Accounted for adequate TENS technique in analysis
Brosseau et al., (2003) Cochrane review	Rheumatoid arthritis	Three RCTs (78 patients) Meta-analysis	Evidence of effect	Low-quality studies with small sample sizes

Table 8.3 (continued) Summary of systematic reviews on TENS

Reference	Condition	Data set and analysis	Reviewers' conclusion	Comment
Abou-Setta et al., (2011)	Pain after hip fracture	83 unique studies (64 RCTs, five non-RCTs, and 14 cohort studies). Two studies on TENS ($n = 2$)	Insufficient evidence to judge	Only two studies on TENS
Robb et al., (2008) Cochrane review	Cancer pain	Two RCTs (64 participants) Descriptive analysis	Insufficient evidence to judge	Low-quality studies with small sample sizes and possibility of under-dosing TENS
Hurlow et al., (2012) Update of Robb et al., (2008)	Cancer pain	Three studies (88 participants) Descriptive analysis	Insufficient evidence to judge	Low-quality studies with small sample sizes and possibility of under-dosing TENS
Kroeling et al., (2009) Cochrane review	Neck disorders (whiplash associated disorders and mechanical neck disorders)	Seven RCTs on TENS (88 patients) Descriptive analysis	Evidence of effect but low quality studies	Low-quality studies with small sample sizes and possibility of under-dosing TENS. Included any surface electrical stimulation including microcurrent devices Insufficient evidence to judge
Bronfort et al., (2004) Cochrane review	Chronic headache	Three RCTs Descriptive analysis	Evidence inconclusive	Low-quality studies with small sample sizes and possibility of under-dosing TENS. Insufficient evidence to judge

Table 8.3 (continued) Summary of systematic reviews on TENS

Reference	Condition	Data set and analysis	Reviewers' conclusion	Comment
Neuropathic pain				
Price & Pandyan (2000) Cochrane review	Post-stroke shoulder pain	Four RCTs (170 patients) of any surface electrical stimulation	Evidence inconclusive	Low-quality studies with small sample sizes and possibility of under-dosing TENS. Two RCTs used TENS to produce muscle contractions. Insufficient evidence to judge
Cruccu et al., (2007)	Various neuropathies	Nine 'controlled trials' (200 patients) Descriptive analysis	Evidence of effect	Low-quality studies with small sample sizes. Insufficient evidence to judge
Mulvey et al., (2010) Cochrane review	Post-amputation pain	No RCTs	No evidence available	Insufficient evidence to judge
Jin et al., (2010)	Painful diabetic neuropathy	Three RCTs (78 patients) Meta-analysis	Evidence of effect	Low-quality studies with small sample sizes. Used non-standard TENS devices
Dubinsky & Miyasaki (2010)	Painful neurological conditions Painful diabetic neuropathy	Three RCTs (two RCTS used in evaluation of 55 patients) Descriptive analysis	Evidence of effect	Low-quality studies with small sample sizes
Pieber et al., (2010)	Painful diabetic peripheral neuropathy	15 studies. Three RCTs and one retrospective analysis of TENS (130 participants)	Evidence of effect (level B)	TENS > placebo three large studies and one small study. Studies used H-wave therapy not TENS

another treatment (Walsh et al., 2009). Of the remaining 163 studies, only 12 RCTs (919 participants) were included for review and meta-analysis was not possible due to insufficient data. Reviewers decided that evidence was inconclusive.

Post-operative pain

In 1996, Reeve and colleagues found that TENS reduced pain to a greater extent than control groups in 12 of 20 RCTs (Reeve et al., 1996). Carroll and colleagues (1996) found that TENS was not superior to placebo TENS in 15 out of 17 RCTs, although TENS was superior to placebo in 17 out of 19 non-RCTs demonstrating that failure to randomize participants to treatment groups overestimated treatment effects. These reviewers concluded that TENS was not effective for post-operative pain. Interestingly, study participants had access to analgesics so they would have been able to titrate analgesic consumption to achieve maximal possible pain relief, biasing outcome towards no difference between TENS and placebo. Furthermore, some RCTs used suboptimal TENS technique and doses. A meta-analysis of 21 RCTs (1350 patients) considered these issues and found that TENS produced larger reductions in analgesic consumption than placebo when adequate TENS technique was used (Bjordal et al., 2003). This was the first review to conduct a subgroup analysis of TENS delivered using 'adequate technique and dosage' defined *a priori* as TENS delivered as 'strong, definite, sub noxious, maximal tolerable . . . within or close to the site of pain'. Only 11 out of 21 RCTs (964 patients) met criteria for adequacy of TENS.

Recently, Freynet and Falcoz (2010) found that TENS was superior to placebo as an adjuvant to opioid analgesics for acute post-thoracotomy pain in seven out of nine RCTs, although only three of these RCTs were double-blind. They concluded that TENS was effective as the sole pain-control treatment in video-assisted thoracoscopy incision (mild post-thoracotomy pain), and useful as an adjunct to analgesics for muscle-sparing thoracotomy incision (moderate post-thoracotomy pain). TENS was ineffective as a stand-alone therapy for posterolateral thoracotomy incision (severe post-thoracotomy pain). Sbruzzi and colleagues (2012) conducted at meta-analysis of 11 RCTs and found that TENS combined with analgesics reduced thoracotomy or sternotomy pain more than placebo TENS combined with analgesics, although there was no improvement in forced vital capacity suggesting that TENS was not beneficial for pulmonary function.

Labour pain

Reeve and colleagues (1996) found no differences between TENS and placebo TENS or conventional pain management in seven out of nine RCTs. Since then systematic reviews have failed to find evidence supporting efficacy, although RCT findings may be contaminated with the effects of concurrent medication in a similar manner to that seen for post-operative pain RCTs. Carroll and co-workers (1997b) found that the effects of TENS were no different to control groups in five out of eight RCTs. An updated review found no differences between TENS and controls in seven out of nine RCTs, although the odds ratio suggested that analgesic intervention was less likely with TENS (Carroll et al., 1997a). However, the number needed to treat was 14 suggesting that 14 patients needed to be treated with TENS before one obtained clinically meaningful benefit. It was noted that RCTs with high methodological scores reported no differences between active and placebo TENS for pain relief or additional analgesic intervention.

The most recent Cochrane review included 19 studies (1671 women) (Dowswell et al., 2009). TENS was applied to the lower back in 15 RCTs, to acupuncture points in two RCTs, and to the cranium in two RCTs. There were no differences between TENS and controls (mostly placebo TENS) for pain ratings or on other interventions and outcomes in labour. Reviewers stressed that the use of TENS at home in early labour was not evaluated. The data was refined to include 14 studies (1256 women) but the conclusion remained the same (Bedwell et al., 2011). In two RCTs that failed to detect differences between TENS and placebo, women receiving TENS reported that they would use TENS again in a future labour when response was taken following childbirth yet still under double-blind conditions (Harrison et al., 1987; Thomas et al., 1988). A meta-analysis of 9 studies (1076 women) found no differences between TENS and no TENS treatment or placebo TENS for pain relief during labour or the need of additional analgesia (Mello et al., 2011). Measuring self-reports of pain in the delivery suite when participants are experiencing fluctuating physical and emotional conditions during childbirth is likely to introduce measurement error. Clinical guidelines on intrapartum care of healthy women and their babies during childbirth developed by the National Collaborating Centre for Women's and Children's Health and published by NICE concluded that TENS should not be offered to women in established labour, although it may be beneficial in the early stages of labour (National Institute for Health and Clinical Excellence, 2007).

Dysmenorrhoea

A Cochrane review of seven RCTs (213 participants) on TENS for primary dysmenorrhoea found that high- but not low-frequency TENS was superior to placebo TENS for pain relief, although there were inconsistencies in RCT findings and TENS technique (Proctor et al., 2003). Reviewers concluded that there was weak evidence supporting beneficial effects for TENS. More recently, Wang and colleagues (2009) found that high-frequency conventional TENS reduced pain intensity and autonomic symptoms compared with placebo TENS in women with primary dysmenorrhoea. Tugay and colleagues (2007) found that 20 minutes of conventional TENS (120 pps, 100 μs or interferential therapy (0–100 pps and 90–100 pps) applied to low back and proximal gluteal muscle reduced symptoms of primary dysmenorrhoea with no difference in efficacy between methods. Wu and colleagues (2012) found that non-invasive acupoint stimulation using currents at frequencies of 1000–10,000 Hz applied at LI4 (Hegu) and SP6 (Sanyinjiao) points twice weekly for eight weeks reduced pain associated with primary dysmenorrhoea in 66 women. However, there were no differences in outcome when currents were administered to acupuncture or non-acupuncture points.

Angina

Early RCTs with small sample sizes by Mannhiemer and co-workers found that TENS with electrodes placed directly over the painful area of the chest improved pain, exercise tolerance, ST segment depression, nitrate usage, and ischaemic episodes in patients with angina (for reviews, see Borjesson, 1999; Moore & Chester, 2001). Recent evidence suggests that TENS provides long-term benefit for angina pectoris-like chest pains in individuals refractory to medication (de Vries et al., 2007). However, there are no systematic reviews to date and NICE concluded that current evidence was weak and insufficient to judge the effectiveness and therefore TENS should not be recommended for stable angina until new evidence demonstrates clinical and cost-effectiveness (National Institute for Health and Clinical Excellence, 2011).

Miscellaneous

Published reports on the use of TENS for other acute pain conditions are plentiful and generally positive for reductions in pain associated with lacerations, fractures, hematomas, contusions, and dental procedures although good-quality RCTS are lacking (Hansson & Ekblom, 1984; Morrish, 1997; Meechan et al., 1998; Oncel et al., 2002).

Chronic pain

The most recent Cochrane review of TENS for chronic pain ($\leq$ 3 months duration) included 25 RCTs (1281 patients) published between 1978 and 2006 (Nnoaham & Kumbang, 2008). There were wide variations in TENS technique and methodological quality between RCTs so meta-analysis was not possible. TENS was superior to inactive TENS controls in 13 out of 22 studies and superior in eight out of 15 studies using multiple-dose TENS treatment comparisons. There were no differences in pain outcome in comparisons of high-frequency and low-frequency TENS.

Musculoskeletal pain

The largest meta-analysis of TENS to date evaluated the efficacy of percutaneous electrical nerve stimulation (PENS) or TENS for the relief of chronic musculoskeletal pain and included 29 RCTs (1227 participants, six studies on PENS, Johnson & Martinson, 2007). Nine RCTs scored <3 out of 5 on the Jadad scale of methodological quality, with 335 participants receiving placebo, 474 participants receiving TENS or PENS, and 418 participants crossed over to receive both placebo and electrical nerve stimulation. There were 38 comparisons of which 32 were on TENS (19 high-frequency TENS, six low-frequency TENS, one very high-frequency TENS, four AL-TENS, and two of unspecified frequency). Electrical nerve stimulation was superior to placebo in 24 comparisons, with pain relief approximately three times the pain relief provided by placebo (Figure 8.2). The review was criticized for combining multiple diseases at the expense of homogeneity, although this approach did increase statistical power of the analysis.

Back, neck, and shoulder pain

Low back pain

The most recent Cochrane review of TENS for chronic low back pain was published in 2008 and included four high-quality RCTs (585 patients) (Khadilkar et al., 2008). A qualitative synthesis of three RCTs that administered TENS to 110 participants and placebo TENS to 87 participants was inconclusive for pain outcomes. TENS did not

Principal investigator (year)

Standard difference in mean (95% CI)

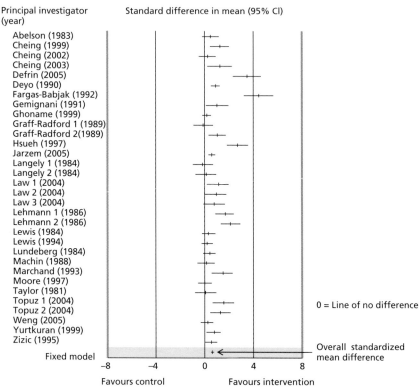

Fig. 8.2 Forest plot of TENS comparisons for chronic musculoskeletal pain created using data provided in supplementary appendices of the published report of Johnson and Martinson (2007). For each study the standardized mean difference is represented by a vertical line and the 95 per cent confidence interval by the horizontal line. The cumulative result of TENS studies is represented by the cross in the 'fixed model' row. Original reference citations can be found in the original article.

Source: data from Johnson, M. and Martinson, M., Efficacy of electrical nerve stimulation for chronic musculoskeletal pain: a meta-analysis of randomized controlled trials, *PAIN®*, Volume 130, Issue 1, pp. 157–165, Supplementary Materials, Copyright © 2007 International Association for the Study of Pain. Published by Elsevier Inc. All rights reserved. Acknowledgement: Dr Osama Tashani.

improve back-specific functional status based on two RCTS (TENS = 271 participants, placebo = 95 participants). Inadequate stimulation intensity was used in at least two RCTs administering AL-TENS. In 2009, a meta-analysis by Machado and colleagues (2009) of two trials of acute back pain and two of chronic back pain (178 participants) found that pain relief from TENS was comparable to 10–20 per cent reduction of pain from baseline. In 2011, van Middelkoop and colleagues (2011) evaluated the effectiveness of TENS for chronic low back pain from six RCTs, although some TENS interventions did not use standard TENS devices. Five RCTs compared TENS with placebo TENS with only two RCTs having a low risk of bias. Outcomes between RCTs were inconsistent, and pooled, weighted, mean differences for pain or disability had wide confidence intervals that crossed the line of no effect suggesting no differences between groups. Reviewers concluded that evidence had serious limitations due to a large degree of heterogeneity.

There are also many systematic reviews of evidence conducted by clinical guideline development teams. In 2001, the Philadelphia Panel that developed evidence-based clinical practice guidelines on rehabilitation interventions for chronic low back pain concluded TENS did not reduce pain and claimed that this was based on level I(A) evidence (Panel, 2001). European guidelines for the management of chronic non-specific low back pain published in 2006 suggested that there was strong (level A) evidence that TENS was no more effective than placebo (Airaksinen et al., 2006), and in 2007 the American College of Physicians and the American Pain Society concluded that TENS had not been proven to be effective for chronic low back pain (Chou & Huffman, 2007). In 2008, Poitras and Brosseau (2008) conducted a systematic review, on behalf of the North American Spine Society, that included six RCTs with 375 participants receiving TENS and 192 receiving placebo TENS. They claimed that evidence suggested that TENS reduced pain intensity in the immediate short term but not in the long term. In 2009, the UK National Institute for Health and Clinical Excellence evaluated three RCTs, conducted by two investigating teams, with 331 participants receiving TENS and 168 receiving placebo TENS and concluded that it was not possible to judge the effectiveness of TENS for early management of persistent non-specific low back pain (National Institute for Health and Clinical Excellence, 2009b). It was recommended that TENS should not be offered as part of the treatment package for persistent non-specific low back pain. In 2010, Practice Guidelines for Chronic Pain Management: An Updated Report by the American Society of Anesthesiologists Task Force on Chronic Pain Management and the American Society of Regional Anesthesia and Pain Medicine published in April 2010 recommended that 'TENS should be used as part of a multimodal approach to pain management for patients with chronic back pain and may be used for other pain conditions (e.g. neck and phantom limb pain)' (American Society of Anesthesiologists, 2010).

There are more systematic reviews on TENS for chronic low back than there are methodologically robust RCTs.

Reasons for the inconsistency in recommendations can be demonstrated by critical evaluation of the review process. In 2010, the Therapeutics and Technology Assessment Subcommittee of the American Academy of Neurology (AAN) conducted a systematic review and concluded that there was level A evidence from two good-quality RCTs that TENS should not be recommended for the relief of chronic low back pain (Dubinsky & Miyasaki, 2010). The aim of the review was to assess 'clinical trials . . . for well-defined painful neurologic disorders' although it is debatable that low back pain is a well-defined painful neurological disorder as it is usually considered as a mixed pain pattern even when radiculopathy is present. Further scrutiny of review methodology revealed serious limitations in reviewers' claims that the recommendation for low back pain was based on level A evidence because only 114 patients had received TENS and 87 had received placebo in the dataset (Johnson & Walsh, 2010). One of the two RCTs included in the review by Deyo and colleagues (1990a) was criticized at the time of publication for clinical heterogeneity, use of a suboptimal TENS technique, and the concurrent use of hot packs which may have masked the effects of TENS. Moreover, placebo TENS on its own was associated with improvements in pain that lasted up to two months following intervention. The other RCT included in the review sampled a population of patients with multiple sclerosis and despite a lack of statistical difference between active and placebo groups, the original trial authors argued that clinically important effects from TENS may have been masked because some participants in the placebo TENS group were taking additional analgesics (Warke et al., 2006).

Recently, RCTs have been published that were not included in systematic reviews. A prospective, randomized, single-blind study that recruited 236 adults consulting for chronic low back pain, with or without radicular pain, in 21 pain centres in France found that TENS (n = 117) given in four, one-hour, daily treatment sessions for three months did not improve functional status or the use of analgesic and anti-inflammatory medication compared with placebo TENS (n = 119) (Buchmuller et al., 2012). There was an improvement in pain measured using visual analogue scales at the first and last assessments. A single-blind randomized controlled trial that recruited 150 patients attending a physiotherapy department in Brazil found that there was a superior reduction of pain measured using visual analogue scales in patients receiving ten 30-minute sessions of either TENS or interferential current therapy, compared with a no-treatment control group, although there were no differences between TENS and interferential current therapy (Facci et al., 2011). The failure to include a placebo control means that it is not possible to determine whether the beneficial effects were due to TENS per se.

'. . . the conclusion that "TENS is established as ineffective" for chronic low back pain was based on an analysis of two Class I RCTs with a total of 114 participants who received TENS and 87 participants who received sham TENS (no current) . . . It seems unreasonable that the effectiveness of TENS, and subsequent clinical recommendations, can be "established" from studies with so few participants'. Reproduced from Johnson and Walsh, 2010, p. 314, with permission from Elsevier.

Neck and shoulder pain

A Cochrane review on electrotherapy for whiplash-associated disorders and mechanical neck disorders included seven RCTs (88 patients) on TENS, including microcurrent devices, and the descriptive analysis suggested evidence of effect although the methodological quality of studies was low with small sample sizes and possibility of underdosing TENS (Kroeling et al., 2009).

Non-inflammatory rheumatic diseases

Osteoarthritis and related conditions

The most recent Cochrane review on the efficacy of TENS on osteoarthritic knee pain, conducted in 2009, included 18 RCTs (813 patients) (Rutjes et al., 2009).

Eleven RCTs compared the effects of TENS (275 participants) with placebo or no intervention (190 participants), and the remaining RCTs investigated interferential current therapy ($n = 4$), TENS and interferential current therapy ($n = 1$), or pulsed electrostimulation ($n = 2$). Meta-analysis of the effect of any type of surface electrical nerve stimulation on pain outcome included 16 RCTs and 18 comparisons (726 patients) and found a large standard mean difference corresponding to a reduction of pain of 21 mm on a 100 mm visual analogue scale in favour of surface electrical nerve stimulation compared with control with no differences in the magnitude of effects between the different types of electrical nerve stimulation (Figure 8.3). Comparisons of TENS found a large, standard mean difference approximately 20 mm on a visual analogue scale. Inadequate sample sizes, blinding, selective, and inadequate reporting of outcomes and variability in intervention technique caused a high degree of heterogeneity in the analysis. Unrealistically large, standardized mean differences up to three times the magnitude expected for total joint replacement was found in four of the included studies. When meta-regression techniques were used to minimize biases associated with small trials of questionable quality the predicted effect sizes became negligibly small. As a consequence the reviewers decided that evidence was inconclusive.

An earlier systematic review of 36 RCTs (2434 participants) investigating a variety of physical interventions for osteoarthritic knee pain found that TENS, electroacupuncture, and low-level laser therapy provided clinically relevant short-term pain relief when administered at optimal doses within an intensive 2–4 week treatment regimen (Bjordal et al., 2007). The meta-analysis of seven RCTs on TENS found reductions in pain of 22.2 mm (95 per cent confidence interval (CI): 18.1–26.3) on a 100 mm visual analogue scale compared with placebo. The most recent RCT found that a single treatment with high- and low-frequency TENS increased pressure pain threshold in participants with osteoarthritis of the knee compared with placebo (no current) TENS although there were no differences in pain reduction at rest or on movement between active and placebo TENS (Vance et al., 2012). In the UK, the National Institute for Health and Clinical Excellence recommended that TENS should be offered as an adjunct to core treatment for short-term relief of osteoarthritic knee pain (National Institute for Health and Clinical Excellence, 2008).

Bone fractures and osteoporosis

The findings of early studies suggested that conventional TENS over the site of rib fracture reduced pain and improved function including increases in ventilation and arterial oxygen concentrations compared with placebo and analgesic medication, although a systematic review of a variety of pain management interventions for hip fracture found two RCTs on TENS and one on non-invasive interactive neurostimulation and insufficient evidence to judge the effectiveness (Gorodetskyi et al., 2007; Lang et al., 2007; Abou-Setta et al., 2011). RCTs have found that TENS alleviated pain and trismus (limited mouth opening) caused by muscle spasm in patients undertaking jaw exercise treatment for fractures of the mandible (Fagade et al., 2005). Interferential current therapy reduced chronic low back pain due to multiple vertebral osteoporotic fractures

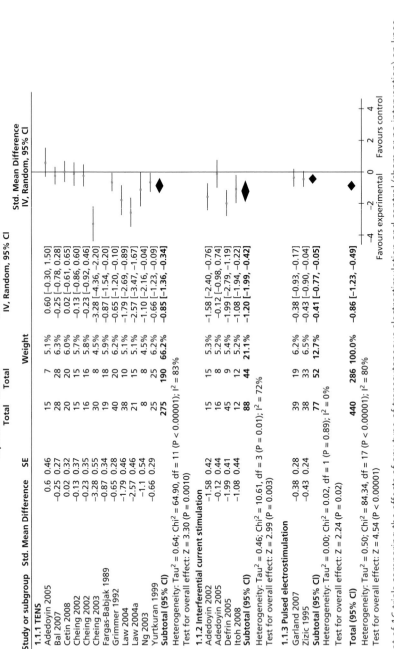

Fig. 8.3 Forest plot of 16 trials comparing the effects of any type of transcutaneous electrostimulation and control (sham or no intervention) on knee pain. Standardized mean differences are represented by squares and the 95 per cent confidence interval by the horizontal line. The cumulative result of studies is represented by the diamonds. Std. = standard; SE = Standard Error; CI = confidence interval.

Reproduced with permission from Rutjes, A.W.S., et al., Transcutaneous electrostimulation for osteoarthritis of the knee, *Cochrane Database of Systematic Reviews*, Issue 1, 2010, Copyright © 2010 The Cochrane Collaboration. Published by John Wiley & Sons, Ltd; available at: <http://www.thecochranelibrary.com>.

when added to a standard exercise program (Zambito et al., 2007). A systematic review and meta-analysis of 11 RCTs found that various types of electromagnetic stimulation reduced pain in only one of four RCTs and did not improve delayed unions or un-united long-bone fractures, although the quality of available research was low (Mollon et al., 2008).

There has been little research on the effectiveness of TENS on osteoporosis. A systematic review of non-pharmacological treatments to prevent bone loss after spinal cord injury found beneficial effects to trabecular bone in the distal femur or proximal tibia following early-phase electrical stimulation (five studies), and variable results for chronic-phase electrical stimulation (14 studies, including mixed periods after injury) (Biering-Sorensen et al., 2009). Higher frequencies and intensities were more effective. An RCT using 150 women receiving therapeutic exercise found that the addition of interferential current therapy (30 minutes per day, five days per week for two weeks) or Horizontal® Therapy (a TENS-like device similar to interferential current therapy, see: <http://www.hakomed.it/ht.php>) was superior to placebo Horizontal® Therapy in alleviating pain and disability in patients with chronic back pain due to previous multiple vertebral osteoporotic fractures (Saggini et al., 2004).

Fibromyalgia and myofascial pain syndromes

There are no systematic reviews or meta-analysis on the effectiveness of TENS for fibromyalgia syndrome or myofascial pain syndrome. Recent RCTS have found beneficial effects from TENS. Lauretti et al., (2013) found that TENS of the lower back improved pain and fatigue in fibromyalgia compared with placebo TENS, and that using two TENS devices simultaneously over the back and neck improved symptoms further. Dailey et al., (2013) found that TENS a single treatment of TENS provided short-term relief of symptoms of fibromyalgia. Carbonario and colleagues (2013) found that high-frequency TENS (150 Hz) on bilateral tender points of trapezium and supraspinatus improved pain, work performance, fatigue, stiffness, anxiety, and depression associated with fibromyalgia when given as an adjuvant to aerobic and stretching exercises. Other RCTs on fibromyalgia have found comparable pain relief from TENS and superficial warmth (42 °C) (Lofgren & Norrbrink, 2009), and the addition of TENS to a 12-week exercise program improved tender point count and painful symptoms (Mutlu et al., 2013).

RCTs on myofascial pain syndrome are generally positive. Rodriguez-Fernandez and colleagues (2011) found that ten minutes of low-frequency TENS (burst pattern 2 Hz, 200 μs, 100 pps) increased referred pressure pain threshold over latent myofascial trigger points in the trapezius muscle, and increased ipsilateral cervical range of motion. Gemmell and Hilland (2011) found that electric point stimulation using TENS was superior to placebo TENS at reducing pain associated with latent upper trapezius trigger points. Hou and colleagues (2002) found that TENS combined with hot pack, range of motion, and ischaemic compression, or hot pack, active range of motion, and stretch with spray, more efficacious than therapy combinations that did not include TENS. However, Gul and Onal (2009) found that Botulinum toxin-A injection provided better pain control than TENS or trigger-point injection with lidocaine or 20 sessions of low level laser therapy. An early study (Graff-Radford et al., 1989) found that high-frequency TENS (100 pps) was superior to low-frequency TENS (2 Hz) in reducing myofascial pain.

Inflammatory rheumatic diseases

Rheumatoid arthritis and ankylosing spondylitis

The most recent Cochrane review of TENS for rheumatoid arthritis of the hand was published in 2003 and included three RCTs (78 patients), and only two of these compared TENS (27 patients) against a placebo (27 patients) (Brosseau et al., 2003). Evidence was inconclusive because of a limited number of RCTs. The Ottawa Panel Evidence-Based Clinical Practice Guidelines and NICE recommended that TENS should be used as an adjunct to core treatment for short-term relief of rheumatoid arthritis of the hand (Ottawa Panel, 2004; National Institute for Health and Clinical Excellence, 2009a).

Soft-tissue periarticular disorders

A systematic review of various electrophysical techniques for the treatment of medial and lateral epicondylitis (Dingemanse et al., 2013) included only one RCT on TENS that found that low- or high-frequency TENS on acupuncture points improved pain when compared with placebo TENS, with no differences between high-frequency and low-frequency TENS (Weng et al., 2005). A pragmatic randomized controlled trial of TENS for the management of tennis elbow found that there was no additional benefit when TENS was used as an adjunct to primary-care management of tennis elbow, although this may have been due in part to poor adherence to TENS treatment protocols (Chesterton et al., 2013).

Neuropathic pain

There are no Cochrane reviews evaluating the effectiveness of TENS for neuropathic pain (Johnson & Bjordal, 2011), although a Cochrane protocol has been published (Claydon et al., 2010). The European Federation of Neurological Societies Task Force for neuro-stimulation therapy for neuropathic pain conducted a review of nine controlled trials with data extracted for 200 patients and found that TENS was superior than placebo, although the methodological quality of RCTs was low, with no adequately powered prospective, randomized trials with masked outcome assessment (Cruccu et al., 2007). It was recommended that TENS may be useful as a preliminary or add-on therapy because it was non-invasive, safe, and could be self-administered (level C evidence).

Peripheral neuropathic pain conditions

Diabetic peripheral neuropathy

The authors of a meta-analysis of three RCTs claimed that TENS was superior to placebo (no current) TENS at reducing mean pain scores and overall neuropathic symptoms associated with diabetic peripheral neuropathy (Jin et al., 2010). However, TENS-like devices (H-wave therapy and Salutaris TENS) rather than a standard TENS device were included and only 78 patients were included in the analysis with 45 receiving an active intervention. The Therapeutics and Technology Assessment Subcommittee of the American Academy of Neurology claimed that TENS was 'probably effective' (level B evidence, i.e. at least one RCT) for painful diabetic neuropathy based on the findings of three RCTs. One of the included RCTs was not included in the meta-analysis by Jin et al. (2010), and only 31 participants received active TENS and 24 placebo TENS (Dubinsky & Miyasaki, 2010).

Post-herpetic and trigeminal neuralgias

There are no systematic reviews on TENS for post-herpetic and trigeminal neuralgias and very few RCTs. An RCT of 30 participants with post-herpetic neuralgia found that TENS reduced pain intensity and sleep interference when combined with pregabalin (Barbarisi et al., 2010), and a small RCT found that TENS provided no benefit for post-herpetic neuralgia compared with acupuncture (Rutgers et al., 1988).

Amputation and complex regional pain syndrome

A Cochrane review found that there were no RCTs to judge the efficacy of TENS for phantom pain and/or stump pain (Mulvey et al., 2010), and there are no systematic reviews on TENS for complex regional pain syndrome.

Central neuropathic pain conditions

Stroke

A Cochrane review on various forms of electrical stimulation for post-stroke shoulder pain included four trials on TENS (170 patients) (Price & Pandyan, 2001). Three of these trials used TENS to deliver functional electrical stimulation by generating muscle contractions to improve motor function, and the remaining trial found that high-intensity TENS (100 pps, three times the sensory threshold) was superior to sensory threshold or placebo TENS for management of hemiplegic shoulder pain and passive range of motion for flexion (Leandri et al., 1990). A meta-analysis of eight RCTs found that functional electrical stimulation and TENS improved gait speed in post-stroke patients although there was variation in the type of stimulation device, location of electrodes, and dose between the studies (Robbins et al., 2006). In general, there are very few clinical trials on the use of TENS for central neuropathic pain, and most are non-randomized or lacking control groups.

Multiple sclerosis

The National Institute for Health and Clinical Excellence in the UK recommended that any person with multiple sclerosis with unresolved secondary musculoskeletal pain should be considered for TENS, although this was based on evidence from a Cochrane review on chronic pain (Carroll et al., 2001) that did not include any RCTs on multiple sclerosis (National Institute for Health and Clinical Excellence & Conditions, 2003). Since then Warke and colleagues (2006) conducted a placebo-controlled RCT on chronic low back pain in a multiple sclerosis population and found that TENS did not produce any statistically significant effects on pain and functional outcomes, although 'clinically important' differences were observed. Miller and colleagues (2007) compared TENS (100 pps, 125 μs) administered for 60 minutes a day with TENS administered for eight hours a day for two weeks in patients with multiple sclerosis, and found that TENS administered for eight hours daily reduced Penn muscle-spasm scores and pain compared with 60 minute daily treatments, although there were no differences in global spasticity scores.

Spinal cord injuries

A systematic review on the use of physical therapies for neuropathic pain in spinal cord injuries which included two case series, one questionnaire survey, and one cross-sectional descriptive study suggested that TENS may be beneficial but there were no RCTs to make a judgement (Fattal et al., 2009). Since the review, a prospective RCT on 33 patients with neuropathic pain following spinal cord injury found that 30 minutes of low-frequency TENS given daily for ten days reduced pain intensity compared with placebo TENS (Celik et al., 2013). A cross-over study on 24 patients who self-administered TENS three times each day for two weeks found no differences in ratings of pain intensity, mood, coping, or sleep quality between high (80 Hz) and low (2 Hz bursts) frequency (Norrbrink, 2009). Engholm and Leffler (2010) found that high-frequency TENS reduced pain but did not alter sensory functions in patients with long-term, unilateral, painful, traumatic, peripheral, partial-nerve injury.

Cancer pain

The most recent Cochrane review on TENS for cancer-related pain found three small studies (88 participants) with insufficient data to judge effectiveness (Hurlow et al., 2012). An RCT using 45 women with chronic pain associated with breast cancer treatment found that neither TENS nor transcutaneous spinal electroanalgesia (TSE) were superior to placebo TSE although 15 women preferred to continue TENS treatment compared to five for TSE and six for placebo (Robb et al., 2008). A feasibility study suggested that TENS may improve bone pain on movement, although the study was not designed to investigate intervention effect (Bennett et al., 2010). A case series of 16 patients found that daily treatment with electrical stimulation using a TENS-like device (MC5-A Calmare, see: <http://www.calmarett.com>) reduced pain associated with refractory chemotherapy-induced peripheral neuropathy (Smith et al., 2010).

Miscellaneous

A Cochrane review on non-invasive physical treatments for chronic/recurrent headache included three low-quality RCTs on TENS but insufficient evidence to judge effectiveness (Bronfort et al., 2004).

There are no systematic reviews on TENS for wound pain. An RCT found that conventional TENS on healthy subjects was as effective as acetaminophen (300–600 mg) with codeine (30–60 mg) (Ordog, 1987), and a small study found that auricular TENS was superior to placebo pill for pain relief during wound-dressing changes (Lewis et al., 1990). Evidence from case series suggests that TENS may be beneficial for burn pruritus. Improvements in vulvar pain and dyspareunia during the postpartum period related to perineal trauma caused by episiotomy have been reported in an open-label study without a control group during weekly applications of intravaginal TENS with myofascial stretching and pelvic-floor exercises (Dionisi & Senatori, 2011).

Comparison with other pain-relieving treatments

Machado and colleagues (2009) compared the effect size of 34 treatments (76 RCTs) for non-specific, chronic low back pain and found that 17 treatments had statistically significant pain-relieving effects. Effect sizes were less than ten points on a 100–point scale for 47 per cent of treatments, between 10 and 20 points for 38 per cent of treatments, and greater than 20 points for 15 per cent of treatments (Figure 8.4). The effect size of TENS was 10–20 points based on four trials (178 participants), of which two were assessing acute pain. The effect size for TENS was comparable in magnitude to a wide range of other treatments including muscle relaxants and NSAIDs.

It is remarkable that the uncertainty about the effectiveness of TENS has persisted for so many decades despite a constant stream new RCTs.

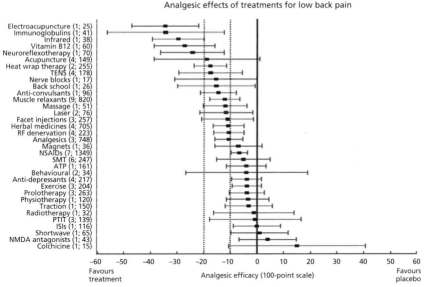

Analgesic effects of treatments for low back pain

Fig. 8.4 Pain-relieving efficacy of 34 treatments for non-specific low back pain of any duration (number of trials: total number of participants). Pooled estimates of random effects (multiple trials) or means (single trials) are shown as squares with 95 per cent confidence intervals. Dotted lines represent magnitude of effects as large (>20 points), moderate (between 10 and 20 points) or small (<10 points). Key: ATP: adenosine triphosphate; ISIs: Intradiscal steroid injections; NMDA: N-methyl-D-aspartate. PTIT: percutaneous thermocoagulation intradiscal techniques; RF: radiofrequency; SMT: spinal manipulative therapy.

Methodological shortcomings in TENS research

Methodological shortcomings in RCT design and conduct are the likely cause for the conflicting evidence. Bennett and colleagues (2011) quantified sources of bias from 38 RCTs from Cochrane reviews on TENS for acute, chronic, and cancer pain, and found bias towards negative outcomes and underestimation of TENS effects. Many RCTs used inadequate TENS technique and infrequent treatments of insufficient duration leading to underdosing. Investigators often failed to measure TENS effects *during* stimulation (i.e. they measured outcomes before and after TENS), and often failed to monitor concurrent medication which would contaminate TENS effects. The blinding and design of an authentic placebo TENS, necessary to isolate specific effects associated with TENS, has also been problematic. Placebo TENS interventions used in RCTs include:

- sham TENS devices with no current output
- active TENS devices delivering currents below sensory-detection threshold
- active TENS devices delivering currents at sensory-detection threshold (barely perceptible TENS)
- transient sham TENS devices that deliver currents to produce a TENS sensation for a short period of time before fading away to zero current output (Rakel et al., 2010)

It is impossible to blind participants to whether or not they receive a strong, non-painful TENS sensation. However, bias can be reduced if the participant is uncertain whether a strong, non-painful TENS sensation is a prerequisite for pain relief (i.e. participant naivety). Instructions and background information orientating participants to study aims and procedures can be used to raise uncertainty in participants' minds. For example, the participant information sheet can include the following statements: 'The best way to administer TENS is not known' . . . 'Some types of TENS do not produce sensations whereas others produce a tingling sensation on the skin and some cause muscle contractions' . . . 'You may receive an intervention that is a placebo'. Discouraging the participant to disclose their sensory experience during the intervention will facilitate assessor blinding. Furthermore, recent evidence suggests that study participants do not adhere to instructions given for self-administered TENS in unsupervised settings in RCTs (Pallett et al., 2013). Adherence and implementation monitoring of self-administered TENS can be monitored using data capture systems time-linked to TENS use and should be used in future studies to ensure treatment fidelity. The requirements for a robust RCT on TENS are discussed in detail in Chapter 12.

Summary

1 The largest meta-analyses of RCTS on TENS found that TENS was superior to placebo for chronic musculoskeletal pain and for post-operative pain.

2 Many systematic reviews reveal insufficient good-quality RCTs on which to make a judgement.

3 Systematic reviews with inclusion criteria for adequacy of TENS technique and dosage are more positive than those that do not.

4   Recommendations about the use of TENS from professional and government bodies are inconsistent.

5   Present evidence supports continued use of TENS as an adjunct to core treatment until methodologically robust evidence is produced that is not superior to placebo.

Further reading

- Claydon, L., and Chesterton, L. (2008) Does transcutaneous electrical nerve stimulation (TENS) produce 'dose-responses'? A review of systematic reviews on chronic pain. *Physical Therapy Reviews*, **13**, 450–63.

- Bjordal, J.M., Johnson, M.I., and Ljunggreen, A.E. (2003) Transcutaneous electrical nerve stimulation (TENS) can reduce postoperative analgesic consumption. A meta-analysis with assessment of optimal treatment parameters for postoperative pain. *Eur J Pain*, **7**, 181–8.

- Johnson, M., and Martinson, M. (2007) Efficacy of electrical nerve stimulation for chronic musculoskeletal pain: a meta-analysis of randomized controlled trials. *Pain*, **130**, 157–65.

- Johnson, M.I., and Walsh, D.M. (2010) Pain: continued uncertainty of TENS' effectiveness for pain relief. *Nat Rev Rheumatol*, **6**, 314–16.

- Nnoaham, K.E., and Kumbang, J. (2008) Transcutaneous electrical nerve stimulation (TENS) for chronic pain. *Cochrane Database Syst Rev*, CD003222.

- Walsh, D.M., Howe, T.E., Johnson, M.I., and Sluka, K.A. (2009) Transcutaneous electrical nerve stimulation for acute pain. *Cochrane Database Syst Rev*, CD006142.

In Chapter 9 the physiological evidence contributing to knowledge about the physiological and pharmacological actions of TENS is explored.

Chapter 9

Mechanism of action of TENS

Introduction

In 1965, *Pain mechanisms: a new theory* provided a physiological explanation of how stimulating the skin using electricity could relieve pain (Melzack & Wall, 1965). Since then a large amount of research evidence has been gathered that supports Melzack and Wall's physiological explanation for how TENS could relieve pain. The intention of using conventional TENS and AL-TENS is to activate distinct populations of peripheral nerve fibres to mediate physiological actions at peripheral, spinal, and supraspinal levels of the nervous system. The purpose of this chapter is to discuss research evidence that has contributed to our knowledge about the physiological and pharmacological actions of TENS by covering:

◆ The mechanism of action of conventional TENS and AL-TENS

◆ Peripheral mechanisms of TENS

◆ Central mechanisms of TENS

◆ Findings from inflammatory and neuropathic models of pain

◆ The neuropharmacology of TENS hypoalgesia and TENS tolerance

Mechanism of action of conventional TENS (low-intensity TENS)

The purpose of conventional TENS is to selectively activate large-diameter myelinated low-threshold peripheral afferents (A-β fibres) without simultaneously exciting higher-threshold nociceptive afferents (A-δ fibres). Strong, non-painful sensations during conventional TENS result from activity in A-β afferents with some contributions from A-α and A-δ afferents. Low-threshold A-β peripheral afferents enter the spinal cord and ascend in the fasciculus gracilis and the fasciculus cuneatus of the posterior (dorsal) columns to terminate in the nucleus gracilis and the nucleus cuneatus in the medulla (Figure 9.1). Both pathways conduct nerve impulses from sensory receptors associated with fine touch, pressure, and proprioception. The gracilis pathway conducts nerve impulses from the lower part of the body, including the legs, and the cuneatus pathway from the upper part of the body, including the arms. These pathways give rise to collaterals (branches) within the spinal cord which synapse with inhibitory interneurones. The axon terminals of the inhibitory interneurones synapse with the axon terminals of peripheral nociceptive afferents (i.e. A-δ and C-fibres) and the dendrites of neurones involved in onward transmission of central nociceptive information. The interneurones

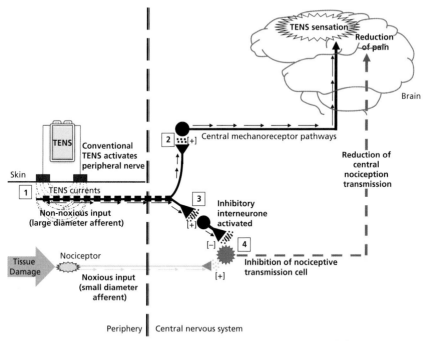

Fig. 9.1 Mechanism of action of conventional TENS. (1) TENS activates low-threshold afferents, which transmit information along central transmitting pathways to the brain (2) resulting in TENS sensation. Collaterals excite inhibitory interneurones (3) that inhibit activity of central nociceptive cells in the spinal cord (4). Key: [+] = excitatory neurotransmitter, [−] = inhibitory neurotransmitter.

release inhibitory neurotransmitters, including gamma-amino-butyric acid (GABA), that inhibit activity in peripheral nociceptive afferents (presynaptic) and central nociceptive transmission cells (post-synaptic). The neural circuitry mediating these effects is located segmentally which explains why the effects of conventional TENS are optimal when electrodes are placed within the same dermatomes as the origin of the pain. In addition, TENS-induced A-β afferent activity will block afferent impulses arising from natural stimuli that are also being conducted in low threshold A-β afferents.

Mechanism of action of AL-TENS (high-intensity TENS)

The purpose of AL-TENS is to activate small-diameter myelinated afferents (A-δ) that have higher thresholds of activation than A-β afferents. The literature is unclear as to whether the primary purpose of AL-TENS is to generate impulses in cutaneous or muscle afferents or both. Small-diameter myelinated cutaneous afferents have high thresholds of activation and conduct nerve impulses related to the transduction of cold, pressure, and noxious stimuli. A large proportion of small-diameter myelinated muscle afferents are mechanoreceptors that are activated by muscle contraction and convey information about the status of muscle (Mense, 1993). Other small-diameter myelinated muscle afferents are nociceptive and elicit pain if directly activated. The most efficient way to activate small-diameter myelinated mechanoreceptive muscle afferents is to stimulate large-diameter myelinated efferent motor neurones (A-α) that have low thresholds of activation. The resultant muscle twitch generates impulses in small-diameter myelinated mechanoreceptive muscle afferents. A simple way of stimulating large-diameter myelinated efferent motor neurones (A-α) is via AL-TENS using burst patterns of stimulation (Cox et al., 1993) (Figures 9.2 and 3.13). Muscle afferents branch as they enter the spinal cord and form pre- and post-synaptic connections with non-noxious and noxious central nervous transmission neurones in various laminae of the spinal cord. During AL-TENS, users experience strong, non-painful muscle contractions and pulsating sensations with kinaesthesia resulting from simultaneous activation of cutaneous afferents and proprioceptors.

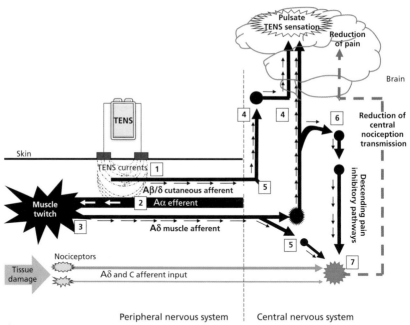

Fig. 9.2 Mechanism of action of AL-TENS. TENS activates low- and possibly high-threshold cutaneous afferents (1), and also motor neurones (2), resulting in a muscle twitch (3). This causes muscle-afferent input to the brain (4) resulting in sensations of TENS and muscle twitching. Collaterals from muscle afferents excite central transmission pathways activate descending pain-inhibitory pathways (6) that feed back to the spinal cord to inhibit activity of central nociceptive cells (7) i.e. via supraspinal mechanisms. Also, collaterals from cutaneous (not shown) and muscle afferents excite inhibitory interneurones (5) that inhibit (7) activity of central nociceptive cells in the spinal cord (7) i.e. via spinal mechanisms.

It is also possible that AL-TENS activates some small-diameter myelinated cutaneous afferents (A-δ) and generates sensations at, or just below, pain threshold. Cutaneous A-δ afferents branch as they enter laminae I and II of the spinal cord and synapse with inhibitory interneurones that synapse with second-order nociceptive specific neurones (Waldeyer cells) forming spinothalamic tracts conveying information related to pin-prick pain. TENS-induced activity in small-diameter cutaneous and muscle afferents leads to excitation of inhibitory interneurones that release inhibitory neurochemicals including GABA and met-enkephalin, causing post-synaptic inhibition of substantia gelatinosa cells and preventing onward transmission of nociceptive information. This explains observations of segmental effects of AL-TENS.

In addition, TENS-induced activity in small-diameter cutaneous and muscle afferents excites central transmission neurones of ascending neuronal tracts whose collaterals synapse in regions of the brain that are part of the descending pain-inhibitory pathways forming a feedback loop to the spinal cord to prevent further transmission of noxious information (i.e. closing the pain gate). The regions of the brain forming this supraspinal loop include the periaqueductal grey in the mid brain and nucleus raphe magnus. Axons forming the supraspinal loop have collaterals that synapse with inhibitory interneurones at all levels of the spinal cord. The inhibitory interneurones inhibit onward transmission of nociceptive information and this action explains some of the extrasegmental effects observed during AL-TENS. In addition, impulses in cutaneous A-δ peripheral afferents generated during AL-TENS block conduction of impulses generated from natural stimuli associated with tissue damage also travelling in cutaneous A-δ peripheral afferents.

Peripheral mechanisms of TENS

Blockade of afferent impulses during TENS

During TENS, antidromic impulses generated in afferents travel towards the sensory receptor and will collide and extinguish orthodromic impulses travelling towards the central nervous system that have been generated during activation of sensory receptor cells by natural stimuli (Figure 9.3). Ignelzi and Nyquist (1976) demonstrated that percutaneous electrical nerve stimulation of A-δ afferents reduced the conduction velocity and amplitude of A-α, A-β, and A-δ components of the compound action potential of isolated cat nerves with largest reductions observed in A-δ components. However, in clinical practice current amplitudes used during conventional TENS activate low-threshold cutaneous afferent axons (i.e. A-β), but are not sufficiently high to activate higher-threshold cutaneous afferents (i.e. A-δ or C-fibres). In order to extinguish orthodromic impulses arising from nociceptors TENS would need to be administered at amplitudes sufficient to excite A-δ and/or C-fibres and this would be painful for patients (Ignelzi & Nyquist, 1979; Swett & Law, 1983). Furthermore, a microneurographic study on healthy human participants, demonstrated that when TENS was administered to excite A-δ afferents at painful intensities, reductions in pain were not due to transmission failure in A-δ fibres, although intermittent blocking of nerve conduction of impulses to noxious stimuli did occur (Janko & Trontelj, 1980).

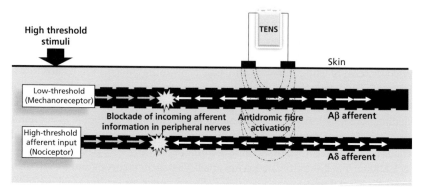

Fig. 9.3 Antidromic activation of a peripheral nerve. Arrows indicate direction of nerve impulses.

Orthodromic impulses travelling in low-threshold afferents as a consequence of tissue damage would be extinguished by antidromic impulses in A-β axons during TENS. This 'busy line' effect in low-threshold afferents in peripheral nerves has been reflected in studies recording latencies and amplitudes of components of compound action potentials from peripheral nerves and somatosensory evoked spinal and cortical potentials (Nardone & Schieppati, 1989; Walsh et al., 1998). For example, conventional TENS delivered to the median nerve reduced the amplitude and increased the latency of peripheral, spinal, and late cortical components of somatosensory-evoked potentials (e.g. N9, P14, N18), demonstrating modulation of non-noxious input in peripheral nerves and at the level of the cuneatus nucleus within the brainstem (Nardone & Schieppati, 1989).

Axon reflexes

Axon reflexes occur in response to peripheral nerve stimulation, when impulses travel in afferent axons towards the periphery. Axon reflexes are not true reflexes as they do not involve a complete reflex arc and are mediated by activity in high-threshold afferents. Antidromic activity generated in high-threshold afferents during high-intensity TENS could generate axon reflexes resulting in the release of various substances at the distal ends of sensory receptors that influence activity in blood vessels, sweat glands, and mast cells. The release of substance P and calcitonin gene-related peptide (CGRP) triggers a local inflammatory response resulting in vasodilation and erythema. Axon reflexes have been suggested as a mechanism for tissue-healing effects of TENS (Burssens et al., 2005), although there has been little research on the role of axon reflexes in TENS hypoalgesia.

TENS sensations and nerve fatigue

At low frequencies TENS generates pulsate sensations and afferents are able to generate a nerve impulse following each electrical pulse (i.e. they can follow the pulse frequency). At higher frequencies the electrical pulse falls within the relative and absolute refractory period of the axon and the axon is unable to generate an action potential (i.e. the frequency of TENS is beyond the following frequency of the axon). This results in abnormal spacio-temporal patterns of neural activity within and between axons creating sensations of electrical paraesthesiae. Studies using microelectrodes inserted into nerve fascicles before and after ten minutes of electrical-conditioning stimuli (TENS, 200 pps), have found progressive increases in neural activity immediately after stimulation with individual afferents becoming spontaneously active and discharging in high-frequency bursts, causing post-stimulation paraesthesiae (Burke & Applegate, 1989). Sensations of electrical paraesthesiae result from ectopic impulse generation in peripheral nerves with low-threshold axons being more excitable, although some ectopic activity also occurs in central nerves (Macefield & Burke, 1991; Kiernan et al., 1997).

When an axon is driven to fire beyond its maximal frequency for a prolonged period of time it is likely to fatigue, making it harder for subsequent stimuli to generate a nerve impulse. Evidence suggests that prolonged high-frequency TENS reduces the excitability of axons and this can result in post-stimulation hypoesthesia (Applegate & Burke, 1989). In addition, post-stimulation hypoaesthesia is due in part to stimulation-induced refractoriness at central synapses (Burke & Applegate, 1989). Evidence suggests that synaptic fatigue is predominantly a pre-synaptic phenomenon that can result from temporary depletion of synaptic vesicles, although post-synaptic changes may also contribute including desensitization of receptor efficacy.

There do not appear to be any studies that have directly measured the following frequency of cutaneous afferents in response to different frequencies of TENS. Such studies would be useful because they would provide insights into optimal pulse frequencies for TENS. In principle, higher frequencies of TENS would generate more nerve impulses providing a stronger afferent input to the central nervous system, thereby producing stronger segmental inhibition of second-order nociceptive transmission-cell neurones. However, the theoretical relationship between TENS frequency and fibre response breaks down in practice because of the dispersion of currents in underlying tissue.

Action on efferent axons

The action of TENS on efferent axons is often overlooked because the primary purpose of TENS is to generate afferent input to the central nervous system. Whenever currents permeate the skin they are likely to excite efferent fibres such as low-threshold, A-α motor neurones innervating skeletal muscle, and parasympathetic and sympathetic autonomic efferents innervating smooth muscle and glands. In principle activation of sympathetic nerves will produce physiological responses associated with 'fight–flight–fright' which tend to be systemic such as cardiovascular system responses, whereas activation of parasympathetic nerves will generate physiological responses that are associated with changes in discrete organ function, such as bowel and bladder function. Interestingly, research on the physiological action of TENS on the autonomic nervous system is limited. Research on the use of peripheral-nerve stimulation techniques to target autonomic nerves is more complete.

Studies on the effects of TENS on the sympathetic division of the autonomic nervous system are conflicting. Reeves and colleagues (2004) investigated the effects of 20 minutes of TENS on experimental pain and sympathetic function in healthy volunteers and found that neither low-frequency/high-intensity nor high-frequency/low-intensity TENS affected measures of heart rate, digital pulse volume, and skin conductance when compared with placebo TENS. In contrast, Olyaei and colleagues (2004) found that 20 minutes of TENS (2 pps, 250 µs, over the median nerve) decreased the amplitude and increased the latency of the sympathetic skin response compared with placebo TENS suggesting that TENS inhibited sympathetic nerve activity. Interestingly, there were no differences between TENS over the median nerve and over the acupuncture point HT7 (Heart 7) of the hand. Sommer and colleagues (2011) suggest that the axonal properties of sympathetic efferent and nociceptive afferent fibres differ. They found a positive correlation between sweat output and TENS intensity with sweat output peaking when TENS amplitude was 10 mA and rated as painful by participants. When TENS was delivered at 7.5 mA sweat output was highest at 20 pps without further increases at 50 pps or 100 pps.

Afferent activation and central nervous system response

There is strong evidence that electrical stimulation of cutaneous A-fibres inhibits noxious-evoked activity of centrally nociceptive transmission cells in the same dermatome with more profound inhibition occurring when A-δ fibres are recruited. (Sjölund, 1988) found that maximal inhibition of C-fibre-evoked flexor responses to noxious stimulation in anaesthetized cats occurred during low-frequency bursts of low-intensity TENS which activated muscle afferents rather than cutaneous afferents with recruitment of small-diameter GIII (A-δ) muscle afferents strengthening the inhibitory effect. Radhakrishnan and Sluka (2005) used a rat model of inflammatory hyperalgesia and found that TENS at both 4 pps and 100 pps reversed hyperalgesia in controls and when cutaneous afferents from skin around the inflamed joint were blocked using EMLA cream. However, hyperalgesia was not reversed when large-diameter input from deeper knee-joint afferents was blocked using 2 per cent lidocaine gel suggesting that deep afferents mediated hypoalgesia during TENS. In humans, Duranti and colleagues (1988) found no differences in hypoalgesia during AL-TENS-induced muscle contractions using surface electrodes, or muscle contractions induced by intramuscular electrodes that bypassed the skin, suggesting activity in GIII (A-δ) muscle afferents, rather than cutaneous afferents, was the important factor in hypoalgesia.

Central mechanisms of TENS

The neurophysiology and neuropharmacology associated with TENS and acupuncture within the central nervous system is complex and summarized in Figure 9.4.

Spinal and supraspinal mechanisms of TENS: evidence from animal studies

There is strong electrophysiological evidence from studies on anesthetized cats, rats, and monkeys that TENS inhibits activity in spinal nociceptive-specific and wide-dynamic-range neurones (i.e. central nociceptive transmission cells) that are either

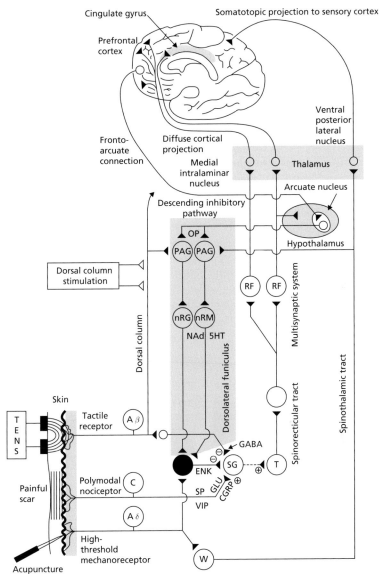

Fig. 9.4 Generalized overview of neurophysiological and neuropharmacological mechanisms associated with TENS and acupuncture. Key: W = Waldeyer cell; VIP = vasoactive intestinal polypeptide; SP = substance P; ENK = enkephalin; SG = substantia gelatinosa; T = nociceptive transmission cell; GABA = gamma-amino-butyric acid; NAd = noradrenaline; 5HT = 5-hydroxytryptamine (serotonin); nRG = nucleus reticularis gigantocellularis; nRM = nucleus raphe magnus; PAG = periaqueductal grey; OP = opioid; RF = reticular formation; [+] = excitatory neurotransmitter; [−] = inhibitory neurotransmitter.

spontaneously active or responding to evoked noxious stimuli. The neural circuitry is located at the first synapse between the peripheral afferent and the central transmission neurone (i.e. spinal) and also in the brain (i.e. supraspinal). A series of studies on anesthetized cats using microelectrodes to record extracellular action potentials found that TENS applied to somatic receptive fields reduced activity in 65 per cent of spontaneously active dorsal horn cells with 30 per cent of the spontaneously active cells not responding to TENS and 5 per cent increasing activity during TENS (Garrison & Foreman, 1994). TENS reduced activity of cells noxiously evoked using manual pinch or manual clamp techniques (Figure 9.5). Inhibition was not affected by spinal cord transection at T12 suggesting that supraspinal mechanisms were not involved (Garrison & Foreman, 1996). Ipsilateral TENS was superior to contralateral TENS (Garrison & Foreman, 2002). Likewise, Hanai (2000) found that responses of dorsal horn wide-dynamic-range neurones to C-fibre input elicited by superficial peroneal nerve stimulation in anesthetized cats were reduced during electrical nerve stimulation of posterior tibial and sciatic peripheral nerves. The findings of other investigating teams are similar (Ignelzi et al., 1981; Chung et al., 1984a; Chung et al., 1984b). Ma and Sluka (2001) confirmed the findings in an inflammatory model of pain and found that high- and low-frequency TENS reduced innocuous and noxious evoked responses of wide-dynamic-range and high-threshold dorsal horn neurones immediately after

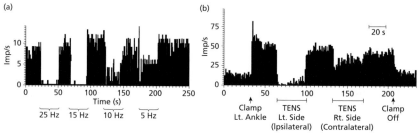

Fig. 9.5 Examples of the findings of studies that have recorded the activity of central nociceptive transmission cells during TENS in anaesthetised cats. (a) The activity of a spontaneously active high-threshold dorsal horn neurone was reduced during various frequencies of TENS (60 mA, 100 μs, continuous pattern). (b) A greater reduction in noxiously evoked dorsal horn activity from a mechanical clamp continuously applied to the left ankle is observed for ipsilateral compared with contralateral TENS (45 mA, 125 pps, 100 μs, continuous pattern).

and one hour after TENS had been ceased. They measured spontaneous activity and response to innocuous and noxious mechanical stimulation of dorsal horn neurones after 20 minutes of either high- (100 pps) or low-frequency (4 pps) TENS (100 µs) applied to the inflamed paw of anesthetized rats at intensity just above motor threshold. TENS had no effect on activity of non-noxious low-threshold dorsal horn neurones.

More profound inhibition of central nociceptive transmission cells occurs when the amplitude of TENS currents is increased beyond that usually used in clinical practice. Chung and colleagues found that inhibition of nociceptive spinothalamic tract neurones in anesthetized monkeys by electrical stimulation of A-α and A-β afferents was increased and prolonged when A-δ and C-fibre afferents were recruited (Chung et al., 1984a; Chung et al., 1984b). Sjölund (1985) found that electrical stimulation of dissected skin nerves in lightly anesthetized rats at amplitudes that recruited A-β and A-δ fibres generated more powerful inhibition of C-fibre evoked nociceptive reflex responses than activating A-β fibres on their own, with stimulation frequencies of 80 pps generating greatest effects. Sandkühler and colleagues (1997) demonstrated that low-frequency stimulation (1 pps) of peripheral A-δ afferents (10 V, 100 µs) produced long-term depression of excitatory post-synaptic potentials in substantia gelatinosa neurones in the rat spinal cord. The inhibition lasted for more than two hours post-stimulation and was reversible and not due to damage of individual synapses. These effects remain following spinalization in some studies but not others suggesting that some of the circuitry may be supraspinal.

TENS at noxious intensities applied to remote body sites not related segmentally to the site of nociception (i.e. counter-irritation) also inhibits activity of centrally transmitting neurones. The physiological process of a painful stimulus applied at a distant site on the body reducing pain at another body site is termed 'diffuse noxious inhibitory controls', or 'conditioned pain modulation'. Early studies by Le Bars and colleagues (1979) demonstrated that noxious TENS administered to the tail of anaesthetized spinally intact rats could inhibit activity of lumbar dorsal horn neurone cells responding to noxious stimuli. Inhibition persisted post-stimulation and was related to the duration of TENS. Morton and colleagues (1988) demonstrated that lumbar dorsal horn neurones excited by noxious heat of the hind paw of anaesthetized cats could also be inhibited by electrical stimulation administered at remote body sites using in repetitive trains at intensities activating small, myelinated, or unmyelinated fibres.

There is strong evidence from animal studies that brainstem structures that form descending pain-inhibitory pathways including the periaqueductal grey matter and nucleus raphe magnus are involved in hypoalgesia during TENS, especially at higher intensities. Studies in the 1980s demonstrated that the response to TENS was diminished following spinal transection. For example, Woolf and colleagues (1980) found that the flexor withdrawal response in rats following immersion of the tail in hot water was reduced during high-frequency TENS at intensities causing fibrillation of tail muscles (100 pps, 200 µs), and the effect was reversed following spinal transection at T10–T11. More recently, Maeda and colleagues (2007) suggested that approximately 50 per cent of the hypoalgesic effects of high-frequency TENS remains after spinal transection.

Kalra and colleagues (2001) found that microinjection of naloxone into the rostral ventral medulla at doses sufficient to block µ-opioid receptors prevented the antihyperalgesic effect of low-frequency (4 pps) but not high-frequency (100 pps) TENS, whereas injection of naltrindole at doses sufficient to block δ-opioid receptors prevented the antihyperalgesic effect of high- but not low-frequency TENS. DeSantana and colleagues (2009) found that 20 minutes of high- (100 pps) or low-frequency (4 pps) TENS increased paw withdrawal threshold in rats with knee joint inflammation (3 per cent kaolin/carrageenan) and that this effect was prevented by pre-TENS microinjection of cobalt chloride into the ventrolateral periaqueductal grey but not the dorsolateral periaqueductal grey. This suggests that TENS effects are mediated through the ventrolateral periaqueductal grey, sending projections through the rostral ventral medulla to the spinal cord to produce opioid-mediated hypoalgesia.

Studies measuring nociceptive reflex response in humans

Further evidence for the involvement of central neuronal circuitry is provided by studies using healthy human participants that have shown that conventional TENS increases the threshold to elicit nociceptive reflexes to noxious (electrical) stimulation during and after TENS. Danziger and colleagues (1998) found that low-intensity TENS within the receptive field of the noxious stimulus reduced spinal nociceptive cell response with short-lived post-stimulation effects, whereas high-intensity TENS initially increased spinal nociceptive cell response which was followed by prolonged post-TENS inhibition. They measured the RIII reflex response elicited by sural nerve stimulation at the ankle before, during, and after two minutes of TENS administered segmentally on the sural nerve or non-segmentally (heterotopically) on the contralateral hand. Segmental high-frequency, non-noxious TENS (100 pps, 2 mA, 100 μs) inhibited the RIII reflex during stimulation but not post-stimulation, whereas segmental low-frequency, noxious TENS (3 pps, 20 mA, 2 ms) enhanced the RIII reflex during stimulation and inhibited the RIII reflex post-stimulation. Non-segmental low-frequency, noxious TENS (3 pps, 20 mA, 2 ms) inhibited the RIII reflex during and post-stimulation possibly via diffuse noxious-inhibitory controls. Similar findings have been reported in patients with chronic intractable pain where RIII reflexes were inhibited and pain relieved by spinal cord stimulation or TENS with very little effect on other cutaneous, non-nociceptive responses (Garcia-Larrea et al., 1989). In contrast, a study using 70 healthy participants Cramp and colleagues (2000b) found that 15 minutes of TENS (5 pps, or 100 pps, or 200 pps) or interferential current therapy (5 Hz, or 100 Hz, or 200 Hz) applied segmentally did not affect RIII, H-reflexes, or subjective pain intensity.

Studies measuring somatosensory evoked potentials in humans

There is evidence that TENS reduces amplitudes and increases latencies of spinal and supraspinal components of somatosensory-evoked potentials. This demonstrates that TENS causes central modulation (gating) of afferent input at all levels of the central nervous system, although effects are sometimes variable and unreliable (Fernandez-Del-Olmo et al., 2008). Somatosensory-evoked potentials are measured as a series of positive and negative voltage waves (P and N waves) reflecting the nervous system's response to stimuli presented to the surface of the body (see Figure 4.10). Potentials

Table 9.1 Cortical components of somatosensory evoked potentials to stimulation of the median nerve

Component	Physiological correlate (reflecting location of impulses)
N9	Peripheral sensory fibres and motor fibres to the shoulder
N13	Mid-cervical cord
P14	Cervicomedullary junction and lemniscal decussation
N18	Medial lemniscus to upper midbrain and thalamus
N20	Traversing the internal capsule and arrival of impulses at the contralateral primary somatosensory region
N25, P60, N80	Initial processing in the primary somatosensory cortex
P100, N140	Processing by the secondary somatosensory cortex, posterior parietal, and frontal cortices

are usually recorded using surface electrodes on the scalp (i.e. cortical potentials) with the latency of the wave relative to the evoking stimulus measured in milliseconds and reflecting the location of the afferent volley of impulses (Table 9.1).

Findings from somatosensory-evoked potential studies suggest that conventional TENS modulates non-noxious input at the first synaptic relay in the central nervous system (e.g. cuneate nucleus) with maximal effects derived when it is administered to skin overlying the same peripheral nerve as that eliciting the somatosensory-evoked potential (Golding et al., 1986; Nardone & Schieppati, 1989; Macefield & Burke, 1991; Akyuz et al., 1995; Urasaki et al., 1998; Torquati et al., 2003). Studies using CO_2-laser to activate cutaneous A-δ and C-fibre afferents provide evidence that conventional TENS also modulates cutaneous noxious input. For example, Timofeeva and colleagues (2011) found that ten minutes of non-noxious TENS (90 pps) of the posterior surface of the neck decreased laser-induced potentials evoked from the same dermatome, and Krabbenbos and colleagues (2009) found that ten minutes of non-noxious TENS (110 pps) at the dorsolateral forearm reduced the amplitudes of laser-evoked potentials evoked to noxious heat stimuli to the dorsum of the right hand. De Tommaso and colleagues (2003) found that low- (10 pps) and high-frequency (100 pps) TENS reduced the amplitude of CO_2-laser-evoked potentials and the subjective rating of noxious heat stimuli, with high frequency producing larger effects. Hoshiyama and Kakigi (2000) measured pain-related brain responses to painful electrical finger stimulation using electroencephalography and magnetoencephalography and found that 30 minutes of TENS (50 pps) produced a post-stimulation reduction in the amplitudes of pain-related brain responses but that this was not enough to relieve the subjective painful feeling. Torquati and colleagues (2007) found that low-frequency, low-intensity TENS (7 pps, 200 μs) of the median nerve reduced the amplitude of late (35 ms) but not early (20 ms) somatosensory-evoked field response in healthy humans, suggesting a delayed 'gating' effect from the primary and secondary somatosensory cortices. These effects were more prolonged in secondary somatosensory cortices reflecting its integrative role in sensory processing of electrical nerve stimulation.

Studies measuring brain activity in humans

Brain imaging studies provide evidence that TENS affects pain-related cortical activation. Kara and colleagues (2010) used functional magnetic resonance imaging (fMRI) in patients with carpal tunnel syndrome and found that TENS, but not placebo-TENS, decreased the pain-related cortical activations in contralateral somatosensory and motor cortices, and in parahippocampal, lingual, and superior temporal gyri. Effects persisted up to 35 minutes after TENS (Figure 9.6). Murakami and colleagues (2010) recorded movement-related cortical magnetic field potentials associated with voluntary, self-paced finger movement before and after high-frequency TENS to the forearm muscle and found that TENS modulated the excitability of the primary somatosensory cortex and motor cortex in a different manner. Meesen and colleagues (2011) investigated the long-term effect of TENS on reorganization of the motor cortex in healthy individuals using transcranial magnetic stimulation. An increase in cortical motor representation of muscles was observed following a three-week intervention of TENS when compared with controls suggesting that there are persistent neuroplastic changes in the human cerebral cortex following TENS.

TENS effects on experimental models of inflammatory pain

Sluka and colleagues have provided a substantial contribution to the understanding of the mechanism of action of TENS. Their electrophysiological and behavioural studies using models of joint inflammation in rats provide evidence that TENS reduces primary and secondary hyperalgesia (for review, see DeSantana et al., 2008c). They have demonstrated that TENS at motor threshold reduced flexion reflexes and increased tail-flick latencies to noxious heat and mechanical stimuli (King et al., 2005; Radhakrishnan & Sluka, 2005; Sluka et al., 2006; Vance et al., 2007), although TENS did not reduce oedema in this inflammatory model (Resende et al., 2004).

Sluka and colleagues (1998) found that 20 minutes of either high- (100 pps) or low-frequency (4 pps) TENS increased paw withdrawal latency to radiant heat (secondary hyperalgesia) but not spontaneous pain behaviours or joint circumference produced by injection of kaolin and carrageenan into the knee joint of the rat causing inflammation. High-frequency TENS effects lasted > 24 hours and low-frequency TENS lasted > 12 hours. Vance and colleagues (2007) found that high- (100 pps) or low-frequency (4 pps) TENS reversed compression withdrawal thresholds when administered 24 hours or two weeks after the onset of inflammation of the knee joint induced by intra-articular injection of a mixture of 3 per cent kaolin and 3 per cent carrageenan, but not when administered four hours after the induction of inflammation. The findings suggested that the reduction in primary hyperalgesia by TENS depended on when TENS was administered during the development of acute and chronic stages of inflammation. Gopalkrishnan and Sluka (2000) found that 20 minutes of high- (100 pps) but not low-frequency (4 pps) TENS reduced primary hyperalgesia to heat and mechanical stimuli and spontaneous pain-related behaviours compared with no-TENS control or low-frequency TENS. Varying intensity above motor threshold versus above sensory-detection threshold, or pulse duration (100 µs, 250 µs) had no effect on the magnitude of antihyperalgesia produced. A similar study by King and Sluka (2001) found

Post-TENS versus baseline

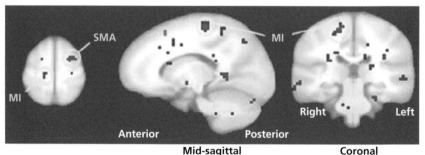

Post-placebo TENS versus baseline

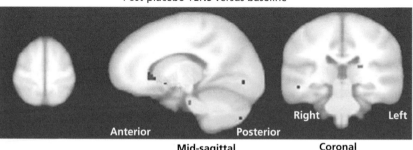

Fig. 9.6 Images are the differences in brain activation patterns measured by functional magnetic resonance imaging (fMRI) for median nerve-innervated second digit before and 20 minutes after 30 minutes of strong, non-painful TENS below motor threshold or placebo (no-current) TENS over the median nerve (100 Hz, 200 μs) in patients with carpaltunnel syndrome. For active TENS there was decreased fMRI activation (dark regions) in the ipsilateral motor cortex (MI), contralateral supplementary motor cortex (SMA) and contralateral cerebellum, and in the contralateral secondary somatosensory cortex, contralateral parahippocampal gyrus, contralateral lingual gyrus, and bilateral superior temporal gyrus. Differences were not seen in the placebo TENS group. Abbreviations: M1, primary motor cortex; SMA, supplementary motor cortex.

Adapted from *Archives of Physical Medicine and Rehabilitation*, Volume 91, Issue 8, Murat Kara et al, Quantification of the Effects of Transcutaneous Electrical Nerve Stimulation with Functional Magnetic Resonance Imaging: A Double-Blind Randomized Placebo-Controlled Study, pp. 1160–65, Copyright © 2010 American Congress of Rehabilitation Medicine, with permission from Elsevier, http://www.sciencedirect.com/science/journal/00039993.

that low- (4 pps) and high-frequency (100 pps) TENS and sensory (just below motor threshold) or motor (2 × threshold for motor contraction) TENS reduced secondary mechanical hyperalgesia associated with acute joint inflammation.

Antihyperalgesic effects appear to persist longer for low-frequency TENS compared with high-frequency TENS (Sabino et al., 2008), but there were no differences between asymmetric biphasic square, and symmetric biphasic square waveforms during high-frequency TENS (Hingne & Sluka, 2007). TENS applied to a contralateral uninjured limb was shown to reduce hyperalgesia in an inflamed limb (Ainsworth et al., 2006; Sabino et al., 2008).

TENS effects on experimental models of neuropathic pain

Nerve injury creates a state of persistent amplification of normal sensory input via peripheral and central sensitization, ectopic impulse generation due to expression of ion channels (Na^+), neurotransmitters and receptors, and re-organization of neural connections. Leem and colleagues (1995) used a rat model of peripheral neuropathy induced by a tight ligation of L5–L6 nerves and found that low-frequency, high-intensity TENS (2 Hz, 4–5 mA) applied to the somatic receptive field reduced the response of sensitized, wide-dynamic-range neurones to brush-and-pinch stimuli with post-TENS effects persisting for 30–45 minutes for brush stimuli and 60–90 minutes for pinch. Low-frequency, high-intensity TENS was also shown to reduce injury-induced mechanical allodynia but not cold hyperalgesia in rats with nerve injury with endogenous opioids involved (Nam et al., 2001). Studies using chronic constriction injuries to the sciatic nerve of rats demonstrated that daily applications of high-frequency TENS prevented thermal and mechanical allodynia when delivered contralaterally to the site of injury (Somers & Clemente, 1998; 2006b).

There is tentative evidence that TENS parameters affect the responsiveness and neuropharmacology of the central nervous system to allodynia in different ways, and that early intervention with TENS contralateral to a nerve injury with high- and low-frequency TENS combined may reduce allodynia in humans with neuropathic pain. Nam and colleagues (2001) found that antinociceptive effects associated with low-frequency, high-intensity TENS depended on sympathetic activity. They measured behavioural signs of mechanical allodynia and cold hyperalgesia in rats with nerve injury using paw-withdrawal frequency from repetitive application of von Frey hairs and paw-lift duration at a cold temperature, respectively. After a unilateral nerve injury, both paw-withdrawal frequency and paw-lift duration increased in the injured hind paw. Low-frequency, high-intensity TENS of the injured paw reduced mechanical allodynia but not cold hyperalgesia. The effect of TENS on mechanical allodynia was reversed by naloxone, suggesting that opioids played a role in the antinociceptive effects. Intraperitoneal administration of phentolamine, a non-specific alpha-adrenergic antagonist, reduced cold hyperalgesia but not mechanical allodynia, suggesting that cold hyperalgesia was mediated by sympathetic activity. Sun and colleagues (2004) demonstrated that low-frequency (2 Hz), peripheral electrical nerve stimulation using an implanted electrode reduced proxy measures of neuropathic pain following spinal-nerve ligations in rats, and prevented expression of NMDA receptor 1 involved in central sensitization and the development of mechanical allodynia.

Neuropharmacology of TENS

The neuropharmacology of TENS is complex with many neurotransmitters and neuro-modulators implicated (Table 9.2). Neurotransmitters are released from axon terminals

Table 9.2 Neurochemicals implicated in the mechanism of action of TENS

Neurochemical	Low frequency	High frequency
Opioids	μ-opioid receptors (spinal and supraspinal)	δ-opioid receptors (spinal and supraspinal)
Gamma-amino butyric acid (GABA)	Elevation of GABA	Elevation of GABA
		GABA(A) receptors (spinal)
Glycine	No effect	No effect
Serotonin	Elevation of 5-HT levels	
	5-HT(2) and 5-HT(3) receptors (spinal)	
Noradrenaline	Alpha(2) receptors (peripheral)	Alpha(2) receptors (peripheral)
Acetylcholine	Muscarinic(1) and Muscarinic(3) receptors (spinal)	Muscarinic(1) and Muscarinic(3) receptors (spinal)
Aspartate and Glutamate		Reduction in glutamate and aspartate
		Elevations when high and low frequency TENS combined

and they transmit signals to another neurone or an effector by binding to and activating their respective neurotransmitter membrane receptor. Neurotransmitter effects are rapid, localized, and restricted to neuronal connections, although some neural connections may form a distinct system that may influence regions of the brain distant from origin of the neurone. Examples of neurotransmitters include acetylcholine, noradrenaline, glutamate, dopamine, serotonin (5-hydroxytryptamine), and gamma-aminobutyric acid (GABA). Some chemical neurotransmitters act as neuromodulators that diffuse across large areas of the nervous system to regulate diverse populations of neurons simultaneously. Examples include dopamine, serotonin, acetylcholine, histamine, opioids (including endorphins, enkephalins, and dynorphins), and endocannabinoids. Many neurotransmitters are also neuromodulators.

Opioids

Opiates are extracted from the resin of the opium poppy (Papaver somniferum) and have been used for medicinal purposes, including pain relief, since early times. Opioids are peptide molecules that include opiates and their synthetic derivatives, and their endogenous equivalents are found in the peripheral and central nervous system. Endogenous opioids have a range of physiological actions including analgesia, sedation, respiratory depression, constipation, cough suppression, and euphoria. Opioids have been implicated the mechanism of action of TENS since the publication of the gate control theory of pain in 1965.

Evidence that opioids were involved in TENS analgesia emerged in the 1970s when Sjölund and Eriksson (1976) reported that intravenous injection of naloxone hydrochloride (0.2–0.8 mg), but not saline (placebo), reversed AL-TENS analgesia in three out of five pain patients. Naloxone reversed analgesia associated with AL-TENS (2 bps) in six out of ten patients, but none out of ten patients using high-frequency, conventional TENS (50–100 pps) (Sjölund & Eriksson, 1979). Naloxone is a competitive antagonist for μ-opioid receptors that are known to mediate analgesic effects via their action on the central nervous system, although it also has a lower affinity for κ- and δ-opioid receptors. Early claims that low-frequency, high-intensity TENS but not high-frequency, low-intensity TENS was mediated by opioids was based on inconsistent research evidence (Pertovaara et al., 1982; Hansson et al., 1986). Chapman and Benedetti (1977) originally reported that AL-TENS was partially reversed by naloxone, and then withdrew their claim as their original report reflected a type I error (Chapman et al., 1983).

The findings of studies measuring opioid levels in plasma before, during, and after TENS, were also conflicting (Facchinetti et al., 1984; O'Brien et al., 1984). Plasma opioid measurements reflect release from peripheral sites as centrally released opioids are unlikely to cross the blood–brain barrier due to poor lipophilic properties and the large size of opioids. β-endorphin levels in cerebrospinal fluid were found to increase after AL-TENS (Sjölund et al., 1977) and high-frequency TENS (40–60 pps, 40–80 mA, 'tingling sensation, without pain') (Salar et al., 1981) in individuals with chronic pain, although there were no placebo controls in these studies. Han and colleagues (1991) found an increase in Met-enkephalin-Arg-Phe but not dynorphin following 30 minutes of AL-TENS (2 pps, with accompanying muscle contractions) to acupuncture points in 37 individuals in pain, and an increase in dynorphin A but not Met-enkephalin-Arg-Phe following high-frequency TENS (100 pps, muscle contractions). In the last decade, Sluka and colleagues have demonstrated that the effects of high- and low-frequency TENS are mediated by different opioid receptors.

Sluka and colleagues (1999) used microdialysis to administer opioid antagonists to the spinal cord of rats with inflammation of the knee joint induced by kaolin and carrageenan, and measured withdrawal latency to heat stimuli. Low-dose naloxone (μ-opioid receptor antagonism) blocked low-frequency (4 pps) TENS-induced antihyperalgesia, whereas high doses of naloxone (δ- and κ-opioid receptor antagonism) blocked high-frequency (100 pps) TENS-induced antihyperalgesia. Spinal blockade of δ-opioid receptors using naltrindole diminished high-frequency TENS antihyperalgesia in a dose-dependent manner whereas blockade of κ-opioid receptors using norbinaltorphimine had no effect on low- or high-frequency TENS effects. High-frequency (100 pps) TENS fully reversed secondary hyperalgesia from knee joint inflammation induced by kaolin and carrageenan in morphine-tolerant rats induced by subcutaneous implantation of morphine pellets over ten days (Sluka et al., 2000). Knee joint inflammation was unaffected by low-frequency TENS. The findings suggested that low-frequency TENS action was via μ-opioid receptors whereas high-frequency TENS via spinal δ-opioid receptors. Kalra and colleagues (2001) found that blockade of μ-opioid receptors in the rostral ventral medulla diminished the antihyperalgesic effects of low-frequency (4 pps) but not high-frequency (100 pps) TENS, whereas antagonism of δ-opioid receptors diminished the antihyperalgesic effect of high- but not low-frequency

TENS. Sabino and colleagues (2008) found that 20 minutes of either high- or low-frequency (10 pps) TENS reduced hyperalgesia in an inflammation model produced by the injection of carrageenan in rat paws, and that intraplantar administration of naltrexone reversed the antihyperalgesic effect of low-frequency but not high-frequency TENS, suggesting that low-frequency TENS effect were mediated by local release of endogenous opioids. Thus, these findings suggest that high-frequency TENS mediates effects via δ-opioid receptors, whereas low-frequency TENS mediates effects via μ-opioid receptors.

Gamma-amino-butyric acid (GABA)

Gamma-amino-butyric acid (GABA) and glycine are amino acids which act as inhibitory neurotransmitters in the central nervous system. Glycine also has a co-agonist role with glutamate for NMDA receptors leading to increased central sensitization. GABA has been shown to have a role in centrally mediated hypoalgesia during TENS and spinal cord stimulation. Duggan and Foong (1985) were the first to demonstrate inhibition of spinal nociceptive neurones by dorsal column stimulation in anaesthetized cats was reversed by bicuculline (GABA(A) receptor antagonist) administered intravenously or electrophoretically from micropipettes. Recently, Barchini and colleagues (2012) found that hypoalgesia during spinal cord stimulation in a neuropathic rat model of nociception was reduced by GABA(A) and GABA(B) antagonist drugs.

Jeong and colleagues (1995) found that high-frequency, high-intensity, electrical peripheral nerve stimulation reduced spontaneous activity of lumbosacral dorsal horn neurones, and the effect was reversed during the iontophoretic application of naloxone (opioid antagonist), picrotoxin (GABA(A) receptor antagonist), and strychnine (glycine and acetylcholine receptor antagonist), suggesting that opioid and GABA-ergic systems were involved. Maeda and colleagues (2007) used microdialysis techniques to sample the extracellular fluid of rats with and without knee joint inflammation induced by intra-articular injection of kaolin and carrageenan and found increased extracellular concentrations of GABA in spinal segments following high-frequency TENS. Blockade of GABA(A) receptors with bicuculline prevented high-frequency antihyperalgesia. In contrast, low-frequency TENS did not alter extracellular GABA concentrations in spinal segments. Blockade of GABA(A) receptors reduced the antihyperalgesia generated during low-frequency TENS although investigators speculated that this may have been due in part to the use of anaesthetic during collection. No increases in glycine in response to low- or high-frequency TENS were observed. Somers and Clemente (2009) found that contralateral high-frequency or a combination of high- and low-frequency TENS administered daily for one hour administered to reduced mechanical but not thermal allodynia in the right hind-paw of neuropathic rats with a right-sided chronic constriction injury. High-frequency TENS elevated the synaptosomal content of GABA in the dorsal horn bilaterally, and a combination of high- and low-frequency TENS elevated the dorsal horn content of aspartate, glutamate, and glycine bilaterally. When taken together these findings suggested that high-frequency TENS increased GABA levels in the spinal cord which may be due to increased neuronal or glial release, or decreased neuronal reuptake.

Serotonin

Serotonin (5-hydroxytryptamine, 5-HT) is a monoamine neurotransmitter that is considered to be pain-producing at the site of tissue damage, and pain-reducing in the central nervous system. Woolf and colleagues (1980) demonstrated that systemic administration of parachlorphenylalanine, a serotonin depletor reduced the effect of TENS (100 pps, 200 μs, slight fibrillation of tail muscles) in intact rats, but not in rats with transection at the 10th or 11th thoracic vertebra, suggesting that the supraspinal mechanisms of TENS were mediated by serotonin. Radhakrishnan and colleagues (2003) found that intrathecal administration of Methysergide (5-HT(1) and 5-HT(2) receptor antagonist) and MDL-72222 (5-HT(3) antagonist) blocked antihyperalgesia of low-frequency but not high-frequency TENS. Ketanserin (5-HT(2A) antagonist) reduced the effect of low-frequency TENS whereas NAN-190 (5-HT(1A) antagonist) had no effect. Twenty minutes of low-frequency TENS (4 pps, sensory intensity, 100 μs), but not high-frequency TENS (100 pps), or placebo TENS, increased serotonin concentrations during and immediately after treatment measured using high-performance liquid chromatography with coulemetric detection from samples of cerebrospinal fluid taken from the dorsal horn of the spinal cord in rats with knee joint inflammation (Sluka et al., 2006). Thus, spinal 5-HT(2) and 5-HT(3) receptors are involved in antihyperalgesia generated by low-, but not high-frequency TENS.

Noradrenaline

In the periphery, noradrenaline and adrenaline influence sympathetic effector activity associated with the fight–flight–fright response by activating α and β adrenoceptors. Alpha(2A) receptors are expressed on primary afferent neurones and macrophages near injured tissue. In the central nervous system, noradrenaline and adrenaline mediate arousal, reward, and antinociception. Stimulation of spinal and supraspinal α(2) receptors located on axon terminals results in presynaptic inhibition of the release of noradrenaline. This negative feedback mechanism controls noradrenaline and adrenaline levels in the central nervous system. Alpha(2A) and α(2C) receptors mediate antinociception when activated by noradrenaline, and they have a synergistic action with opioid receptor activation.

Clonidine, a centrally acting α(2) receptor agonist, has synergistic effects when combined with opioids and was found to enhance the reduction in primary hyperalgesia associated with inflammation of the rat hind paw produced during low- (4 pps) or high-frequency (100 pps) TENS (Sluka & Chandran, 2002). Intrathecal administration of yohimbine (α(2) receptor antagonist) did not reverse antihyperalgesia associated with low- (4 pps) or high-frequency (100 pps) TENS at sensory intensities (Radhakrishnan et al., 2003). The effect of low- and high-frequency TENS in reducing in secondary heat hyperalgesia to intra-articular injection of a mixture of carrageenan/kaolin (3 per cent) was diminished in mice that lacked functional α(2A) receptors compared with normal mice (King et al., 2005). Moreover the reduction in secondary heat hyperalgesia produced by TENS was reversed by SK&F 86466, (α(2) receptor antagonist) administered intra-articularly (peripheral), but not intrathecally (spinal), or intracerebroventricularly (supraspinal). Thus, spinal and supraspinal α(2) receptors appear not to be involved in TENS antihyperalgesia in rats.

Acetylcholine

In the central nervous system, acetylcholine acts via nicotinic and muscarinic receptors to mediate learning, short-term memory, arousal, and reward. Activation of spinal cholinergic receptors is antinociceptive with interactions with opioid and serotonin receptors. The antihyperalgesic effects of low- and high-frequency TENS applied to the inflamed knee in rats are diminished by intrathecal administration of various muscarinic antagonists (e.g. atropine, a non-selective muscarinic antagonist; pirenzepine, a muscarinic 1 receptor antagonist; and 4-DAMP, a muscarinic 3 receptor antagonist) but not by a muscarinic 2 receptor antagonist (methoctramine) or a non-selective nicotinic antagonist (mecamylamine) (Radhakrishnan & Sluka, 2003). Thus, spinal muscarinic receptor subtypes 1 and 2 appear to be involved in TENS antihyperalgesia.

Aspartate and glutamate

Aspartate and glutamate are excitatory amino acids released at afferent terminals in response to noxious stimulation. All have a critical role in pain states through actions on NMDA and non-NMDA receptors such as α-amino-3-hydroxy-5-methyl-4-isoxazolepropionic acid (AMPA) receptors, and metabotropic and kainite receptors. There are considerable amounts of glutamate in the dorsal horn released from A-δ and C-nociceptive afferents which not only generates painful sensations but also contributes to the induction and maintenance of sensitization of central nociceptive transmission cells.

High- (100 pps) but not low-frequency (4 pps) TENS has been shown to reduce the release of aspartate and glutamate in the dorsal horn of rats with joint inflammation (Sluka et al., 2005). The mechanism appears to be mediated via release of endogenous opioids because naltrindole (δ-opioid receptor antagonist) reduced glutamate and aspartate associated with high-frequency TENS. In contrast, and surprisingly, a combination of high- and low-frequency TENS elevated aspartate, glutamate, and glycine bilaterally in the dorsal horn of rats with a right-sided chronic constriction injury, although reductions in mechanical allodynia were observed (Somers & Clemente, 2009). The investigators suggested that the effect of combining high- and low-frequency TENS may result in elevated glutamate acting via group II and III metabotropic glutamate receptors which are known to reduce mechanical allodynia after nerve injury.

Neuropharmacology of TENS tolerance

Studies using animal models of nociception have provided insights into the mechanism of tolerance to repeated application of TENS. Chandran and Sluka (2003) demonstrated that repeated daily application of TENS resulted in tolerance to the antihyperalgesia to inflammation produced by TENS with a corresponding cross-tolerance to μ- and δ-opioid agonists. They induced knee joint inflammation (3 per cent carrageenan) in rats and administered low- (4 Hz) or high-frequency (100 Hz) TENS 20 minutes per day for six days to the inflamed knee joint. There was a reduction in the ability of TENS to reduce secondary mechanical hyperalgesia by the fourth day. Animals were also tested for tolerance to morphine, a μ-opioid agonist, and SNC-80, a δ-opioid agonist, administered intrathecally. When compared to a group of rats that did not receive

TENS it was found that the effects of morphine were reduced in the low- but not the high-frequency TENS group, suggesting cross-tolerance to μ-opioid agonists. The effects of SNC-80 were reduced in the high- but not the low-frequency TENS group suggesting cross-tolerance to δ-opioid agonists. This demonstrated a role for spinal opioid receptors in tolerance to TENS analgesia.

Cholecystokinin and NMDA receptors also have a role. Cholecystokinin is a peptide hormone that stimulates digestion of fat and protein, and is involved in the induction of drug tolerance to opioids and pain hypersensitivity during opioid withdrawal. Systemic and spinal blockade of cholecystokinin receptors using proglumide prevented tolerance to high- (100 pps) and low-frequency (4 pps) TENS in rats with knee joint inflammation (3 per cent kaolin/carrageenan) (DeSantana et al., 2010). Blockade of spinal cholecystokinin(B) receptors prevented cross-tolerance at spinal μ-opioid receptors during repeated application of low-frequency TENS whereas blockade of spinal cholecystokinin(A) prevented cross-tolerance at spinal δ-opioid receptors with high-frequency TENS. Blockade of NMDA receptors using MK-801 prevented tolerance to antihyperalgesia by repeated high- (100 pps) or low-frequency (4 pps) TENS (20 minutes daily, for four days) in rats with knee joint inflammation (Hingne & Sluka, 2008). As NMDA receptor blockade is likely to prevent tolerance at spinal opioid receptors it was suggested that TENS tolerance may be prevented by co-administration of ketamine or dextromethorphan.

Summary

1 There is strong evidence from electrophysiological and behavioural studies using animals and healthy humans that conventional TENS activates large-diameter, low-threshold afferents which inhibits central nociceptive transmission with gamma-amino-butyric acid (GABA) and opioids playing a key role.

2 The neural circuitry is located at spinal and supra-spinal sites. Activation of small-diameter, deep-seated afferents is more likely to trigger descending-pain inhibitory pathways arising from the periaqueductal grey and nucleus raphe magnus that form feedback loops to the spinal cord.

3 Direct stimulation of small-diameter cutaneous and muscle afferents may be painful so TENS can be delivered to stimulate low-threshold motor efferents to generate muscle twitches resulting in muscle afferent input (i.e. AL-TENS).

4 Antidromic impulses generated during TENS will cause peripheral blockade of afferent impulses arising from sensory receptors.

5 At intensities below motor threshold low-frequency TENS acts via μ-opioid serotonin and noradrenaline receptors whereas high-frequency TENS acts via δ-opioid receptors. Opioids, cholecystokinin, and NMDA receptors have a role in TENS tolerance.

Further reading

♦ DeSantana, J.M., Walsh, D.M., Vance, C., Rakel, B.A., and Sluka, K.A. (2008) Effectiveness of transcutaneous electrical nerve stimulation for treatment of hyperalgesia and pain. *Curr Rheumatol Rep*, **10**, 492–9.

In Chapter 10 the use of TENS to manage non-painful conditions is discussed.

Chapter 10

The use of TENS for non-painful conditions

Introduction

Clinicians have tried electrical nerve stimulation techniques, including TENS, to treat a range of non-painful conditions. The purpose of this chapter is to provide an overview of the mechanism of action, the clinical use, and the clinical efficacy of TENS when used to manage non-painful conditions by covering:

- TENS of the autonomic nervous system
- Circulatory effects of TENS
- TENS for tissue regeneration
- TENS for psychomotor conditions
- TENS for incontinence, constipation, and ileus
- TENS for post-surgical symptoms
- Antiemetic effects of TENS (PC6 stimulation)

TENS of the autonomic nervous system

The autonomic nervous system controls visceral processes mediated by smooth muscle, cardiac muscle, and glands including digestion, excretion, and cardiovascular function. The parasympathetic division of the autonomic nervous system is involved with rest, repose, and reproduction, and the sympathetic division is involved with fight–flight–fright responses. Parasympathetic nerves are a primary target for many invasive and non-invasive peripheral electrical nerve stimulation techniques because they exert local reflex control over many visceral functions (Chapter 4, Table 4.1). The sympathetic division exerts generalized control of visceral functions associated with mobilizing energy, resulting in more widespread physiological actions. Sympathetic nerves and ganglia are a target when there is a need to regulate sympathetic tone and in pain medicine the goal is often to inhibit sympathetic activity using techniques such as the injection of local anaesthetic. Research on the effect of TENS on sympathetic tone is conflicting, with increases, decreases, and no change in tone all reported (Olyaei et al., 2004; Reeves et al., 2004). In general, the effect of TENS on physiological function will depend on whether electrodes are positioned over sympathetic or parasympathetic nerves. Preganglionic and postganglionic autonomic fibres are classified as B axons

(Chapter 2, Table 3.4) and have higher thresholds of excitation than the A-β somatosensory fibres activated during conventional TENS. Preganglionic and postganglionic autonomic fibres are located in deeper tissue, and are more difficult to stimulate precisely using surface electrodes than with percutaneous and implanted nerve stimulation techniques.

Circulatory effects of TENS

TENS and blood flow in ischaemic tissue

Studies using healthy human participants have found that high-frequency, strong, non-painful TENS increases (Wikstrom et al., 1999), decreases (Casale et al., 1985), or does not change (Cramp et al., 2000a; Chen et al., 2007) blood flow in healthy humans. The findings of studies using low-frequency TENS are more consistent, with TENS increasing blood flow providing intensities are above motor threshold (Cramp et al., 2002). Phasic muscle contractions elicited by AL-TENS and neuromuscular electrical stimulation (NMES) have been used to increase regional blood flow and to improve oxygenation of tissue in arterial insufficiency and claudication due to arterial and neuropathic diseases, although the Canadian Physiotherapy Association recommends that NMES is contraindicated in the presence of severe arterial disease (Chapter 5, 106–108). Kaada (1982) pioneered the use of low-frequency TENS (burst pattern, internal frequency of 100 pps) to generate widespread and prolonged cutaneous vasodilation to manage peripheral ischaemia and the symptoms of Reynaud's syndrome. The cathode was positioned between the first and second metacarpal and the anode on the ulnar edge of the same hand to twitch the fingers and the thumb, and it was found that this technique increased plasma serotonin (5-HT), calcitonin gene-related peptide (CGRP), and vasoactive intestinal peptide (VIP) Recently, it has been suggested that TENS might be useful to prevent venous stasis during surgical treatment as TENS of the peroneal nerve increased peak venous velocity and flow volume in the popliteal vein in the limbs of healthy participants (Izumi et al., 2010).

TENS has been used to reduce tissue necrosis (death), especial in the transfer of tissue (skin and fat, muscle, nerve, bone) and its associated blood supply from one site of the body (donor) to another (recipient), termed 'free flaps'. Daily treatment with high-(80 pps) and low-frequency (2 pps) TENS has been shown to increase the viability of ischaemic skin flaps in rats, with 15 mA demonstrating largest effects (Liebano et al., 2006; 2008). An RCT of 173 post-mastectomy breast cancer patients found that fewer patients had skin flap necrosis and ecchymosis when high-frequency, low-intensity conventional TENS (70 pps, 2 mA) was applied to areas of flap ecchymosis and necrosis (Atalay & Yilmaz, 2009).

TENS and healing of open wounds

In 1999, a meta-analysis of 15 studies and 24 interventions of a variety of types of electrical stimulation using surface electrodes and 15 controls found that the rate of healing of chronic wounds for electrical stimulation was 22 per cent per week compared with 9 per cent (95 per cent CI: 3.8–14 per cent) for controls, with stimulation most effective for pressure ulcers (Gardner et al., 1999). There were no differences in the rate of healing between different types of electrical stimulation, with net increases in rate of healing being 10.87 per cent for TENS (three studies), 12.59 per cent for continuous direct current (seven studies), and 15.50 per cent for pulsed direct current (13 studies). In 2011, a systematic review found evidence that electrical stimulation with usual physiotherapy reduced local acute oedema after burn injury and increased active hand motion (Edgar et al., 2011).

TENS may accelerate wound healing by increasing regional blood flow in ischaemic tissue. Khalil and Merhi (2000) found that low-frequency TENS of the sciatic nerve (20 V, 5 Hz for one minute) improved the vascular response of the hind-footpad of rats measured using laser Doppler flowmetry. In healthy humans, Wikstrom and colleagues (1999) found that blood flow measured by laser Doppler imaging increased by 23 per cent during low-frequency TENS (2 Hz), and by 17 per cent during high-frequency TENS (100 pps) when applied around blister wounds on the lower leg. In patients, low-frequency TENS (2 Hz, 10–45 mA, 60 minutes) increased blood flow by 35 per cent in chronic lower-leg ulcers at the end of stimulation, and by 15 per cent in the intact skin surrounding the ulcer, and it remained elevated at 29 per cent in the ulcer and 9 per cent in surrounding skin 15 minutes post-stimulation (Cosmo et al., 2000). However, Kim and colleagues (2010) measured regional transcutaneous oxygen tension or pressure distribution over gluteal muscles of six participants with motor paralysis following complete spinal cord injury and failed to detect differences between TENS administered below motor threshold, and placebo TENS.

TENS for tissue regeneration

Electrical stimulation techniques have a direct effect on the regeneration of nerve, soft tissue, skin, and bone. Electrical stimulation (2 pps or 20 pps) via implanted or percutaneous electrodes has been shown to accelerate axon outgrowth from proximal nerve stumps to distal nerve stumps in studies using rat models of sciatic nerve injury. The time for muscle re-innervation was accelerated and facilitation of spinal motor response was reduced, with tyrosine kinase B receptors and their ligands involved (English et al., 2007; Geremia et al., 2007; Vivo et al., 2008). Low-frequency stimulation of proximal nerves has been shown to regenerate median nerves after carpal tunnel release surgery so that they re-innervate thenar muscles within 6–8 months, with failure to re-innervate thenar muscles in non-treated individuals (Gordon et al., 2009).

It is claimed that the milliampere currents used during TENS are too large to facilitate tissue repair directly and that microampere currents are more appropriate (Chapter 11). Lu and colleagues (2009) found that low-frequency (2 Hz) percutaneous electrical stimulation administered at 1 mA and 2 mA increased proximal and distal nerve stump regeneration, whereas 4 mA hindered regeneration, suggesting that a therapeutic window for current amplitude for regeneration of nerve fibres may exist. Animal studies have found that microcurrent electrical stimulation (20 Hz, 2 µA, 30 minutes) improves functional and sensory recovery, with improvements in sciatic functional index, mean conduction velocity, the number of retrogradely labelled sensory neurones, axon counts, and myelin thicknesses (Alrashdan et al., 2010).

Few studies have investigated the effect of TENS using a standard device on nerve regeneration. Baptista and colleagues (2008) induced a crush lesion in mice and delivered high- and low-frequency TENS at or just below motor threshold for five weeks at 30 minutes per day, five days per week. TENS impaired nerve regeneration, producing more axons with dark axoplasm, greater signs of oedema, less organized cytoarchitecture, and fewer and thinner myelinated fibres when compared with a no-stimulation control. Interestingly, Static Sciatic Index values did not differ between the groups. Gigo-Benato and colleagues (2010) used sciatic nerve crush injuries in rats, and found that TENS at amplitudes to induce a visible contraction increased muscle fibre atrophy and decreased muscle excitability and functional recovery at day 14 post-injury compared with no stimulation. TENS was administered from three days post-injury on the tibialis anterior muscle every other day using a variety of electrical characteristics.

A review of systematic reviews on electrical stimulation for fracture healing found four published meta-analyses and concluded that evidence tended to support benefits from electrical stimulation (Goldstein et al., 2010). There is also tentative evidence that electrical stimulation may be of benefit in the prevention and treatment of osteoporosis if given early after spinal cord injury (Biering-Sorensen et al., 2009). However, these reviews on electrical stimulation have found that there has been little research on TENS per se.

TENS for psychomotor conditions

A systematic review provided evidence that TENS improved memory and affect, somatosensory functioning, visuo-spatial abilities, and postural control and acceleration in a variety of conditions including Alzheimer's disease and neglect due to stroke (van Dijk et al., 2002). TENS may also improve awakening in coma due to traumatic brain injury.

Dementia

A Cochrane review of eight trials, of which three were included in a meta-analysis, found evidence that TENS had short-lived improvements for certain aspects of memory in people with early and mid-stage Alzheimer's disease dementia, although it was not possible to draw definitive conclusions (Cameron et al., 2003). Much of the research has been conducted by Scherder and colleagues, and suggests that muscular twitches induced by low-frequency TENS between T1 and T5 on the spine (burst patterns, 2 bps, asymmetric biphasic square waves, 100 μs, 30 minutes per day) improves verbal long-term memory, verbal fluency, visual memory, mood, alertness, and social contacts in individuals at the early stage of Alzheimer's disease (Scherder et al., 2000). Effects were less prominent in individuals with mid-stage Alzheimer's but still occurred in elderly individuals without dementia. TENS improved rest–activity rhythm and night-time restlessness in individuals with early and mid-stage Alzheimer's disease by strengthening the coupling of circadian rest–activity rhythm to external cues that synchronize the individual's endogenous bodyclock to the daily light/dark cycle (i.e. Zeitgebers). TENS also increased neural input to areas of the brain affected by dementia and aging such as the dorsal Raphe nucleus, the locus coeruleus, the septo-hippocampal region, and the hypothalamus (Scherder et al., 2003).

Neuromuscular conditioning

Non-invasive electrical stimulation techniques provide therapeutic improvements in neuromuscular functional condition through strengthening muscles, increasing motor control, reducing spasticity, decreasing pain, and increasing range of motion (therapeutic electrical stimulation). These techniques also provide functionally useful movements during stimulation to aid limb, hand, and foot function whilst standing, walking, and grasping (functional electrical stimulation) (Schuhfried et al., 2012). A systematic review of 15 studies found evidence that strong, non-painful TENS improved force production of the ankle dorsiflexors and timed up-and-go tests when used in combination with active training (Laufer & Elboim-Gabyzon, 2011). Evidence also suggests that TENS or functional neuromuscular electrical stimulation improves muscle strength and function during rehabilitation for soft-tissue injuries following surgical or conservative treatment after anterior cruciate ligament reconstruction and meniscectomy (Imoto et al., 2011). TENS-induced muscle contractions have also been reported to reduce reflex excitability and to restore voluntary limb movement of patients including reach-to-grasp, walking, and drop foot with hemiplegia, although some RCTs have failed to find beneficial effects. Early intervention may be necessary to achieve a positive long-term outcome.

Post-stroke

The Ottawa Panel for the management of adults with hemiplegia or hemiparesis following ischaemic or haemorrhagic stroke recommend TENS and transcutaneous neuromuscular electrical stimulation for post-stroke rehabilitation. Evidence suggests that TENS reduces spasticity in patients with spinal cord injury or post-stroke (Sadowsky, 2001; Ping Ho Chung & Kam Kwan Cheng, 2010). Conventional high-frequency TENS (100 pps) over peripheral nerves of the affected limb has improved stretch reflex activity in spasticity in patients with hemiplegia, with benefits to activities of daily living (Tekeoglu et al., 1998). Low-frequency TENS of acupuncture points (ST36 (Stomach 36, Zusanli), LV3 (Liver 3, Taichong), GB34 (Gall bladder 34, Yanglinquan), and BL60 (Bladder 60, Kunlun)) in the affected limb decreased post-stroke spasticity, and increased strength and walking capability (Ng & Hui-Chan, 2009; Yan & Hui-Chan, 2009). Evidence also suggests that TENS is beneficial for other post-stroke symptoms. Low-frequency TENS (burst pattern, internal frequency 80 pps, below motor threshold) in front of the mylohyoid muscles improves swallowing coordination in patients with oropharyngeal dysphagia (Gallas et al., 2010), and strong, non-painful TENS of ipsilateral and contralateral upper limbs reduced hemispatial neglect (Schroder et al., 2008). TENS may also reduce severe anosognosia in some patients but not emotional status or cognitive functioning (Rorsman & Johansson, 2006).

Epilepsy

There is a fear that electrical nerve stimulation may trigger seizures in susceptible individuals (Chapter 5, 105–106), although electrical stimulation of the vagus nerve has been used to manage drug-resistant epilepsy (Beekwilder & Beems, 2010). Besio and co-workers have found that focal TENS (200–750 pps, 50 mA or 60 mA, symmetrical biphasic waveforms, 200–200 μs) administered via bipolar concentric ring electrodes at

CZ on the scalp reduced electrographic and behavioural seizure activity in pilocarpine-induced status epilepticus in experimental rats if administered five minutes after the onset of the seizure, although pulse frequency and amplitude were higher than conventional TENS (Besio et al., 2007). The investigators suggested that this type of stimulation may be pacing or defibrillating the brain in a similar manner to that observed for the heart. Studies using the technique on humans are yet to be conducted.

Sleep, fatigue, depression, and coma

TENS-like devices have been used to improve sleep quality, fatigue, and depression, although standard TENS devices are rarely used for direct actions on sleep. TENS of the genioglossus muscle decreased snoring, respiratory disturbance, and neural respiratory drive in patients with obstructive sleep apnoea (Steier et al., 2011), and transcutaneous vagal nerve stimulation of the left outer auditory canal decreased activity in limbic brain with improvements in well-being in healthy humans (Kraus et al., 2007). Auricular TENS has been used to reduce major depression and to improve cognitive functions in children with attention deficit hyperactivity disorder. TENS of the median nerve has been used to arouse persons with reduced levels of consciousness and acute coma after traumatic brain injury (Cooper et al., 2005).

TENS for incontinence, constipation, and ileus

Electrical stimulation has been used for incontinence, constipation, and ileus, although there are difficulties in targeting visceral nerves and tissue using surface electrodes. Percutaneous techniques overcome this problem but they are more expensive and pose greater risk. Systematic reviews have found evidence of efficacy for sacral nerve stimulation for faecal incontinence and constipation, anorectal function, faecal incontinence associated with an anal sphincter lesion, lower urinary tract dysfunction, urinary urge incontinence, and overactive bladder. There is tentative evidence for reductions in pain and improvements in quality-of-life measures of overactive bladder syndrome and faecal incontinence during percutaneous tibial nerve stimulation. A review of research literature by members of the International Children's Continence Society on therapeutic interventions for congenital neuropathic bladder and bowel dysfunction in children found no research studies on the use of TENS, although studies using percutaneous nerve stimulation found beneficial effects (Rawashdeh et al., 2012).

Faecal incontinence

TENS has been used to manage faecal incontinence with reports of success when administered over sacral nerves, posterior tibial nerves, posterior genital nerves, and via anal probes (transmucosal stimulation). Interferential current therapy has also been shown to be beneficial. A Cochrane review found tentative evidence that electrical stimulation combined with biofeedback may be beneficial compared with electrical stimulation or anal sphincter exercises on their own in the management of faecal incontinence (Norton & Cody, 2012). Most included studies used electrical muscular stimulation of smooth muscle fibres using anal probes and current amplitudes high enough to achieve perineal contractions. For example, strong, non-painful TENS (burst pattern, three seconds on and three seconds off, internal frequency 30–40 pps, 200 μs) with transmucosal stimulation delivered using a Neuro Trac ETS device (e.g. see <http://www.neurotracpelvitone.co.uk>) and an anal probe (Anuform) for 20 minutes, twice daily for eight weeks, improved subjective perception of post-delivery anal incontinence control, although neither technique improved incontinence scores, quality of life, or faecal incontinence quality of life scores (Naimy et al., 2007). An RCT not included in the Cochrane review failed to detect superiority of TENS of the posterior tibial nerve for three months over placebo on the number of incontinence and urgency episodes, although a larger proportion of patients receiving active TENS reported a decrease in faecal incontinence severity scores (Leroi et al., 2012). Interestingly, physicians rated active TENS more effective than placebo TENS.

Urinary incontinence (enuresis) and dysfunction

There is increasing use of electrical stimulation of sacral nerves, pudendal nerves, and tibial nerves to manage stress incontinence and overactive bladder syndrome. Sacral stimulation is used to stimulate pelvic floor muscles to generate adequate muscle contraction, and to modulate activity in nerves innervating the bladder, sphincter, and pelvic floor which help to restore the coordination of sacral reflexes. Originally, currents were delivered at 10–50 pps to stimulate pelvic floor muscles to reduce detrusor muscle instability, although some investigators have used much higher frequencies when treating pelvic pain in conditions associated with bladder dysfunction such as interstitial cystitis. In recent years, sacral nerve stimulation has been achieved using tibial nerve stimulation via electrode leads placed in the lower tibia or above the ankle.

Indrekvam and Hunskaar (2003) found that over a two-year period between 1992 and 1994, TENS for use at home for urinary incontinence was requested by 429 general practitioners and 147 gynaecologists, and that prescribers of TENS were proactive in treating urinary incontinence. Early reports suggested improvements in stress incontinence, bladder over-activity syndrome, and detrusor instability could be achieved using TENS with electrodes placed on perianal skin, the base of the penis, the suprapubic region, the posterior tibial nerve, and parasacral, although most studies lacked control groups. The magnitude of effect has been reported to be similar to oral oxybutynin (Soomro et al., 2001).

A systematic review that included seven studies on the use of parasacral TENS to manage non-neurogenic lower urinary tract dysfunctions found evidence that daily strong, non-painful TENS treatment was superior to placebo in treating overactive bladder syndrome in children (Barroso et al., 2011). The proportion of patients with complete resolution of symptoms ranged from 73 per cent to 13 per cent, although optimal TENS parameters could not be determined because pulse frequencies used by study investigators ranged from 2 pps to 150 pps. Low-frequency currents of less than 20 pps were commonly used. TENS (continuous, 10 pps, 200 μs) of the posterior tibial nerve with electrodes placed on the ankle behind the internal malleolus was found to improve urge urinary incontinence due to multiple sclerosis, spinal cord injury, and Parkinson's disease, and when added to pelvic floor muscle exercises in elderly women (Schreiner et al., 2010).

Constipation

Percutaneous sacral nerve stimulation with electrodes in the third sacral foramen has been used to modulate reflexes inhibiting large bowel function in individuals with idiopathic slow and normal transit constipation. TENS with electrodes placed over the abdomen, lumbosacral region, or acupuncture points is a viable option, although most research to date has investigated interferential current therapy because currents permeate to deep-seated structures. Studies by Robertson and colleagues suggest daily self-administered treatment with interferential current therapy (one hour per day, sine waveform, 4 kHz carrier frequency, 80–160 Hz beat frequency, intensity < 33 mA), with two electrodes positioned over the epigastrium and two positioned over the kidneys improves colonic transit, with increased defecation in children with idiopathic slow transit constipation (Ismail et al., 2009). Long-term follow-up studies found that children were able to self-administer interferential current therapy daily for up to six months, with over 50 per cent of children reporting perceived improvements in soiling frequency, defecation frequency, wetter stools, and abdominal pain with associated reductions in laxative use (Leong et al., 2011).

A study without a control comparison found that parasacral stimulation using two electrodes placed either side of S2 and S4 using a TENS-like device (961 Dualpex Uro; 10 pps, 20 minutes × three times per week, 700 ms, strong, non-painful intensity without muscle contraction) improved constipation symptoms in 85.7 per cent of children including faecal incontinence and stool retention (Veiga et al., 2012).

Ileus and gastrointestinal discomfort

TENS has been used for ileus since the 1970s but there are few studies of note. Xiao and Liu (2004) found that acupoint TENS (bidirectional square waves, 300 μs, 100 pps, 26–30 mA, LI4 (Large intestine 14, Hegu), ST36 (Stomach 36, Zusanli point), BL57(Bladder 57, Chenshan)) generating visible contraction of the underlying muscle increased rectal sensory threshold, increased stool times, decreased abdominal pain, and elevated psychological scores in 24 patients with diarrhoea-predominant irritable bowel syndrome. Koklu and colleagues (2010) found that a four-week course of interferential current therapy (beat frequency sweep of 80–150 Hz) using vacuum electrodes applied to the paravertebral area of T10–T12 reduced upper gastrointestinal system symptoms including epigastric discomfort, pyrosis, bloating, early satiation, and postprandial fullness in 44 individuals with drug-refractory functional dyspepsia.

Studies on animals have found that hemodynamic responses to colon distension were lessened during TENS, and this may prove useful in various conditions including autonomic dysreflexia in paraplegic and quadriplegic individuals, and for gastrointestinal symptoms associated with stress in conditions such as irritable bowel syndrome. Yoshimoto and colleagues (2012) found that TENS applied to the bilateral hind limbs of rats every other day reduced accelerated colonic transit from chronic heterotypic stress. The effect of TENS was prevented by injection of an oxytocin antagonist into the central nervous system, and the investigators suggested that TENS up-regulated hypothalamic expression of oxytocin which is known to inhibit corticotropin releasing factor responsible for colonic dysmotility.

TENS for post-surgical symptoms

TENS has been shown to have beneficial effects on a variety of post-surgical symptoms including atelectasis (collapse or closure of the lung) that causes diminished gaseous exchange (for review, see Johnson & Bagley, 2009). Evidence is conflicting but tends towards TENS reducing post-operative pulmonary dysfunction following chest and upper abdominal surgery including improvements in peak expiratory flow rates and forced vital capacity post-operatively following cardiac surgery, and improved forced expiratory volume, forced vital capacity, PaO_2, $PaCO_2$, and tolerance of chest physical therapy following thoracotomy (Erdogan et al., 2005). These effects are likely to be due to TENS-induced reductions in movement-evoked pain during deep breathing post-operatively (Rakel & Frantz, 2003).

Antiemetic effects of TENS (PC6 stimulation)

Non-pharmacological treatments are recommended as adjuncts to medication to manage nausea and vomiting (emesis). Dundee and colleagues pioneered the use of TENS of acupuncture points PC6 (Pericardium 6, Neiguan), ST36 (Stomach 36, Zu San Li), and CV12 (Conception Vessel 12, Zhong Wan), to reduce nausea and vomiting. TENS-like devices that deliver transcutaneous electrical acupoint stimulation to PC6 acupoint on the wrist are commercially available to alleviate nausea associated with cancer, side effects of treatment, pregnancy, and motion/travel sickness (e.g. ReliefBand device, see <http://reliefband.com.au>, and Chapter 11, 201). Ezzo and colleagues (2006) evaluated the results of Cochrane systematic reviews and concluded that PC6 stimulation was beneficial for post-operative and chemotherapy-induced nausea and vomiting, although results for pregnancy-related nausea and vomiting were mixed. However, transcutaneous electrical acupoint stimulation was not effective for chemotherapy-induced nausea and vomiting. A Cochrane review of 40 trials (4858 patients) found that PC6 acupoint stimulation reduced nausea, vomiting, and the need for rescue antiemetics compared with placebo controls, with no differences between invasive and non-invasive stimulation techniques (Lee & Fan, 2009). TENS (5 Hz, 50 ms, 0.5–4.0 mA) administered to the trapezoid area using one electrode applied to the neck and two electrodes applied to the mastoid area was found to reduce post-operative nausea and vomiting following laparoscopic cholecystectomy (Cekmen et al., 2007).

Summary

1 The use of TENS to manage various non-painful conditions is supported by evidence from the basic sciences.

2 Autonomic nervous system effects depend on whether sympathetic or parasympathetic nerves are targetted during TENS, with the latter having most clinical utility.

3 Evidence suggests that TENS may be beneficial for ischaemic tissue, skin flaps, and wound healing, but definitive studies are needed.

4 Moderate evidence is available to support the use of TENS to manage nausea, bladder and bowel dysfunction, and motor recovery following stroke, although

acupuncture, peripheral electrical nerve stimulation, and neuromuscular electrical stimulation techniques may be more efficacious.

5   Evidence is growing to support the use of TENS to improve neuro-cognitive functioning in dementia, epilepsy, sleep, fatigue, depression, and coma.

Further reading

◆ Barroso, U., Jr., Tourinho, R., Lordelo, P., Hoebeke, P., and Chase, J. (2011) Electrical stimulation for lower urinary tract dysfunction in children: a systematic review of the literature. *Neurourol Urodyn*, **30**, 1429–36.

◆ Laufer, Y., and Elboim-Gabyzon, M. (2011) Does sensory transcutaneous electrical stimulation enhance motor recovery following a stroke? A systematic review. *Neurorehabil Neural Repair*, **25**, 799–809.

◆ Lee, A., and Fan, L.T. (2009) Stimulation of the wrist acupuncture point P6 for preventing postoperative nausea and vomiting. *Cochrane Database Syst Rev*, CD003281.

◆ van Dijk, K.R., Scherder, E.J., Scheltens, P., and Sergeant, J.A. (2002) Effects of transcutaneous electrical nerve stimulation (TENS) on non-pain related cognitive and behavioural functioning. *Rev Neurosci*, **13**, 257–70.

Chapter 11 discusses the use of self-administered TENS-like devices to manage painful and non-painful ailments.

TENS-like devices

Introduction

Electrotherapy using non-invasive techniques has its roots in physiotherapy and rehabilitation medicine where treatment took place in the clinic under the supervision of a trained therapist using large, costly, non-portable devices. Technological advances have resulted in reductions in the size and cost of electrotherapeutic devices with increasing varieties of self-administered, hand-held TENS-like devices available to practitioners and the general public. TENS-like devices deliver electrical currents across the intact surface of the skin using pulse generators with technical output specifications that differ from a standard TENS device (for review, see Johnson, 2001a; Johnson, 2001b). The purpose of this chapter is to provide a snapshot of the characteristics, the mechanism of action, and the effectiveness of some commercially available TENS-like devices.

> A TENS-like device delivers electrical currents across the intact surface of the skin but has design features and/or technical output specifications that differ from a standard TENS device.

Categorizing TENS-like devices

TENS-like devices could be categorized according to:

1 Technical output characteristics of the device

2 Type and position of electrodes used. For example, hand-held pen-like or baton-like devices that deliver currents using a single-point electrode or treatment head with or without lead wires

3 Principles of action including stimulating central nervous system, peripheral nervous system, acupuncture points, or areas of low skin resistance

4 Clinical indications such as pain relief, wound healing, and improving circulation.

Most commonly, categorization is made according to broad, technical output characteristics of the device. Some TENS-like devices are considered to be electrotherapeutic modalities in their own right (e.g. interferential current therapy, neuromuscular electrical stimulation, high-voltage pulsed current, microcurrent electrical therapy), and are used for specific purposes (Table 11.1) However, other TENS-like devices have design features that are unique to the device (e.g. transcutaneous spinal electoanalgesia, transcutaneous piezoelectric current, and non-invasive interactive neurostimulation

Table 11.1 Clinical utility of broad categories of TENS-like devices

Device	Utility
Interferential current therapy	Deep tissue (muscle) stimulation, e.g. pelvic floor therapy
Transcutaneous neuromuscular electrical stimulation	Muscle strengthening and prevention of muscle atrophy and functional mobility
High-voltage pulsed current	Wound healing and the management of swelling
Microcurrent electrical therapy	Tissue healing
Low-intensity transcutaneous cranial electrical stimulation	Psychomotor conditions

(InterX®)), or are similar to a standard TENS device (e.g. Pain Doctor, Action Potential Simulation (APS), H-Wave Therapy).

Interferential current therapy

Interferential current therapy delivers two out-of-phase currents (e.g. 2000 Hz and 2100 Hz) which overcome skin impedance and collide to generate an amplitude-modulated interference 'beat' wave (e.g. 100 Hz) within deep-seated tissue (for review, see Palmer & Martin, 2008) (Figure 11.1). Electrodes include self-adhesive hypoallergenic, carbon–rubber surrounded by cloth pads soaked in saline, and vacuum-pump suction electrodes. Generally, interferential current therapy devices are trolley-based units with treatment delivered by practitioners under the constraints of the clinical rota, although portable devices are also marketed to the general public (between GB£50.00 and GB£300.00).

Interferential current therapy is used to manage pain and inflammation, to facilitate tissue repair (including bone healing), and to re-educate muscle, especially for incontinence. It is claimed that the amplitude-modulated wave is the active element of interferential current therapy although a direct action of carrier currents may also contribute to pain relief. Studies measuring experimental pain provide evidence that interferential current therapy is superior to placebo but no different from TENS. Different amplitude-modulated frequencies or swing patterns have not been shown to affect hypoalgesia. There are no systematic reviews covering interferential current therapy for pain relief or for any other condition, although interferential current therapy has been included in systematic reviews of electrotherapies in general. RCTs have found superiority over placebo and equivalence to other treatments for chronic low back pain but not for osteoarthrosis of the knee or jaw pain. Evidence suggests that interferential current therapy may be beneficial for pharyngeal dysphagia, constipation, and faecal and urinary incontinence (Chapter 10, 198–200). There is a lack of good-quality experimental evidence to support claims made in textbooks about the specificity of interferential current therapy protocols for various conditions (Johnson, 1999). When used for pain relief, interferential current therapy is delivered to generate strong, non-painful electrical paraesthesiae at

(a) Interferential current therapy

(b) Microcurrent therapy

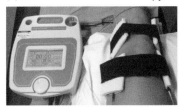

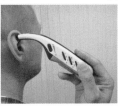

(c) Transcutaneous spinal electroanalgesia (TSE)

(d) Transcutaneous piezoelectric current

(e) Non-invasive interactive neurostimulation

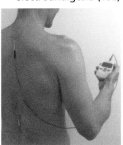

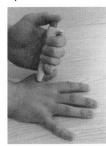

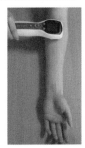

Fig. 11.1 Examples of TENS-like devices. (a) Interferential current therapy, (b) microcurrent electrical therapy, (c) transcutaneous spinal electroanalgesia (TSE), (d) transcutaneous piezoelectric current (Pain®Gone), and (e) non-invasive interactive neurostimulation (InterX®).

the site of pain, an approach comparable with conventional TENS. If there are no differences in the analgesic profiles of TENS and interferential current therapy then it would be wiser to lend a standard TENS device, or a portable interferential current therapy device, to patients so that they can self-administer treatment as frequently as needed.

Transcutaneous neuromuscular electrical stimulation (tNMES)

Neuromuscular electrical stimulation (NMES) uses pulsed electrical currents to stimulate motor nerves to produce a fused tetanic muscle contraction with or without joint movement. This can be achieved transcutaneously (tNMES) or via electrodes implanted to stimulate small, deep muscles and nerves that are difficult to penetrate with transcutaneous currents (for review, see McDonough, 2008). Neuromuscular electrical stimulation is used therapeutically to reduce pain, prevent atrophy, improve tissue oxygenation and cardiopulmonary conditioning. Neuromuscular electrical stimulation is used functionally to aid limb mobility, bladder function, and respiratory control. Some NMES devices are housed in braces and prosthesis with advanced systems harnessing signals from the cerebral cortex to enhance interfacing with a neuroprosthesis to facilitate movement. In general, tNMES is used therapeutically in rehabilitation of spinal cord injury, stroke, brain injury, multiple sclerosis, cerebral palsy, and bladder dysfunction.

An early Cochrane review found benefit for passive humeral lateral rotation but not for post-stroke shoulder pain, although more recent systematic reviews have been inconclusive for patellofemoral pain syndrome and knee osteoarthritis (Giggins et al., 2012). Systematic reviews provide evidence that tNMES improves outcomes for anterior cruciate ligament reconstruction, surgery after ligament and meniscal injuries, knee osteoarthritis, stroke, spinal cord injury, cerebral palsy, chronic heart failure, and chronic obstructive pulmonary disease. Inconclusive reviews exist for hand function and coordination of reach-to-grasp following stroke, post-total knee replacement, and within-cast muscle training.

High-voltage pulsed current (HVPC)

High-voltage pulsed current (HVPC) devices deliver twin-peaked monophasic pulsed current of 10–500 V (500 ohm load) with short pulse durations (microseconds) to increase penetration of tissue to recruit motor nerves in innervated muscle and without discomfort for the patient (for review, see Watson, 2008). Electrodes include sponge, traditional carbon–rubber, and hand-held point electrodes. High-voltage pulsed current is used for wound healing, muscle strengthening, and the management of swelling, with less attention given to its use for pain relief.

A systematic review of 11 pre-clinical studies found that HVPC reduced oedema (Snyder et al., 2010). Evidence suggests that HVPC improves tissue oxygenation and is superior to placebo for healing various types of chronic wounds, although there are no systematic reviews. Studies have found improvements in healing of pressure ulcers associated with spinal cord injury, repetitive stress injuries of the wrist, Bell's Palsy, and Levator ani syndrome, although RCTs found no clinical benefit on return-to-play after lateral ankle sprain or for post-traumatic pain following lateral ankle sprain. Studies using healthy humans failed to detect differences between HVPC and TENS on electrically induced pain threshold and tolerance.

Microcurrent electrical therapy

Microcurrent electrical therapy is low-intensity direct current which delivers monophasic or biphasic pulsed microamperage currents, commonly as adjustable pulse frequencies (0.5–150 pps), with periodic reversals in polarity. Probe, pad, or clip electrodes are used at acupuncture points, trigger points, on the ears, or over the site of pain (Figure 11.1). Microcurrent electrical therapy was developed from claims that a microampere current of injury occurred at the site of tissue damage, and that delivering microampere but not milliampere currents would assist tissue growth and healing (for review, see Poltawski & Watson, 2009).

Microcurrents are 1000 amperes smaller than TENS and do not generate sensations, suggesting that there is limited activation of low-threshold afferent fibres. Evidence suggests that microcurrent electrical therapy promotes protein synthesis, secretion of growth factors, and migration of human dermal and nasal fibroblasts, and reduces bacterial adherence, growth, and survival. Good-quality animal studies in the 1990s found that microcurrent electrical therapy did not accelerate healing of experimentally induced wounds although recently, studies from Medonoca and colleagues using Wistar rats found that microcurrent electrical therapy improved healing of open wounds. A meta-analysis of physical therapies for Achilles tendinopathy found limited evidence of efficacy for microcurrent electrical therapy (Sussmilch-Leitch et al., 2012). Evidence from clinical trials is inconsistent for neck pain, chronic low back pain, diabetic neuropathy, migraine and chronic headaches, wounds, temporomandibular joint, lateral epicondylitis, and spinal cord injury, although recent studies suggest that microcurrent electrical therapy may improve wound healing from burns, post-operative analgesic consumption, and may help promote tendon normalization in chronic tennis elbow.

Low-intensity transcutaneous cranial electrical stimulation

Low-intensity transcutaneous cranial electrical stimulation devices used to stimulate the brain are categorized as either constant current (transcranial direct current stimulation) or low-intensity, non-constant current (for review, see Fregni et al., 2007; Zaghi et al., 2010). Output specifications vary greatly between manufacturers and some devices are sold directly to the general public for self-treatment. Benefits have been reported for tinnitus, stroke-caused motor defects, fibromyalgia, depression, epilepsy, Parkinson's disease, depression, Alzheimer's disease, migraine, and central neuropathic pain. The effects of transcranial direct current stimulation are modified when combined with medication and other neurostimulation techniques, such as repetitive transcranial magnetic stimulation.

Transcranial low-intensity direct current stimulation is often administered in clinics under the supervision of health-care professionals using current amplitudes between 260 μA and 2 mA and sponge-based rectangular pads (25–35 cm^2) placed on the scalp, or electrodes attached (clipped) to the ears. Transcranial low-intensity direct current stimulation does not generate action potentials per se, but instead it polarizes brain tissue by modifying transmembrane neuronal potential which modulates both excitability and the firing rate of neurones. Excitation of cortical tissue occurs beneath the anode and decreased excitability occurs beneath the cathode, and this may cause longer-term synaptic changes.

Non-invasive, low-intensity, non-constant currents are delivered using various techniques including cranial electrotherapy stimulation, Limoge currents, Lebedev currents, and transcranial alternating current stimulation. Putative mechanisms include activation of descending pain-inhibitory mechanisms, modulation of craniospinal nerve activity and neurotransmitter release, suppression of peripheral and central sensitization, interruption of cortical activity by introducing cortical noise, and synchronization of brain activity.

Evidence from clinical research is contradictory but generally positive about potential efficacy of low-intensity transcutaneous cranial electrical stimulation. A Cochrane review with a meta-analysis of five transcranial direct current stimulation trials (83 people) found no differences between active and placebo transcranial direct current stimulation of the motor cortex for chronic pain. A meta-analysis of 18 studies found that transcranial direct current stimulation and repetitive transcranial magnetic stimulation of the primary motor cortex reduced pain (Zaghi et al., 2011).

Transcutaneous direct current stimulation over the spinal cord

Currents normally used in transcutaneous direct current stimulation have been delivered on the skin overlying the spinal cord to modulate spinal excitability in lemniscal, spinothalamic, and motor systems to improve pain and sensory motor disorders (Cogiamanian et al., 2011). There are no RCTs or case reports on the effectiveness of transcutaneous direct current stimulation over the spinal cord.

Transcutaneous spinal electroanalgesia (TSE)

Transcutaneous spinal electroanalgesia (TSE) devices were developed by Macdonald and Coates to deliver high-frequency (600–10,000 pps) pulsed currents at a high voltage (~180 V) and short pulse duration (1.5–4 μs) via electrodes at T1 and T12 or straddling C3–C5 (Figure 11.1). It is claimed that TSE devices reduce central sensitization and are beneficial in the management of various painful conditions including back pain, arthritis, headache, migraine, fibromyalgia and neuralgias, and stress (see <http://www.acticare.com/default.asp>). There are no systematic reviews on the effectiveness of TSE, and small-scale RCTs have failed to detect differences with placebo for chronic pain following breast cancer treatment, chronic low back pain, or chronic critical limb ischaemia (Thompson et al., 2008).

Transcutaneous piezoelectric devices

Transcutaneous piezoelectric devices generate a high-voltage (claimed to be 15 000 V) single rectangular, short-duration, pulsed piezoelectric microampere current (6 μA) by forcing two crystals (piezoelectric elements) together when clicking a plunger button on an oversized pen-like device. Examples include Pain®Gone (e.g. <http://www.medi-direct.co.uk/paingone.html>, Figure 11.1), and Piezo No Needle Acupuncture Pen (e.g. <http://www.masterformula.net/piezo_pen.htm>). Electric charge is delivered through the skin via single-point electrode producing a sensation that resembles a mild pinprick. Research on healthy humans has found long-lasting inhibitory aftereffects of the nociceptive RIII flexion reflex and local neurogenic inflammation of the skin, but no differences in pain outcomes compared with placebo. Case series suggest that piezoelectric stimulation may reduce back and neck pain, cancer pain, chronic musculoskeletal pain, and lateral epicondylitis.

Non-invasive interactive neurostimulation (InterX®)

Non-invasive interactive neurostimulation (InterX®) uses a single electrode head of outer and inner concentric stainless-steel electrodes to deliver currents across the skin without the use of electrode gels (e.g. <http://www.nrg-unlimited.com>, Figure 11.1). Treatment consists of scanning and stimulation. During scanning the electrode head of the non-invasive interactive neurostimulation device is moved across the surface of the skin to search for areas of low impedance. During stimulation, interactive neurostimulation currents are delivered to areas of the skin with low impedance points. Interactive neurostimulation currents are high-amplitude pulsed, damped, biphasic, sinusoidal waveform currents with automatic adjustments of the shape of the current according to 'tissue status'. There is tentative evidence that non-invasive interactive neurostimulation alters levels of biomarkers of respiration, lymphocyte metabolism, and cytokine production, and placebo-controlled trials have found that non-invasive interactive neurostimulation reduced pain associated with knee osteoarthritis, mechanical neck conditions, trochanteric fracture of the femur, AO type-B2 ankle fractures with comminution and total knee replacement surgery (Nigam et al., 2011; Schabrun et al., 2012).

Pain Doctor

Pain Doctor is a baton-sized hand-held device that delivers currents with characteristics similar to TENS including adjustable pulse amplitude and three preset pulse frequencies (i.e. 1 pps, 15 pps, or 22 pps, e.g. <http://www.medi-direct.co.uk/paindoctor.html>). Treatment is administered to the site of pain via a single contact electrode with a carbon–rubber treatment head (2.8 cm × 1.2 cm), with the handle forming the second electrode. The user experiences TENS sensation at the treatment head and in the hand which is holding the device. The treatment-head electrode enables delivery of currents to discrete points on the surface of the body, and enables individuals to 'hunt' for optimal electrode sites by moving the electrode head across the surface of the skin whilst stimulating. Reapplying gel frequently during treatment is critical to prevent skin irritation from the high density of the current. Termination of current can be immediately achieved by lifting the electrode off the skin surface. Pain Doctor also delivers vibration individually or in combination with TENS. The mechanism of action will be similar to conventional TENS, although no experimental studies have been performed. There are no published trials on Pain Doctor.

Cutaneous field stimulation

Cutaneous field stimulation uses a flexible rubber plate with 16 needle-like electrodes (4 × 4 matrix) as a cathode, and a self-adhesive surface electrode (Uni-patch, Re-Ply) as an anode. The intention of cutaneous field stimulation is to stimulate unmyelinated C-fibres to mimic scratching without skin damage (Nilsson et al., 1997). Electrodes on the needle plate are activated consecutively at a frequency of 4 pps, a pulse duration 1.0 ms, and a voltage of less than 10 V (current < 0.8 mA). This voltage is sufficient to stimulate cutaneous nerve fibres because the current density at the sharp electrode tips is high. Cutaneous field stimulation has been used for symptomatic relief of pain and itch associated with dermatitis, and mechanisms include long-term depression of central nociceptive cell transmission. Studies have found that cutaneous field stimulation generates longer-lasting inhibition of acute histamine evoked itch and cutaneous pain than TENS, and reductions in chronic itch due to atopic dermatitis, hereditary localized pruritus, generalized itch, and IgE-mediated allergy without adverse effects on contact dermatitis (Nilsson et al., 2003).

Action potential simulation

Action potential simulation uses a monophasic square wave with exponential decay and a DC offset that remains at 5 V. Pulse durations are 800 μs–6.6 ms and pulse frequencies fixed at ~150 pps, with pulse amplitude adjustable between 0 mA and 24.4 mA into a 500 ohm load. Currents are administered using two electrodes attached close to the site of pain. Treatment protocols focus on treatment times in multiples of eight minutes (e.g. 8 and 16 minutes), although the rationale for this approach is vague. Action potential simulation is indicated to relieve pain, to reduce inflammation and swelling, and to increase mobility and bone growth. Early research was positive and conducted by Berger and colleagues although more recent studies have failed to find differences between action potential simulation, TENS, and interference current therapy on skin temperature and mechanical pain threshold. Randomized controlled clinical trials have failed to detect superiority over placebo for chronic low back pain, mobility and swelling associated with osteoarthritis or fibromyalgia, although the investigators argue that action potential simulation is still a viable treatment (Fengler et al., 2007).

H-Wave Therapy

H-Wave therapy uses a biphasic exponentially decaying waveform pulsed current (~25–35 V) of long duration (4–16 ms) with frequencies of 2 pps or 60 pps delivered via two electrodes placed on the site of pain, acupuncture points, or muscle bellies. H-Wave therapy is indicated for tissue healing, reducing inflammation and oedema, and relieving pain for soft tissue injuries. Blum and colleagues suggest that H-Wave therapy causes small muscle fibre contraction without activation of motor nerves of larger white muscle fibres or small-diameter sensory fibres (e.g. Aδ and C nociceptive fibres). This reduces tetanizing fatigue and discomfort associated with other forms of electrical stimulation. Evidence from animal studies suggests that H-Wave therapy may stimulate red-slow-twitch skeletal muscle fibres and small smooth muscle fibres within the lymphatic vessels leading to fluid shifts and reduced oedema, and also enhancing microcirculation and angiogenesis via a nitric oxide mechanism. Placebo-controlled studies using healthy humans by McDowell and colleagues suggest that H-Wave therapy reduces peripheral nerve conduction and experimental mechanical and ischaemic pain, and increases skin blood flow. A systematic review with meta-analysis of five studies (6535 participants) found that H-Wave therapy decreased analgesic consumption and pain ratings for various chronic soft-tissue inflammation and neuropathic conditions, and improved functionality with no evidence of any adverse effects (Blum et al., 2008).

Transcutaneous electrical acupoint stimulation (TEAS)

The term transcutaneous electrical acupoint stimulation (TEAS) is often used to describe electrical stimulation of classical Chinese acupoints using non-painful pulsed currents alternating between 2 pps with a long pulse duration (e.g. 600 μs) and 15 pps with a shorter pulse duration (e.g. 300 μs), at three-second intervals. Commonly TEAS is administered to the PC6 (Neiguan) acupuncture point using a device worn like a wristwatch, with a pair of gold-plated electrodes that contact the skin between two tendons on the anterior aspect of the wrist over the median nerve delivering intermittent electrical pulses ranging from 10 mA to 35 mA (e.g. Reliefband®; see <http://reliefband.com.au>). Users titrate amplitude to produce a mild tingling sensation radiating into the palm and fingers for 30 minutes each day over a period of weeks (e.g. 12 weeks).

Transcutaneous electrical acupoint stimulation is indicated for nausea and vomiting associated with pregnancy, motion sickness, and medication including chemotherapy, and for fatigue, insomnia, and depression. Outcome is dependent on the acupuncture point stimulated, with PC6, ST36, and CV12 modulating the vomiting centre for antiemetic effects, and LI4, ST36, SP6, and PC6 elevating plasma arginine-vasopressin and oxytocin with improvements in emotional state, fear, and anxiety. Studies using healthy humans found that TEAS reduced experimental pain and enhanced the rate of muscle-force recovery after strenuous knee extension/flexion exercise. Cochrane reviews provide evidence that TEAS at PC6 reduces post-operative nausea and vomiting but not chemotherapy-induced nausea and vomiting, and with mixed results for pregnancy-related nausea and vomiting (Ezzo et al., 2006) (Chapter 10, 201). Evidence from RCTs suggests improvements in pregnancy rate in patients undergoing in vitro fertilisation (IVF); improvement in depressive mood among elders in a nursing home; reduction of fatigue, improvement of sleep quality and depressed mood during routine haemodialysis treatment; and reductions in pain intensity, stress, and stiffness in adults with sub-acute non-specific spinal pain.

Summary

1 The diversity of TENS-like devices available on the market and inconsistency of terminology makes synthesis of information extremely difficult.

2 Interferential current therapy, neuromuscular electrical stimulation, high-voltage pulsed current, and microcurrent electrical therapy have all been used for rehabilitation for many years.

3 Low-intensity transcutaneous cranial electrical stimulation, cutaneous field stimulation, and transcutaneous electrical acupoint stimulation are used to manage psychomotor conditions, itch, and nausea respectively.

4 Evidence supporting efficacy for the variety of self-administered TENS-like devices developed for pain relief is far weaker than that for a standard TENS device.

5 The driving force for the development of some TENS-like devices appears to have been the incorporation of technologically impressive output characteristics rather than a sound physiological rationale.

Further reading

+ Johnson, M. (2001) Transcutaneous Electrical Nerve Stimulation (TENS) and TENS-like devices. Do they provide pain relief? *Pain Reviews*, **8**, 121–8.
+ Luedtke, K., Rushton, A., Wright, C., Geiss, B., Juergens, T.P., and May, A. (2012) Transcranial direct current stimulation for the reduction of clinical and experimentally induced pain: a systematic review and meta-analysis. *Clin J Pain*, **28**, 452–61.

- Palmer, S., and Martin, D. (2008) Interferential Current. In Watson, T. (ed.) *Electrotherapy. Evidence-Based Practice*. Churchill Livingstone Elsevier, Edinburgh, 217–315.
- Robertson, V., Ward, A., Low, J., and Reed, A. (2006) *Electrotherapy Explained: principles and practice*. 4th edn. Butterworth-Heinemann, Oxford.
- Watson, T. (ed.) (2008) *Electrotherapy. Evidence-Based Practice*. Churchill Livingstone Elsevier, Edinburgh. <http://www.electrotherapy.org/modalities>.

Chapter 10 discusses future directions for TENS research and clinical practice.

Chapter 12

Future directions

Introduction

In general, patients and practitioners are satisfied that TENS is a useful adjunct for pain management because it relieves pain and improves the performance of normal daily activities. TENS is inexpensive, safe, and it can be self-administered. However, the findings of the sizable quantity of RCTs are often contradictory causing uncertainty about the efficacy and effectiveness of TENS for some painful conditions. Shortcomings in the design and implementation of RCTs, and confusion about optimal technique for TENS remains a problem. Interestingly, the design of modern-day TENS devices is very similar to that of their original counterparts in the 1970s, despite major advances in technology. One reason for this is that existing TENS devices are an efficient means of stimulating peripheral nerves and they retail at relatively low cost. Nevertheless, the inconvenience of applying electrodes and lead wires and the difficulty of targeting specific nerves remain barriers to effective long-term use. Recently, Gladwell (2013) investigated the experiences of TENS users with chronic musculoskeletal pain and found that they were very strategic in their use of TENS with a broad spectrum of benefits reported including pain relief, reducing sensations of muscle tension and spasm, reducing medication, achieving specific functional goals and enhancing rest periods. Gladwell concluded that TENS was a complex intervention and that outcome measures used in previously published RCTs had only limited capacity to capture benefits reported by patients. Gladwell proposed a context-mechanism-outcome model to assess TENS outcomes in future RCTs. The purpose of this chapter is to explore future directions for TENS research and clinical practice by covering:

- Future developments in TENS technology
- Current status of knowledge
- Future directions for TENS research

Future developments in TENS technology

Finding electrode sites that distribute TENS sensation into the painful area can be difficult because electrodes have to be physically removed from the skin and repositioned to alter the distribution of the currents. Additional electrodes could be used to generate TENS sensation over a larger area although most TENS devices are restricted to two channels, or occasionally, four channels. Often the electrical characteristics for each channel cannot be adjusted independently. Electrode lead wires also prove a hindrance, especially when trying to run lead wires through clothes, and having to take care not to snag the lead wires when holding the TENS device whilst adjusting settings.

TENS devices that clip directly on to one electrode without the need for electrode lead wires have been available for a number of years. These have not been as popular as traditional TENS systems with lead wires, perhaps because the area of stimulation possible using these single-electrode devices is smaller than achieved when using two standard electrodes. Wireless TENS devices for back pain are available and use a pulse generator integrated into a self-adhesive electrode that attaches to the lower back. The pulse generator is controlled using a wireless remote control with a battery life of over 150×30-minute treatment sessions (WiTouch™, ~US$139.00; see <http://www.tensproducts.com/WiTouch-Wireless-TENS-unit-with-remote_p_294.html>: video available at: <http://www.youtube.com/watch?v=SXHFcMAem7w>).

Electrode arrays enable control of the distribution of the electric field and negate the need to move electrodes physically to target stimulation precisely. They are used in implantable electrodes (e.g. spinal cord stimulation and peripheral nerve stimulators). Prototypes for 16-channel and 60-channel (256 pads) electrode sleeves for transcutaneous neuromuscular electrical stimulators have been developed to enable real-time control of the spatial distribution of current to elicit specific movements such as selective finger and wrist extension movements (Keller et al., 2006; Kuhn et al., 2009). Smart electrodes that provide electrical feedback from the skin and communicate with the TENS device without the need for electrode lead wires are also being developed. Kolen and colleagues (2012) manufactured a prototype matrix electrode consisting of 16 small, circular electrode elements, 10 mm in diameter, in a square 4×4 configuration (Figure 12.1). The matrix electrode was held in position using a brace-like garment on the knee. Each electrode element measures skin impedance and delivers current via a single electrode element to this point with all other electrode elements combined as a counter electrode. Bluetooth technology was used to transmit information from the pulse generator to the electrode array. Similarly, cutaneous field stimulation utilizes 16 needle-like electrodes fixed in a 4×4 matrix on a flexible rubber patch to stimulate C-fibres (Chapter 11, 209). Deepwave® is a commercially available system used to deliver currents through the skin directly into deep tissue at the site of pain (see <http://www.biowave.com>). Deepwave® utilizes a 2.5 inch-diameter sterile, single-use disposable patch electrode with 1000 microneedle array (0.74 mm in length) to administer two sine waves of 3858 Hz and 3980 Hz with a amplitude range of 0.0–27.5 Vrms.

In the future it is likely that improvement in electrode array design will enable more precise targeting of currents, including greater depth of penetration, and this is likely to improve efficacy and convenience of application. Such electrode arrays will be integrated into more versatile electrode garments. Smart electrodes that monitor the status of the skin and underlying tissue, and then modify the electrical output characteristics of currents have already been developed, although the assumption that monitoring and modification of output will improve efficacy has not been proven. Voice-activated pulse generators will negate the need to fidget with buttons and dials to adjust electrical characteristics, and usage data will be downloaded into diary software to enable analysis and monitoring of progress. Whether any of these exciting developments lead to substantial improvements in clinical outcome remains to be seen.

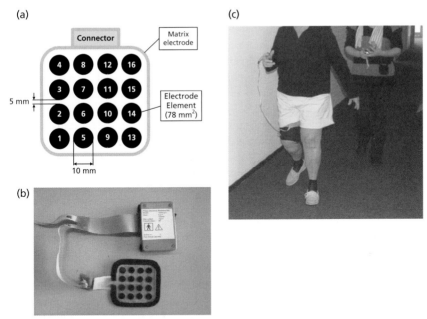

Fig. 12.1 Prototype TENS system using an electrode array to measure skin impedance and to target stimulation spatially. (a) Schematic of the matrix electrode with 16 individual electrode elements with one active electric element and other electrode elements combined as a counter-electrode. (b) Prototype battery-operated electrical pulse generator (above) and matrix electrode (below) and (c) matrix electrode attached to the skin and held in position using a brace-like garment.

Current status of knowledge

The purpose of this book has been to evaluate research findings on TENS to inform safe and appropriate TENS technique in clinical practice. Evidence from basic science and clinical research suggests that conventional TENS is the most effective approach in most instances. This involves using TENS to generate a strong, non-painful TENS sensation within the painful area whenever relief from pain is needed, something that is intuitive to most patients and practitioners.

Research from the basic sciences

There is strong evidence from electrophysiological and behavioural studies using animals and healthy humans that activity in low-threshold cutaneous afferents during strong, non-painful conventional TENS inhibits activity of centrally transmitting nociceptive cells in somatic receptive fields (i.e. segmental), with neural circuitry predominantly located within the spinal cord (i.e. spinal). Recruitment of deeper afferents (e.g. using AL-TENS to produce muscle twitching) may produce stronger and prolonged inhibition with neural circuitry located in the spinal cord and brainstem (i.e. supraspinal). Brainstem structures include the periaqueductal grey and nucleus raphe magnus that form descending pain-inhibitory feedback loops to the spinal cord. Increasing the intensity of TENS to recruit high-threshold cutaneous afferents generates more powerful and prolonged inhibition of central nociceptive transmission cells spreading beyond somatic receptive fields, but stimulation itself is painful is unacceptable for many patients. When used in this way TENS probably acts as a form of counter-irritation (i.e. via diffuse noxious inhibitory controls). In addition, antidromic impulses generated in peripheral afferents during TENS will block orthodromic impulses arising from sensory receptors.

However, this is an oversimplification of the situation. Electrical fields generated during TENS permeate nerve bundles and free nerve endings of many different types of neurones, resulting in activity in a variety of neuronal systems. At intensities below motor threshold, low-frequency conventional TENS predominantly acts via μ-opioid, GABA, serotonin, and noradrenaline receptors, whereas high-frequency conventional TENS predominantly acts via δ-opioid and GABA receptors. Opioids, cholecystokinin, and NMDA receptors appear to have a role in the development of TENS tolerance.

The key determinant of physiological action will be the type of peripheral nerve fibre that is activated during TENS. However, the spatial resolution of TENS in underlying tissue is low because the electric field disperses due to impedance at the electrode–skin interface and the variability in the compostion and density of tissue at different depths of the body. This hinders the ability to target nerve bundles precisely, so in many ways TENS is a blunt instrument. This imprecision has been reflected in the findings of studies using healthy human participants exposed to experimentally induced pain that have investigated the role of specific electrical characteristics and electrode positions for optimal hypoalgesia.

Research from studies on healthy humans

There is strong evidence from studies using healthy humans exposed to experimental pain that TENS needs to be delivered at a strong, non-painful intensity in order to achieve meaningful hypoalgesia. This is achieved by titrating pulse amplitude to recruit low-threshold nerve fibres within a nerve bundle. Evidence from human studies is inconsistent for the effect of pulse frequency, pulse duration, and pulse pattern, and optimal settings for these characteristics have not been found. It is possible that the specific neurophysiological and pharmacological actions associated with specific electrical characteristics of TENS in electrophysiological and behavioural studies in animal models of nociception do not translate into meaningful differences in outcome in humans, or that specific effects are not amenable to generalization. Evidence from neurophysiological studies recording changes in reflex activity and somatosensory evoked potentials in humans suggest that TENS gates nociceptive information in the central nervous system in somatic receptive fields, and not via non-specific mechanisms associated with distraction. However, a definitive systematic study on the effect of electrode position on experimentally induced pain has not been forthcoming.

Evidence from the basic sciences and from studies on healthy humans enables strict control of experimental variables that can confound findings, but research on patients in pain is necessary to confirm that these physiological effects of TENS produce meaningful outcomes in clinical practice.

Research from patients with pain

Evidence suggests that TENS is safe, and the incidence and severity of adverse events are low. There are no reliable predictors of treatment success so any type of pain may respond to TENS. There is tentative evidence that non-responders may have a nervous system non-responsive to sensory stimuli, unrealistic expectations about treatment outcome, and/or a lack of commitment to regularly administer TENS. Over 50 per cent of individuals who try TENS report meaningful improvements in pain, activity level, and analgesic consumption in the short term, but for many, this declines over time. Successful long-term users administer a strong, non-painful TENS sensation within the site of pain but there is no reliable evidence of a relationship between specific combinations of electrical characteristics of TENS and outcome for specific pain types. AL-TENS may be useful when patient response to conventional TENS is sub-maximal.

The largest meta-analyses provide evidence that TENS is efficacious for chronic musculoskeletal pain and post-operative pain, although most systematic reviews are unable to judge efficacy because of insufficient good-quality evidence. Systematic reviews that have set criteria for appropriate technique and dosage tend to be more positive than those that do not. Recommendations about the use of TENS from professional and government bodies are inconsistent. The challenge has been designing and funding large-scale, good-quality research.

> There is sufficient evidence from clinical research to suggest that TENS should remain an adjunct to core treatment for pain management.

Future directions for TENS research

From an evidence-based-medicine perspective, large multi-centred trials are needed. A pragmatic trial on TENS against standard care would determine effectiveness and an RCT would determine clinical efficacy. The Centers for Medicare & Medicaid Services in the USA suggest that a valid placebo-RCT on TENS for chronic low back pain should include a description and confirmation of TENS application, use of a sham (placebo) TENS that is appropriately blinded, standardization of concurrent interventions and standard care, and a sample size adequate to detect an appropriate effect size (Jacques et al., 2012). This approach is not new but to date has failed to deliver a robust RCT. It is ethically unacceptable to continue to conduct clinical trials that align to the attributes of good design yet neglect consideration of specific aspects of operationalizing of these attributes in line with the current status of TENS knowledge. This could be facilitated by the development and publication of:

1 explicit criteria for the delivery of adequate TENS technique and dose in a similar manner to that published for acupuncture and low-level laser therapy (White et al., 2008a).

2 reporting standards for TENS interventions in studies and especially clinical trials based on Consolidated Standards of Reporting Trials (CONSORT) and similar to Standards for Reporting Interventions in Clinical Trials of Acupuncture (STRICTA) guidelines for acupuncture (MacPherson et al., 2010).

These can be used in combination with criteria for judging directions of bias associated with allocation, application, and assessment of TENS interventions in RCTs that have already been published by Bennett and colleagues (2011) (Table 12.1). Importantly, they (Bennett et al., 2011) suggest that at least 200 participants may be required in each trial arm to achieve sufficient statistical power and this can only be achieved from a fully funded large-scale RCTs, as has been achieved in clinical trials on acupuncture.

An enriched enrolment, randomized withdrawal design using a two-stage recruitment process may be more appropriate than a traditional RCT. Participants initially responding to TENS would be identified in stage one and then randomized to receive an active or placebo intervention in stage two. Stage one would provide data on the number of individuals initially responding to TENS or experiencing an adverse event, and stage two would provide data on whether the positive response was due to the TENS or a placebo response. The challenge in designing an enriched enrolment randomized withdrawal trial for TENS is that it may be difficult to reduce expectation bias in stage two because participants would have been instructed to administer TENS at a strong, non-painful intensity in stage one. It is not possible to blind the strong, non-painful TENS sensation to participants, although it is possible to create uncertainty as to whether the intervention was active or inactive (placebo) using prompts given in pre-study instruction (Chapter 8, 170). Participant uncertainty (blinding) can be assessed post-study by asking whether patients believed that the device delivering the intervention was functioning properly (Deyo et al., 1990b).

There is a need to use reliable and valid outcome measures for TENS. Successful TENS users often report that TENS distracts them from their pain rather than relieves their pain. Clearly, the interaction between the sensation from TENS and the sensation of pain compromises estimations of the magnitude of pain reduction. Thus, measures of pain need to be combined with objective measurable outcomes, reflecting changes in normal daily activities, and they need to be meaningful and of relevance to the patient. A context-mechanism-outcome model to assess TENS outcomes as proposed by Gladwell (2013) should be considered in the design of future RCTs. Previous RCTs on TENS may have reported false negatives (type II errors) because investigators report mean outcomes where benefit derived by responders is averaged with absence of benefit from non-responders. As few patients manifest average response to pain-relieving interventions, analysing data using mean values may be inappropriate. It has been suggested that responder analyses that split the data into good response and not-so-good response may be a better approach to analysis, although few studies on TENS have used this approach (Moore et al., 2010).

Table 12.1 Suggested requirements for a methodologically robust clinical trial on TENS

Criterion	Operationalization
Allocation to treatment arm	
Randomized by adequate method	Using computer-generated codes
Adequate sample size per treatment arm	Reliable trials often require >200 patients per arm, although between 50 and 199 patients per arm may be sufficient depending on power calculation for the size of benefit expected within the study context
Allocation independent and blind to outcome assessor	Treatment allocation concealed from investigative team, including the outcome assessor. It may be impossible to blind the therapist, although sophisticated techniques can be used to create uncertainty about which treatment arm is 'active'. For example, 'TENS-naive' assistants can deliver training, and deliver TENS above and below sensory threshold
At least double blind, ideally triple blind	Treatment allocation concealed from patient and outcome assessor (double blind) and, if possible, therapist (triple blind). It is not possible to blind the patient to the sensory experience generated by different types of TENS and placebo (no current) TENS. However, uncertainty about which treatment arm is 'active' can be created (see below) and monitored using post-study questionnaires (Deyo et al., 1990b)
Calibration of patient expectations regarding sensations	In placebo (no current) TENS trials, patients could be told that:
	i) some types of TENS do not produce sensations during stimulation (i.e. microcurrent therapy, transcutaneous spinal electroanalgesia)
	ii) they may or may not experience sensations from the TENS device
	iii) they may or may not receive a placebo intervention
Train patient to self-administer treatment and test competency	Using a systematic approach similar to that used during a supervised trial of TENS on a new patient (Chapter 6, Box 6.1)
Calibration of patient expectations regarding intervention outcome and adherence to self-administered treatment	Use approach similar to a supervised trial of TENS on a new patient (Chapter 6, Box 6.1)
Maintenance of blinding monitored and described	Blinding should be monitored and instances of leakage documented. Measures should be taken to reduce the chance of un-blinding, e.g. patients instructed not to reveal what sensations they have experienced.
	Blinding can be evaluated using post-study questionnaires (Deyo et al., 1990b)

Table 12.1 (continued) Suggested requirements for a methodologically robust clinical trial on TENS

Criterion	Operationalization
Application of treatment	
TENS and placebo interventions administered over pain or segmental area	Electrodes applied over the painful area or proximal to the painful area along neuro-anatomical distribution
Active TENS intervention titrated to 'strong but comfortable'	The intensity of conventional TENS should be strong and non-painful (i.e. within therapeutic window). For AL-TENS, strong, non-painful muscle contractions should be visible
Authentic placebo control TENS device used	The placebo (no current) TENS device should look and behave similarly to the intervention device, including flashing lights and functioning display panel
Placebo control TENS titrated to specified setting	Patients instructed that if they do not feel a sensation, they should set the device at a fixed setting on the display (e.g. just over halfway on the intensity setting) or to vary according to need, although there will be no sensory experience. A transient TENS device may be useful (Rakel et al., 2010)
Intervention self-administered and compliance monitored	Patients shown how to apply, titrate, and remove device. A record of use or assessment of compliance made using a data logger (Pallett et al., 2013)
Duration of TENS applications >30 minutes	Optimal therapeutic effect can be expected after 30 minutes. In home trials, patients should use TENS regularly throughout the day whenever they are in pain, and for at least 30 minutes at a time
Duration of study >six weeks in chronic pain trials	Barriers to effective longer-term TENS use should be carefully assessed and resolved before the start of a trial on chronic pain using a run-in period (e.g. using an enriched enrolment randomised withdrawal design). Acute pain trials should extend to cover the expected duration of pain in that context (e.g. post-operative pain, procedural pain)
Concurrent analgesia standardized and monitored	Consistent doses of regular analgesic medication should be maintained as far as possible during the trial. Use of 'as-needed' analgesia needs to be carefully monitored and assessed for parity between treatment arms
Assessment of outcome	
Consider use of a 'context-mechanism-outcome' model to assess TENS outcomes. Primary outcome is usually pain intensity	Using pain measures recommended by IMMPACT (Initiative on Methods, Measurement, and Pain Assessment in Clinical Trials)

Table 12.1 (continued) Suggested requirements for a methodologically robust clinical trial on TENS

Criterion	Operationalization
Secondary outcomes should be functional and matched with patient expectations of TENS outcome	Use specific measureable functional goals which can be verified with evidence
Outcomes measured during TENS application	While TENS is still applied and switched on
Use responder analyses reporting proportion of responders to treatment arms	Report absolute numbers and percentage of patients in each trial arm achieving good response and poor response (Moore et al., 2010)
For pain, responders defined as >50 per cent or >30 per cent intensity reduction from baseline	Clinically meaningful improvement reported as numbers of patients experiencing >30 per cent reduction in pain intensity, or whose final intensity score is <30 mm
Adverse effects described	Including local reactions, increase in pain, and other adverse events

Clearly, some patients stop using TENS because a disproportionate amount of effort is needed for the amount of pain relief achieved. In Chapter 6 a case was put forward for 'calibrating' new TENS users so that they develop realistic expectations from treatment. There is an urgent need to investigate patients' experiences of using TENS, and especially barriers to effective use, to inform the development of strategies to maximise treatment outcome. Future research should focus on evaluating the effectiveness of calibrating patents' expectations of TENS and their ability to sustain motivation to self-administer treatment. A toolkit to help patients develop skills and knowledge to sustain their motivation to self-administer TENS and troubleshoot declining response is urgently needed.

Summary

Evidence reviewed in this textbook provides a framework of principles on which to administer TENS in clinical practice. However, perhaps more can be learned from trying to synthesize the research rather than examining the specific knowledge it contains. Making sense of research on TENS was at best challenging, and at worst futile. Often, amalgamation of research findings was hindered by inconsistent terminology, variability in clinical technique, and methodologically weak research study design.

Interestingly, evidence for efficacy for many conditions has changed over time and this instability has created uncertainty about whether TENS should be offered and the optimal technique to use in clinical practice. Evidence suggests that prescriptive, over-complicated clinical technique should be avoided despite advances in technology allowing ever-more impressive electronics to be incorporated into device design. Furthermore, the intricacies of neurophysiological mechanisms revealed from the basic sciences, and their relationship to specific characteristics of electrical stimulation may not translate to meaningful variations in clinical outcome in patients experiencing pain. This is because psychosocial factors have a crucial role in treatment outcome for pain relieving treatments.

The synthesis of evidence in this textbook also offers directions for future research and a framework for a methodologically robust clinical trial. It is remarkable that uncertainty about the effectiveness of TENS has persisted for so many decades despite a constant stream of new RCTs. Clinical experience suggests TENS is useful and this is supported by the vast quantity of case series and clinical studies without control groups. However, evidence from RCTs is needed to establish efficacy, and many RCTs are methodologically weak as they use inadequate sample sizes, sub-optimal TENS technique, and inappropriate outcome measurement protocols. Consequently, most systematic reviews find insufficient evidence on which to make a judgement about efficacy, although when sufficient good-quality RCTs are available, outcome tends to be positive, especially if clear criteria for adequacy of TENS technique and dosage were set *a priori*.

In 2004, the advice on analgesic options for the treatment of mild to moderate pain, published by the MHRA following recommendations from their Pain Management Working Group in consultation with the British Pain Society, was that:

Non-drug interventions including TENS [or acupuncture] should be considered for all patients and underpinned by advice on activity and lifestyle (Medicines and Healthcare products Regulatory Agency, 2006).

At present, there seems no reason to change this advice. TENS should remain an adjunct to core treatment for acute and chronic pain, unless evidence from an RCT meeting the requirements of a methodologically robust clinical trial on TENS demonstrates otherwise.

Further reading

- **Sluka, K.A., Bjordal, J.M., Marchand, S., and Rakel, B.A.** (2013) What Makes Transcutaneous Electrical Nerve Stimulation Work? Making Sense of the Mixed Results in the Clinical Literature. *Phys Ther*, Oct;93(10):1427–8.

References

Aarskog, R., Johnson, M.I., Demmink, J.H., Lofthus, A., Iversen, V., Lopes-Martins, R., Joensen, J., and Bjordal, J.M. (2007) Is mechanical pain threshold after transcutaneous electrical nerve stimulation (TENS) increased locally and unilaterally? A randomized placebo-controlled trial in healthy subjects. *Physiother Res Int*, **12**, 251–63.

Abou-Setta, A.M., Beaupre, L.A., Rashiq, S., Dryden, D.M., Hamm, M.P., Sadowski, C.A., Menon, M.R., Majumdar, S.R., Wilson, D.M., Karkhaneh, M., Mousavi, S.S., Wong, K., Tjosvold, L., and Jones, C.A. (2011) Comparative effectiveness of pain management interventions for hip fracture: a systematic review. *Ann Intern Med*, **155**, 234–45.

Ainsworth, L., Budelier, K., Clinesmith, M., Fiedler, A., Landstrom, R., Leeper, B.J., Moeller, L., Mutch, S., O'Dell, K., Ross, J., Radhakrishnan, R., and Sluka, K.A. (2006) Transcutaneous electrical nerve stimulation (TENS) reduces chronic hyperalgesia induced by muscle inflammation. *Pain*, **120**, 182–7.

Airaksinen, O., Brox, J.I., Cedraschi, C., Hildebrandt, J., Klaber-Moffett, J., Kovacs, F., Mannion, A.F., Reis, S., Staal, J.B., Ursin, H., and Zanoli, G. (2006) Chapter 4. European guidelines for the management of chronic nonspecific low back pain. *Eur Spine J*, **15 Suppl 2**, S192–300.

Akyuz, G., Guven, Z., Ozaras, N., and Kayhan, O. (1995) The effect of conventional transcutaneous electrical nerve stimulation on somatosensory evoked potentials. *Electromyogr Clin Neurophysiol*, **35**, 371–6.

Alabas, O.A., Tashani, O.A., Tabasam, G., and Johnson, M.I. (2012) Gender role affects experimental pain responses: a systematic review with meta-analysis. *Eur J Pain*, **16**, 1211–23.

Alon, G., Kantor, G., and Ho, H.S. (1994) Effects of electrode size on basic excitatory responses and on selected stimulus parameters. *J Orthop Sports Phys Ther*, **20**, 29–35.

Alrashdan, M.S., Park, J.C., Sung, M.A., Yoo, S.B., Jahng, J.W., Lee, T.H., Kim, S.J., and Lee, J.H. (2010) Thirty minutes of low intensity electrical stimulation promotes nerve regeneration after sciatic nerve crush injury in a rat model. *Acta Neurol Belg*, **110**, 168–79.

American Society of Anesthesiologists (2010) Practice guidelines for chronic pain management: an updated report by the American Society of Anesthesiologists Task Force on Chronic Pain Management and the American Society of Regional Anesthesia and Pain Medicine. *Anesthesiology*, **112**, 810–33.

Anderson, S.I., Whatling, P., Hudlicka, O., Gosling, P., Simms, M., and Brown, M.D. (2004) Chronic transcutaneous electrical stimulation of calf muscles improves functional capacity without inducing systemic inflammation in claudicants. *Eur J Vasc Endovasc Surg*, **27**, 201–9.

Andersson, S.A., Ericson, T., Holmgren, E., and Lindqvist, G. (1973) Electro-acupuncture. Effect on pain threshold measured with electrical stimulation of teeth. *Brain Res*, **63**, 393–6.

Andersson, S.A., Hansson, G., Holmgren, E., and Renberg, O. (1976) Evaluation of the pain suppressive effect of different frequencies of peripheral electrical stimulation in chronic pain conditions. *Acta Orthop Scand*, **47**, 149–7.

Ansari, A., Ramsey, K.W., and Floyd, D.C. (2006) Rupture of a flexor pollicis longus repair in a body builder through the use of an electronic muscle stimulator. *Br J Sports Med*, **40**, 1009–10.

Applegate, C., and Burke, D. (1989) Changes in excitability of human cutaneous afferents following prolonged high-frequency stimulation. *Brain*, **112 (Pt 1)**, 147–64.

Atalay, C., and Yilmaz, K.B. (2009) The effect of transcutaneous electrical nerve stimulation on postmastectomy skin flap necrosis. *Breast Cancer Res Treat*, **117**, 611–4.

Augustinsson, L.E., Bohlin, P., Bundsen, P., Carlsson, C.A., Forssman, L., Sjoberg, P., and Tyreman, N.O. (1977) Pain relief during delivery by transcutaneous electrical nerve stimulation. *Pain*, **4**, 59–65.

Avramidis, K., Strike, P.W., Taylor, P.N., and Swain, I.D. (2003) Effectiveness of electric stimulation of the vastus medialis muscle in the rehabilitation of patients after total knee arthroplasty. *Arch Phys Med Rehabil*, **84**, 1850–3.

Babu, A.S., Vasanthan, L.T., and Maiya, A.G. (2010) Transcutaneous electrical nerve stimulation to reduce pain in post-op thoracotomy patients: a physical therapists' perspective. *Indian J Anaesth*, **54**, 478.

Baptista, A.F., Gomes, J.R., Oliveira, J.T., Santos, S.M., Vannier-Santos, M.A., and Martinez, A.M. (2008) High- and low-frequency transcutaneous electrical nerve stimulation delay sciatic nerve regeneration after crush lesion in the mouse. *J Peripher Nerv Syst*, **13**, 71–80.

Barbarisi, M., Pace, M.C., Passavanti, M.B., Maisto, M., Mazzariello, L., Pota, V., and Aurilio, C. (2010) Pregabalin and transcutaneous electrical nerve stimulation for postherpetic neuralgia treatment. *Clin J Pain*, **26**, 567–72.

Barchini, J., Tchachaghian, S., Shamaa, F., Jabbur, S.J., Meyerson, B.A., Song, Z., Linderoth, B., and Saade, N.E. (2012) Spinal segmental and supraspinal mechanisms underlying the pain-relieving effects of spinal cord stimulation: an experimental study in a rat model of neuropathy. *Neuroscience*, **215**, 196–208.

Barkana, B.D., Gupta, N., and Hmurcik, L.V. (2010) Two case reports: electrothermal (aka contact) burns and the effects of current density, application time and skin resistance. *Burns*, **36**, e91–5.

Barlas, P., and Lundeberg, T. (2006) Transcutaneous electrical nerve stimulation and acupuncture. In McMahon, S., and Koltzenburg, M. (eds) *Textbook of Pain*. Elsevier Churchill Livingstone, Philadelphia, 583–90.

Barroso, U., Jr., Tourinho, R., Lordelo, P., Hoebeke, P., and Chase, J. (2011) Electrical stimulation for lower urinary tract dysfunction in children: a systematic review of the literature. *Neurourol Urodyn*, **30**, 1429–36.

Bates, J.A., and Nathan, P.W. (1980) Transcutaneous electrical nerve stimulation for chronic pain. *Anaesthesia*, **35**, 817–22.

Bedwell, C., Dowswell, T., Neilson, J.P., and Lavender, T. (2011) The use of transcutaneous electrical nerve stimulation (TENS) for pain relief in labour: a review of the evidence. *Midwifery*, **27**, e141–8.

Beekwilder, J.P., and Beems, T. (2010) Overview of the clinical applications of vagus nerve stimulation. *J Clin Neurophysiol*, **27**, 130–8.

Bennett, M.I., Hughes, N., and Johnson, M.I. (2011) Methodological quality in randomised controlled trials of transcutaneous electric nerve stimulation for pain: low fidelity may explain negative findings. *Pain*, **152**, 1226–32.

Bennett, M.I., Johnson, M.I., Brown, S.R., Radford, H., Brown, J.M., and Searle, R.D. (2010) Feasibility study of transcutaneous electrical nerve stimulation (TENS) for cancer bone pain. *J Pain*, **11**, 351–9.

Berlant, S.R. (1984) Method of determining optimal stimulation sites for transcutaneous electrical nerve stimulation. *Phys Ther*, **64**, 924–8.

Besio, W.G., Koka, K., and Cole, A.J. (2007) Effects of noninvasive transcutaneous electrical stimulation via concentric ring electrodes on pilocarpine-induced status epilepticus in rats. *Epilepsia*, **48**, 2273–9.

Biering-Sorensen, F., Hansen, B., and Lee, B.S. (2009) Non-pharmacological treatment and prevention of bone loss after spinal cord injury: a systematic review. *Spinal Cord*, **47**, 508–18.

Bihari, V., Kesavachandran, C., Pangtey, B.S., Srivastava, A.K., and Mathur, N. (2011) Musculoskeletal pain and its associated risk factors in residents of National Capital Region. *Indian J Occup Environ Med*, **15**, 59–63.

Bittar, R.G., Kar-Purkayastha, I., Owen, S.L., Bear, R.E., Green, A., Wang, S., and Aziz, T.Z. (2005) Deep brain stimulation for pain relief: a meta-analysis. *J Clin Neurosci*, **12**, 515–19.

Bjordal, J.M., Johnson, M.I., and Couppe, C. (2001) *Clinical Electrotherapy. Your guide to optimal treatment.* HoyskoleForlaget Norwegian Academic Press, Kristiansand.

Bjordal, J.M., Johnson, M.I., and Ljunggreen, A.E. (2003) Transcutaneous electrical nerve stimulation (TENS) can reduce postoperative analgesic consumption. A meta-analysis with assessment of optimal treatment parameters for postoperative pain. *Eur J Pain*, **7**, 181–8.

Bjordal, J.M., Johnson, M.I., Lopes-Martins, R.A., Bogen, B., Chow, R., and Ljunggren, A.E. (2007) Short-term efficacy of physical interventions in osteoarthritic knee pain. A systematic review and meta-analysis of randomised placebo-controlled trials. *BMC Musculoskelet Disord*, **8**, 51.

Blum, K., Chen, A.L., Chen, T.J., Prihoda, T.J., Schoolfield, J., DiNubile, N., Waite, R.L., Arcuri, V., Kerner, M., Braverman, E.R., Rhoades, P., and Tung, H. (2008) The H-Wave device is an effective and safe non-pharmacological analgesic for chronic pain: a meta-analysis. *Adv Ther*, **25**, 644–57.

Borjesson, M. (1999) Visceral chest pain in unstable angina pectoris and effects of transcutaneous electrical nerve stimulation. (TENS). A review. *Herz*, **24**, 114–25.

Breivik, H., Collett, B., Ventafridda, V., Cohen, R., and Gallacher, D. (2006) Survey of chronic pain in Europe: prevalence, impact on daily life, and treatment. *Eur J Pain*, **10**, 287–333.

Bronfort, G., Nilsson, N., Haas, M., Evans, R., Goldsmith, C.H., Assendelft, W.J., and Bouter, L.M. (2004) Non-invasive physical treatments for chronic/recurrent headache. *Cochrane Database Syst Rev*, CD001878.

Brosseau, L., Judd, M.G., Marchand, S., Robinson, V.A., Tugwell, P., Wells, G., and Yonge, K. (2003) Transcutaneous electrical nerve stimulation (TENS) for the treatment of rheumatoid arthritis in the hand. *Cochrane Database Syst Rev*, CD004377.

Brown, L., Holmes, M., and Jones, A. (2009) The application of transcutaneous electrical nerve stimulation to acupuncture points (Acu-TENS) for pain relief: a discussion of efficacy and potential mechanisms. *Physical Therapy Reviews*, **14**, 93–103.

Brown, L., Tabasam, G., Bjordal, J.M., and Johnson, M.I. (2007) An investigation into the effect of electrode placement of transcutaneous electrical nerve stimulation (TENS) on experimentally induced ischemic pain in healthy human participants. *Clin J Pain*, **23**, 735–43.

Buchmuller, A., Navez, M., Milletre-Bernardin, M., Pouplin, S., Presles, E., Lanteri-Minet, M., Tardy, B., Laurent, B., and Camdessanche, J.P. (2012) Value of TENS for relief of chronic low back pain with or without radicular pain. *Eur J Pain*, **16**, 656–65.

Bundsen, P., and Ericson, K. (1982) Pain relief in labor by transcutaneous electrical nerve stimulation. Safety aspects. *Acta Obstet Gynecol Scand*, **61**, 1–5.

Burke, D., and Applegate, C. (1989) Paraesthesiae and hypaesthesia following prolonged high-frequency stimulation of cutaneous afferents. *Brain*, **112(Pt 4)**, 913–29.

Burssens, P., Forsyth, R., Steyaert, A., Van Ovost, E., Praet, M., and Verdonk, R. (2005) Influence of burst TENS stimulation on collagen formation after Achilles tendon suture in man. A histological evaluation with Movat's pentachrome stain. *Acta Orthop Belg*, **71**, 342–6.

Cameron, M., Lonergan, E., and Lee, H. (2003) Transcutaneous electrical nerve stimulation (TENS) for dementia. *Cochrane Database Syst Rev*, CD004032.

Cameron, N.E., Cotter, M.A., Robertson, S., and Maxfield, E.K. (1993) Nerve function in experimental diabetes in rats: effects of electrical stimulation. *Am J Physiol*, **264**, E161–6.

Carbonario, F., Matsutani, L.A., Yuan, S.L., and Marques, A.P. (2013) Effectiveness of high-frequency transcutaneous electrical nerve stimulation at tender points as adjuvant therapy for patients with fibromyalgia. *Eur J Phys Rehabil Med*, **49**, 197–204.

Carlson, T., Andrell, P., Ekre, O., Edvardsson, N., Holmgren, C., Jacobsson, F., and Mannheimer, C. (2009) Interference of transcutaneous electrical nerve stimulation with permanent ventricular stimulation: a new clinical problem? *Europace*, **11**, 364–9.

Carroll, D., Moore, A., Tramer, M., and McQuay, H. (1997a) Transcutaneous electrical nerve stimulation does not relieve in labour pain: updated systematic review. *Contemporary Reviews in Obstetrics and Gynecology*, September, 195–205.

Carroll, D., Moore, R.A., McQuay, H.J., Fairman, F., Tramer, M., and Leijon, G. (2001) Transcutaneous electrical nerve stimulation (TENS) for chronic pain. *Cochrane Database Syst Rev*, CD003222.

Carroll, D., Tramer, M., McQuay, H., Nye, B., and Moore, A. (1996) Randomization is important in studies with pain outcomes: systematic review of transcutaneous electrical nerve stimulation in acute postoperative pain. *Br J Anaesth*, **77**, 798–803.

Carroll, D., Tramer, M., McQuay, H., Nye, B., and Moore, A. (1997b) Transcutaneous electrical nerve stimulation in labour pain: a systematic review. *Br J Obstet Gynaecol*, **104**, 169–75.

Casale, R., Gibellini, R., Bozzi, M., and Bonelli, S. (1985) Changes in sympathetic activity during high frequency T.E.N.S. *Acupunct Electrother Res*, **10**, 169–75.

Cekmen, N., Salman, B., Keles, Z., Aslan, M., and Akcabay, M. (2007) Transcutaneous electrical nerve stimulation in the prevention of postoperative nausea and vomiting after elective laparoscopic cholecystectomy. *J Clin Anesth*, **19**, 49–52.

Celik, E.C., Erhan, B., Gunduz, B., and Lakse, E. (2013) The effect of low-frequency TENS in the treatment of neuropathic pain in patients with spinal cord injury. *Spinal Cord*, **51**, 334–7.

Chabal, C., Fishbain, D.A., Weaver, M., and Heine, L.W. (1998) Long-term transcutaneous electrical nerve stimulation (TENS) use: impact on medication utilization and physical therapy costs. *Clin J Pain*, **14**, 66–73.

Chandra, A., Banavaliker, J.N., Das, P.K., and Hasti, S. (2010) Use of transcutaneous electrical nerve stimulation as an adjunctive to epidural analgesia in the management of acute thoracotomy pain. *Indian J Anaesth*, **54**, 116–20.

Chandran, P., and Sluka, K.A. (2003) Development of opioid tolerance with repeated transcutaneous electrical nerve stimulation administration. *Pain*, **102**, 195–201.

Chao, A.S., Chao, A., Wang, T.H., Chang, Y.C., Peng, H.H., Chang, S.D., Chang, C.J., Lai, C.H., and Wong, A.M. (2007) Pain relief by applying transcutaneous electrical nerve stimulation (TENS) on acupuncture points during the first stage of labor: a randomized double-blind placebo-controlled trial. *Pain*, **127**, 214–20.

Chapman, C.R., and Benedetti, C. (1977) Analgesia following transcutaneous electrical stimulation and its partial reversal by a narcotic antagonist. *Life Sci*, **21**, 1645–8.

Chapman, C.R., Benedetti, C., Colpitts, Y.H., and Gerlach, R. (1983) Naloxone fails to reverse pain thresholds elevated by acupuncture: acupuncture analgesia reconsidered. *Pain*, **16**, 13–31.

Charlton, J. (2005) Task Force on Professional Education. Stimulation-produced analgesia. In Charlton, J. (ed.) *Task Force on Professional Education*. IASP Press, Seattle, WA, 93–6.

Chartered Society of Physiotherapy, C. (2006) *Guidance for the clinical use of Electrophysical agents*. Chartered Society of Physiotherapy, London.

Cheing, G.L., and Chan, W.W. (2009) Influence of choice of electrical stimulation site on peripheral neurophysiological and hypoalgesic effects. *J Rehabil Med*, **41**, 412–17.

Cheing, G.L., Tsui, A.Y., Lo, S.K., and Hui-Chan, C.W. (2003) Optimal stimulation duration of TENS in the management of osteoarthritic knee pain. *J Rehabil Med*, **35**, 62–8.

Chen, C., Tabasam, G., and Johnson, M.I. (2008) Does the pulse frequency of transcutaneous electrical nerve stimulation (TENS) influence hypoalgesia? A systematic review of studies using experimental pain and healthy human participants. *Physiotherapy*, **94**, 11–20.

Chen, C.C., and Johnson, M.I. (2009) An investigation into the effects of frequency-modulated transcutaneous electrical nerve stimulation (TENS) on experimentally-induced pressure pain in healthy human participants. *J Pain*, **10**, 1029–37.

Chen, C.C., and Johnson, M.I. (2010a) A comparison of transcutaneous electrical nerve stimulation (TENS) at 3 and 80 pulses per second on cold-pressor pain in healthy human participants. *Clin Physiol Funct Imaging*, **30**, 260–8.

Chen, C.C., and Johnson, M.I. (2010b) An investigation into the hypoalgesic effects of high- and low-frequency transcutaneous electrical nerve stimulation (TENS) on experimentally-induced blunt pressure pain in healthy human participants. *J Pain*, **11**, 53–61.

Chen, C.C., and Johnson, M.I. (2011) Differential frequency effects of strong nonpainful transcutaneous electrical nerve stimulation on experimentally induced ischemic pain in healthy human participants. *Clin J Pain*, **27**, 434–41.

Chen, C.C., Johnson, M.I., McDonough, S., and Cramp, F. (2007) The effect of transcutaneous electrical nerve stimulation on local and distal cutaneous blood flow following a prolonged heat stimulus in healthy subjects. *Clin Physiol Funct Imaging*, **27**, 154–61.

Chesterton, L.S., Barlas, P., Foster, N.E., Lundeberg, T., Wright, C.C., and Baxter, G.D. (2002) Sensory stimulation (TENS): effects of parameter manipulation on mechanical pain thresholds in healthy human subjects. *Pain*, **99**, 253–62.

Chesterton, L.S., Foster, N.E., Wright, C.C., Baxter, G.D., and Barlas, P. (2003) Effects of TENS frequency, intensity and stimulation site parameter manipulation on pressure pain thresholds in healthy human subjects. *Pain*, **106**, 73–80.

Chesterton, L.S., Lewis, A.M., Sim, J., Mallen, C.D., Mason, E.E., Hay, E.M., and van der Windt, D.A. (2013) Transcutaneous electrical nerve stimulation as adjunct to primary care management for tennis elbow: pragmatic randomised controlled trial (TATE trial). *BMJ*, **347**: f5160.

Chiang, C., Chang, C., Chu, H., and Yang, L. (1973) Peripheral afferent pathway for acupuncture analgesia. *Scientia Sinica*, **16**, 210–17.

Chipchase, L.S., Williams, M.T., and Robertson, V.J. (2009) A national study of the availability and use of electrophysical agents by Australian physiotherapists. *Physiother Theory Pract*, **25**, 279–96.

Chou, R. (2010) Low back pain (chronic). *Clin Evid (Online)*; online version of *BMJ Clinical Evidence*, (see: <http://www.clinicalevidence.com>), **2010**.

Chou, R., and Huffman, L.H. (2007) Nonpharmacologic therapies for acute and chronic low back pain: a review of the evidence for an American Pain Society/American College of Physicians clinical practice guideline. *Ann Intern Med*, **147**, 492–504.

Chung, J.M., Fang, Z.R., Hori, Y., Lee, K.H., and Willis, W.D. (1984a) Prolonged inhibition of primate spinothalamic tract cells by peripheral nerve stimulation. *Pain*, **19**, 259–75.

Chung, J.M., Lee, K.H., Hori, Y., Endo, K., and Willis, W.D. (1984b) Factors influencing peripheral nerve stimulation produced inhibition of primate spinothalamic tract cells. *Pain*, **19**, 277–93.

Claydon, L., and Chesterton, L. (2008) Does transcutaneous electrical nerve stimulation (TENS) produce 'dose-responses'? A review of systematic reviews on chronic pain. *Physical Therapy Reviews*, **13**, 450–63.

Claydon, L., Chesterton, L., Johnson, M., Herbison, G., and Bennett, M. (2010) Transcutaneous electrical nerve stimulation (TENS) for neuropathic pain in adults. *Cochrane Database of Syst Rev*, CD008756.

Claydon, L.S., Chesterton, L.S., Barlas, P., and Sim, J. (2008) Effects of simultaneous dual-site TENS stimulation on experimental pain. *Eur J Pain*, **12**, 696–704.

Claydon, L.S., Chesterton, L.S., Barlas, P., and Sim, J. (2011) Dose-specific effects of transcutaneous electrical nerve stimulation (TENS) on experimental pain: a systematic review. *Clin J Pain*, **27**, 635–47.

Cogiamanian, F., Vergari, M., Schiaffi, E., Marceglia, S., Ardolino, G., Barbieri, S., and Priori, A. (2011) Transcutaneous spinal cord direct current stimulation inhibits the lower limb nociceptive flexion reflex in human beings. *Pain*, **152**, 370–75.

Committee of Advertising Practice (2010) Transcutaneous electrical nerve stimulation (TENS) machines. Available at: <http:/copyadvice.org.uk/Ad-Advice/Advice-Online-Database/Transcutaneous-Electrical-Nerve-Stimulation-Machines.aspx>.

Cook, T.M., and Riley, R.H. (1997) Analgesia following thoracotomy: a survey of Australian practice. *Anaesth Intensive Care*, **25**, 520–4.

Cooper, E.B., Scherder, E.J., and Cooper, J.B. (2005) Electrical treatment of reduced consciousness: experience with coma and Alzheimer's disease. *Neuropsychol Rehabil*, **15**, 389–405.

Corazza, M., Maranini, C., Bacilieri, S., and Virgili, A. (1999) Accelerated allergic contact dermatitis to a transcutaneous electrical nerve stimulation device. *Dermatology*, **199**, 281.

Cosmo, P., Svensson, H., Bornmyr, S., and Wikstrom, S.O. (2000) Effects of transcutaneous nerve stimulation on the microcirculation in chronic leg ulcers. *Scand J Plast Reconstr Surg Hand Surg*, **34**, 61–64.

Cottell, J., Edmondson, A.S., Fitzgerald, P., Hartford, T., and Johnson, M.I. (2011) Repeated application of self-adhesive transcutaneous electrical nerve stimulation electrodes: an assessment of skin microflora. *Physiotherapy*, **97**, 267–70.

Cowan, S., McKenna, J., McCrum-Gardner, E., Johnson, M.I., Sluka, K.A., and Walsh, D.M. (2009) An investigation of the hypoalgesic effects of TENS delivered by a glove electrode. *J Pain*, **10**, 694–701.

Cox, P.D., Kramer, J.F., and Hartsell, H. (1993) Effect of different TENS stimulus parameters on ulnar motor nerve conduction velocity. *Am J Phys Med Rehabil*, **72**, 294–300.

Cramp, A.F., Gilsenan, C., Lowe, A.S., and Walsh, D.M. (2000a) The effect of high- and low-frequency transcutaneous electrical nerve stimulation upon cutaneous blood flow and skin temperature in healthy subjects. *Clin Physiol*, **20**, 150–7.

Cramp, F.L., McCullough, G.R., Lowe, A.S., and Walsh, D.M. (2002) Transcutaneous electric nerve stimulation: the effect of intensity on local and distal cutaneous blood flow and skin temperature in healthy subjects. *Arch Phys Med Rehabil*, **83**, 5–9.

Cramp, F.L., Noble, G., Lowe, A.S., Walsh, D.M., and Willer, J.C. (2000b) A controlled study on the effects of transcutaneous electrical nerve stimulation and interferential therapy upon the RIII nociceptive and H-reflexes in humans. *Arch Phys Med Rehabil*, **81**, 324–33.

Crothers, E. (2003) The use of transcutaneous electrical nerve stimulation during pregnancy: the evidence so far. Margie Polden Memorial Lecture. *Journal of the Association of Chartered Physiotherapy in Women's Health*, **92**, 4–14.

Cruccu, G., Aziz, T.Z., Garcia-Larrea, L., Hansson, P., Jensen, T.S., Lefaucheur, J.P., Simpson, B.A., and Taylor, R.S. (2007) EFNS guidelines on neurostimulation therapy for neuropathic pain. *Eur J Neurol*, **14**, 952–70.

Dailey, D.L., Rakel, B.A., Vance, C.G., Liebano, R.E., Amrit, A.S., Bush, H.M., Lee, K.S., Lee, J.E., and Sluka, K.A. (2013) Transcutaneous electrical nerve stimulation reduces pain, fatigue and hyperalgesia while restoring central inhibition in primary fibromyalgia. *Pain*, **154**(11), 2554–62.

Danziger, N., Rozenberg, S., Bourgeois, P., Charpentier, G., and Willer, J.C. (1998) Depressive effects of segmental and heterotopic application of transcutaneous electrical nerve stimulation and piezo-electric current on lower limb nociceptive flexion reflex in human subjects. *Arch Phys Med Rehabil*, **79**, 191–200.

Davey, N.J., Nowicky, A.V., and Zaman, R. (2001) Somatopy of perceptual threshold to cutaneous electrical stimulation in man. *Exp Physiol*, **86**, 127–30.

de Tommaso, M., Fiore, P., Camporeale, A., Guido, M., Libro, G., Losito, L., Megna, M., Puca, F., and Megna, G. (2003) High and low frequency transcutaneous electrical nerve stimulation inhibits nociceptive responses induced by CO_2 laser stimulation in humans. *Neurosci Lett*, **342**, 17–20.

de Vries, J., Dejongste, M.J., Durenkamp, A., Zijlstra, F., and Staal, M.J. (2007) The sustained benefits of long-term neurostimulation in patients with refractory chest pain and normal coronary arteries. *Eur J Pain*, **11**, 360–5.

Defrin, R., Ariel, E., and Peretz, C. (2005) Segmental noxious versus innocuous electrical stimulation for chronic pain relief and the effect of fading sensation during treatment. *Pain*, **115**, 152–60.

Demmink, J.H. (1995) The effect of a biological conducting medium on the pattern of modulation and distribution in a two-circuit static interferential field. In: *Proceedings of the 12th International Conference of the World Confederation for Physical Therapy*, 25–29 June 1995; Washington, DC. 1995, 583.

DeSantana, J.M., Da Silva, L.F., De Resende, M.A., and Sluka, K.A. (2009) Transcutaneous electrical nerve stimulation at both high and low frequencies activates ventrolateral periaqueductal grey to decrease mechanical hyperalgesia in arthritic rats. *Neuroscience*, **163**, 1233–41.

DeSantana, J.M., da Silva, L.F., and Sluka, K.A. (2010) Cholecystokinin receptors mediate tolerance to the analgesic effect of TENS in arthritic rats. *Pain*, **148**, 84–93.

DeSantana, J.M., Santana-Filho, V.J., Guerra, D.R., Sluka, K.A., Gurgel, R.Q., and da Silva, W.M., Jr. (2008a) Hypoalgesic effect of the transcutaneous electrical nerve stimulation following inguinal herniorrhaphy: a randomized, controlled trial. *J Pain*, **9**, 623–9.

Desantana, J.M., Santana-Filho, V.J., and Sluka, K.A. (2008b) Modulation between high- and low-frequency transcutaneous electric nerve stimulation delays the development of analgesic tolerance in arthritic rats. *Arch Phys Med Rehabil*, **89**, 754–60.

DeSantana, J.M., Walsh, D.M., Vance, C., Rakel, B.A., and Sluka, K.A. (2008c) Effectiveness of transcutaneous electrical nerve stimulation for treatment of hyperalgesia and pain. *Curr Rheumatol Rep*, **10**, 492–9.

Deyo, R.A., Walsh, N.E., Martin, D.C., Schoenfeld, L.S., and Ramamurthy, S. (1990a) A controlled trial of transcutaneous electrical nerve stimulation (TENS) and exercise for chronic low back pain. *N Engl J Med*, **322**, 1627–34.

Deyo, R.A., Walsh, N.E., Schoenfeld, L.S., and Ramamurthy, S. (1990b) Can trials of physical treatments be blinded? The example of transcutaneous electrical nerve stimulation for chronic pain. *Am J Phys Med Rehabil*, **69**, 6–10.

Dhindsa, A., Pandit, I.K., Srivastava, N., and Gugnani, N. (2011) Comparative evaluation of the effectiveness of electronic dental anesthesia with 2% lignocaine in various minor pediatric dental procedures: a clinical study. *Contemp Clin Dent*, **2**, 27–30.

Dickie, A., Tabasam, G., Tashani, O., Marchant, P., and Johnson, M.I. (2009) A preliminary investigation into the effect of coffee on hypolagesia associated with transcutaneous electrical nerve stimulation. *Clin Physiol Funct Imaging*, **29**, 293–9.

Dingemanse, R., Randsdorp, M., Koes, B.W., and Huisstede, B.M. (2013) Evidence for the effectiveness of electrophysical modalities for treatment of medial and lateral epicondylitis: a systematic review. *Br J Sports Med*, Jan 18. [Epub ahead of print]

Dionisi, B., and Senatori, R. (2011) Effect of transcutaneous electrical nerve stimulation on the postpartum dyspareunia treatment. *J Obstet Gynaecol Res*, **37**, 750–3.

Dowswell, T., Bedwell, C., Lavender, T., and Neilson, J.P. (2009) Transcutaneous electrical nerve stimulation (TENS) for pain relief in labour. *Cochrane Database Syst Rev*, CD007214.

Dubinsky, R.M., and Miyasaki, J. (2010) Assessment: efficacy of transcutaneous electric nerve stimulation in the treatment of pain in neurologic disorders (an evidence-based review): report of the Therapeutics and Technology Assessment Subcommittee of the American Academy of Neurology. *Neurology*, **74**, 173–6.

Duggan, A.W., and Foong, F.W. (1985) Bicuculline and spinal inhibition produced by dorsal column stimulation in the cat. *Pain*, **22**, 249–59.

Dunn, P.A., Rogers, D., and Halford, K. (1989) Transcutaneous electrical nerve stimulation at acupuncture points in the induction of uterine contractions. *Obstet Gynecol*, **73**, 286–90.

Duranti, R., Pantaleo, T., and Bellini, F. (1988) Increase in muscular pain threshold following low frequency-high intensity peripheral conditioning stimulation in humans. *Brain Res*, **452**, 66–72.

Edgar, D.W., Fish, J.S., Gomez, M., and Wood, F.M. (2011) Local and systemic treatments for acute edema after burn injury: a systematic review of the literature. *J Burn Care Res*, **32**, 334–47.

Elzahaf, R.A., Tashani, O.A., Unsworth, B.A., and Johnson, M.I. (2012). The prevalence of chronic pain with an analysis of countries with a Human Development Index less than 0.9: a systematic review without meta-analysis. *Curr Med Res Opin*, **28**, 1221–9.

Engholm, G., and Leffler, A.S. (2010) Influence of pain reduction by transcutaneous electrical nerve stimulation (TENS) on somatosensory functions in patients with painful traumatic peripheral partial nerve injury. *Eur J Pain*, **14**, 918–23.

Engin-Uml Stun, Y., Korkmaz, C., Duru, N.K., and Baser, I. (2006) Comparison of three sperm retrieval techniques in spinal cord-injured men: pregnancy outcome. *Gynecol Endocrinol*, **22**, 252–5.

English, A.W., Schwartz, G., Meador, W., Sabatier, M.J., and Mulligan, A. (2007) Electrical stimulation promotes peripheral axon regeneration by enhanced neuronal neurotrophin signaling. *Dev Neurobiol*, **67**, 158–72.

Erdogan, M., Erdogan, A., Erbil, N., Karakaya, H.K., and Demircan, A. (2005) Prospective, randomized, placebo-controlled study of the effect of TENS on postthoracotomy pain and pulmonary function. *World J Surg*, **29**, 1563–70.

Eriksson, M., and Sjölund, B. (1976) Acupuncture-like electroanalgesia in TNS resistant chronic pain. In Zotterman, Y. (ed.) *Sensory functions of the skin*. Pergamon Press, Oxford/ New York, 575–81.

Eriksson, M.B., Sjölund, B.H., and Nielzen, S. (1979) Long term results of peripheral conditioning stimulation as an analgesic measure in chronic pain. *Pain*, **6**, 335–47.

Eriksson, M.B., Sjölund, B.H., and Sundbarg, G. (1984) Pain relief from peripheral conditioning stimulation in patients with chronic facial pain. *J Neurosurg*, **61**, 149–55.

Ezzo, J.M., Richardson, M.A., Vickers, A., Allen, C., Dibble, S.L., Issell, B.F., Lao, L., Pearl, M., Ramirez, G., Roscoe, J., Shen, J., Shivnan, J.C., Streitberger, K., Treish, I., and Zhang, G. (2006) Acupuncture-point stimulation for chemotherapy-induced nausea or vomiting. *Cochrane Database Syst Rev*, CD002285.

Facchinetti, F., Sandrini, G., Petraglia, F., Alfonsi, E., Nappi, G., and Genazzani, A.R. (1984) Concomitant increase in nociceptive flexion reflex threshold and plasma opioids following transcutaneous nerve stimulation. *Pain*, **19**, 295–303.

Facci, L.M., Nowotny, J.P., Tormem, F., and Trevisani, V.F. (2011) Effects of transcutaneous electrical nerve stimulation (TENS) and interferential currents (IFC) in patients with nonspecific chronic low back pain: randomized clinical trial. *Sao Paulo Med J*, **129**, 206–16.

Fagade, O.O., Oginni, F.O., and Obilade, T.O. (2005) Comparative study of the therapeutic effect of a systemic analgesic and transcutaneous electrical nerve stimulation (TENS) on post-IMF trismus and pain in Nigerian patients. *Niger Postgrad Med J*, **12**, 97–101.

Fargas-Babjak, A.M., Pomeranz, B., and Rooney, P.J. (1992) Acupuncture-like stimulation with codetron for rehabilitation of patients with chronic pain syndrome and osteoarthritis. *Acupunct Electrother Res*, **17**, 95–105.

Fary, R.E., and Briffa, N.K. (2011) Monophasic electrical stimulation produces high rates of adverse skin reactions in healthy subjects. *Physiother Theory Pract*, **27**, 246–51.

Fattal, C., Kong, A.S.D., Gilbert, C., Ventura, M., and Albert, T. (2009) What is the efficacy of physical therapeutics for treating neuropathic pain in spinal cord injury patients? *Ann Phys Rehabil Med*, **52**, 149–66.

Fengler, R.K., Jacobs, J.W., Bac, M., van Wijck, A.J., and van Meeteren, N.L. (2007) Action potential simulation (APS) in patients with fibromyalgia syndrome (FMS): a controlled single subject experimental design. *Clin Rheumatol*, **26**, 322–9.

Fernandez-Del-Olmo, M., Alvarez-Sauco, M., Koch, G., Franca, M., Marquez, G., Sanchez, J.A., Acero, R.M., and Rothwell, J.C. (2008) How repeatable are the physiological effects of TENS? *Clin Neurophysiol*, **119**, 1834–9.

Fillingim, R.B., King, C.D., Ribeiro-Dasilva, M.C., Rahim-Williams, B., and Riley, J.L., 3rd (2009) Sex, gender, and pain: a review of recent clinical and experimental findings. *J Pain*, **10**, 447–85.

Filshie, J., and Hester, J. (2006) Guidelines for providing acupuncture treatment for cancer patients—a peer-reviewed sample policy document. *Acupunct Med*, **24**, 172–82.

Fishbain, D.A., Chabal, C., Abbott, A., Heine, L.W., and Cutler, R. (1996) Transcutaneous electrical nerve stimulation (TENS) treatment outcome in long-term users. *Clin J Pain*, **12**, 201–14.

Fishman, S.M. (2012) *Listening to pain: A clinician's guide to improving pain management through better communication.* Oxford University Press, Oxford.

Ford, K.S., Shrader, M.W., Smith, J., McLean, T.J., and Dahm, D.L. (2005) Full-thickness burn formation after the use of electrical stimulation for rehabilitation of unicompartmental knee arthroplasty. *J Arthroplasty*, **20**, 950–3.

Forst, T., Pfutzner, A., Bauersachs, R., Arin, M., Bach, B., Biehlmaier, H., Kustner, E., and Beyer, J. (1997) Comparison of the microvascular response to transcutaneous electrical nerve stimulation and postocclusive ischemia in the diabetic foot. *J Diabetes Complications*, **11**, 291–7.

Francis, R.P., and Johnson, M.I. (2011) The characteristics of acupuncture-like transcutaneous electrical nerve stimulation (acupuncture-like TENS): a literature review. *Acupunct Electrother Res*, **36**, 231–58.

Francis, R.P., Marchant, P., and Johnson, M.I. (2011a) Conventional versus acupuncture-like transcutaneous electrical nerve stimulation on cold-induced pain in healthy human participants: effects during stimulation. *Clin Physiol Funct Imaging*, **31**, 363–70.

Francis, R.P., Marchant, P.R., and Johnson, M.I. (2011b) Comparison of post-treatment effects of conventional and acupuncture-like transcutaneous electrical nerve stimulation (TENS): a randomised placebo-controlled study using cold-induced pain and healthy human participants. *Physiother Theory Pract*, **27** (8), 578–85.

Fregni, F., Freedman, S., and Pascual-Leone, A. (2007) Recent advances in the treatment of chronic pain with non-invasive brain stimulation techniques. *Lancet Neurol*, **6**, 188–91.

Freynet, A., and Falcoz, P.E. (2010) Is transcutaneous electrical nerve stimulation effective in relieving postoperative pain after thoracotomy? *Interact Cardiovasc Thorac Surg*, **10**, 283–8.

Gallas, S., Marie, J.P., Leroi, A.M., and Verin, E. (2010) Sensory transcutaneous electrical stimulation improves post-stroke dysphagic patients. *Dysphagia*, **25**, 291–7.

Garcia-Larrea, L., Sindou, M., and Mauguiere, F. (1989) Nociceptive flexion reflexes during analgesic neurostimulation in man. *Pain*, **39**, 145–56.

Gardner, S.E., Frantz, R.A., and Schmidt, F.L. (1999) Effect of electrical stimulation on chronic wound healing: a meta-analysis. *Wound Repair Regen*, 7, 495–503.

Garrison, D., and Foreman, R. (2002) Effects of transcutaneous electrical nerve stimulation (TENS) electrode placement on spontaneous and noxiously evoked dorsal horn cell activity in the cat. *Neuromodulation*, 5, 231–7.

Garrison, D.W., and Foreman, R.D. (1994) Decreased activity of spontaneous and noxiously evoked dorsal horn cells during transcutaneous electrical nerve stimulation (TENS). *Pain*, **58**, 309–15.

Garrison, D.W., and Foreman, R.D. (1996) Effects of transcutaneous electrical nerve stimulation (TENS) on spontaneous and noxiously evoked dorsal horn cell activity in cats with transected spinal cords. *Neurosci Lett*, **216**, 125–8.

Gemmell, H., and Hilland, A. (2011) Immediate effect of electric point stimulation (TENS) in treating latent upper trapezius trigger points: a double blind randomised placebo-controlled trial. *J Bodyw Mov Ther*, **15**, 348–54.

Geng, B., Yoshida, K., Petrini, L., and Jensen, W. (2012) Evaluation of sensation evoked by electrocutaneous stimulation on forearm in nondisabled subjects. *J Rehabil Res Dev*, **49**, 297–308.

Geremia, N.M., Gordon, T., Brushart, T.M., Al-Majed, A.A., and Verge, V.M. (2007) Electrical stimulation promotes sensory neuron regeneration and growth-associated gene expression. *Exp Neurol*, **205**, 347–59.

Giggins, O., Fullen, B., and Coughlan, G. (2012) Neuromuscular electrical stimulation in the treatment of knee osteoarthritis: a systematic review and meta-analysis. *Clin Rehabil*, **26**, 867–81.

Gigo-Benato, D., Russo, T.L., Geuna, S., Domingues, N.R., Salvini, T.F., and Parizotto, N.A. (2010) Electrical stimulation impairs early functional recovery and accentuates skeletal muscle atrophy after sciatic nerve crush injury in rats. *Muscle Nerve*, **41**, 685–93.

Gildenberg, P.L. (2006) History of electrical neuromodulation for chronic pain. *Pain Med*, 7 **Suppl 1**, S7–S13.

Giuffrida, O., Simpson, L., and Halligan, P.W. (2010) Contralateral stimulation, using TENS, of phantom limb pain: two confirmatory cases. *Pain Med*, **11**, 133–41.

Gladwell, P.W. (2013) Focusing outcome measurement for transcutaneous electrical nerve stimulation evaluation: incorporating the experiences of TENS users with chronic musculoskeletal pain [Thesis]. University of the West of England, 2013.

Golding, J.F., Ashton, H., Marsh, R., and Thompson, J.W. (1986) Transcutaneous electrical nerve stimulation produces variable changes in somatosensory evoked potentials, sensory perception and pain threshold: clinical implications for pain relief. *J Neurol Neurosurg Psychiatry*, **49**, 1397–406.

Goldstein, C., Sprague, S., and Petrisor, B.A. (2010) Electrical stimulation for fracture healing: current evidence. *J Orthop Trauma*, **24 Suppl 1**, S62–65.

Gopalkrishnan, P., and Sluka, K.A. (2000) Effect of varying frequency, intensity, and pulse duration of transcutaneous electrical nerve stimulation on primary hyperalgesia in inflamed rats. *Arch Phys Med Rehabil*, **81**, 984–90.

Gordon, T., Udina, E., Verge, V.M., and de Chaves, E.I. (2009) Brief electrical stimulation accelerates axon regeneration in the peripheral nervous system and promotes sensory axon regeneration in the central nervous system. *Motor Control*, **13**, 412–41.

Gorodetskyi, I.G., Gorodnichenko, A.I., Tursin, P.S., Reshetnyak, V.K., and Uskov, O.N. (2007) Non-invasive interactive neurostimulation in the post-operative recovery of patients with a trochanteric fracture of the femur. A randomised, controlled trial. *J Bone Joint Surg Br*, **89**, 1488–94.

Graff-Radford, S.B., Reeves, J.L., Baker, R.L., and Chiu, D. (1989) Effects of transcutaneous electrical nerve stimulation on myofascial pain and trigger point sensitivity. *Pain*, **37**, 1–5.

Grond, S., Radbruch, L., Meuser, T., Sabatowski, R., Loick, G., and Lehmann, K.A. (1999) Assessment and treatment of neuropathic cancer pain following WHO guidelines. *Pain*, **79**, 15–20.

Gul, K., and Onal, S.A. (2009) [Comparison of non-invasive and invasive techniques in the treatment of patients with myofascial pain syndrome]. *Agri*, **21**, 104–12.

Hallen, K., Hrafnkelsdottir, T., Jern, S., Biber, B., Mannheimer, C., and DuttaRoy, S. (2010) Transcutaneous electrical nerve stimulation induces vasodilation in healthy controls but not in refractory angina patients. *J Pain Symptom Manage*, **40**, 95–101.

Hamza, M.A., White, P.F., Ahmed, H.E., and Ghoname, E.A. (1999) Effect of the frequency of transcutaneous electrical nerve stimulation on the postoperative opioid analgesic requirement and recovery profile. *Anesthesiology*, **91**, 1232–8.

Han, J., Chen, X., Sun, S., Xu, X., Yuan, Y., Yan, S., Hao, J., and Terenius, L. (1991) Effect of low- and high-frequency TENS on Met-enkephalin-Arg-Phe and dynorphin A immunoreactivity in human lumbar CSF. *Pain*, **47**, 295–8.

Hanai, F. (2000) Effect of electrical stimulation of peripheral nerves on neuropathic pain. *Spine (Phila Pa 1976)*, **25**, 1886–92.

Hansson, P., and Ekblom, A. (1984) Afferent stimulation induced pain relief in acute oro-facial pain and its failure to induce sufficient pain reduction in dental and oral surgery. *Pain*, **20**, 273–8.

Hansson, P., Ekblom, A., Thomsson, M., and Fjellner, B. (1986) Influence of naloxone on relief of acute oro-facial pain by transcutaneous electrical nerve stimulation (TENS) or vibration. *Pain*, **24**, 323–9.

Harreby, K.R., Sevcencu, C., and Struijk, J.J. (2011) The effect of spinal cord stimulation on seizure susceptibility in rats. *Neuromodulation*, **14**, 111–16.

Harrison, R.F., Shore, M., Woods, T., Mathews, G., Gardiner, J., and Unwin, A. (1987) A comparative study of transcutaneous electrical nerve stimulation (TENS), entonox, pethidine + promazine and lumbar epidural for pain relief in labor. *Acta Obstet Gynecol Scand*, **66**, 9–14.

Hartkopp, A., Murphy, R.J., Mohr, T., Kjaer, M., and Biering-Sorensen, F. (1998) Bone fracture during electrical stimulation of the quadriceps in a spinal cord injured subject. *Arch Phys Med Rehabil*, **79**, 1133–6.

Herman, E., Williams, R., Stratford, P., Fargas-Babjak, A., and Trott, M. (1994) A randomized controlled trial of transcutaneous electrical nerve stimulation (CODETRON) to determine its benefits in a rehabilitation program for acute occupational low back pain. *Spine*, **19**, 561–8.

Hettrick, H.H., O'Brien, K., Laznick, H., Sanchez, J., Gorga, D., Nagler, W., and Yurt, R. (2004) Effect of transcutaneous electrical nerve stimulation for the management of burn pruritus: a pilot study. *J Burn Care Rehabil*, **25**, 236–40.

Hingne, P.M., and Sluka, K.A. (2007) Differences in waveform characteristics have no effect on the anti-hyperalgesia produced by transcutaneous electrical nerve stimulation (TENS) in rats with joint inflammation. *J Pain*, **8**, 251–5.

Hingne, P.M., and Sluka, K.A. (2008) Blockade of NMDA receptors prevents analgesic tolerance to repeated transcutaneous electrical nerve stimulation (TENS) in rats. *J Pain*, **9**, 217–25.

Holmgren, C., Carlsson, T., Mannheimer, C., and Edvardsson, N. (2008) Risk of interference from transcutaneous electrical nerve stimulation on the sensing function of implantable defibrillators. *Pacing Clin Electrophysiol*, **31**, 151–8.

Hoshiyama, M., and Kakigi, R. (2000) After-effect of transcutaneous electrical nerve stimulation (TENS) on pain-related evoked potentials and magnetic fields in normal subjects. *Clin Neurophysiol*, **111**, 717–24.

Hoshiyama, M., Kakigi, R., and Tamura, Y. (2004) Temporal discrimination threshold on various parts of the body. *Muscle Nerve*, **29**, 243–7.

Hou, C.R., Tsai, L.C., Cheng, K.F., Chung, K.C., and Hong, C.Z. (2002) Immediate effects of various physical therapeutic modalities on cervical myofascial pain and trigger-point sensitivity. *Arch Phys Med Rehabil*, **83**, 1406–14.

Houghton, P., Nussbaum, E., and Hoens, A. (2010) Electrophysical agents. Contraindications and precautions: an evidence-based approach to clinical decision making in physical therapy. *Physiother Can*, **62**, 5–80

Howson, D.C. (1978) Peripheral neural excitability. Implications for transcutaneous electrical nerve stimulation. *Phys Ther*, **58**, 1467–73.

Hughes, N., Bennett, M.I., and Johnson, M.I. (2013) An investigation into the magnitude of the current window and perception of transcutaneous electrical nerve stimulation (TENS) sensation at various frequencies and body sites in healthy human participants. *Clin J Pain*, **29**, 146–53.

Hurlow, A., Bennett, M.I., Robb, K.A., Johnson, M.I., Simpson, K.H., and Oxberry, S.G. (2012) Transcutaneous electric nerve stimulation (TENS) for cancer pain in adults. *Cochrane Database Syst Rev*, 3, CD006276.

Ignelzi, R.J., and Nyquist, J.K. (1976) Direct effect of electrical stimulation on peripheral nerve evoked activity: implications in pain relief. *J Neurosurg*, **45**, 159–65.

Ignelzi, R.J., and Nyquist, J.K. (1979) Excitability changes in peripheral nerve fibers after repetitive electrical stimulation. Implications in pain modulation. *J Neurosurg*, **51**, 824–33.

Ignelzi, R.J., Nyquist, J.K., and Tighe, W.J., Jr. (1981) Repetitive electrical stimulation of peripheral nerve and spinal cord activity. *Neurol Res*, **3**, 195–209.

Imoto, A.M., Peccin, S., Almeida, G.J., Saconato, H., and Atallah, A.N. (2011) Effectiveness of electrical stimulation on rehabilitation after ligament and meniscal injuries: a systematic review. *Sao Paulo Med J*, **129**, 414–23.

Indrekvam, S., and Hunskaar, S. (2003) Home electrical stimulation for urinary incontinence: a study of the diffusion of a new technology. *Urology*, **62**, 24–30.

Ismail, K.A., Chase, J., Gibb, S., Clarke, M., Catto-Smith, A.G., Robertson, V.J., Hutson, J.M., and Southwell, B.R. (2009) Daily transabdominal electrical stimulation at home increased defecation in children with slow-transit constipation: a pilot study. *J Pediatr Surg*, **44**, 2388–92.

Izumi, M., Ikeuchi, M., Mitani, T., Taniguchi, S., and Tani, T. (2010) Prevention of venous stasis in the lower limb by transcutaneous electrical nerve stimulation. *Eur J Vasc Endovasc Surg*, **39**, 642–5.

Jacques, L., Jensen, T., Rollins, J., Burton, B., Hakim, R., and Miller, S. (2012) Decision Memo for Transcutaneous Electrical Nerve Stimulation for Chronic Low Back Pain (CAG-00429N) In Services, Centers for Medicare and Medicaid (ed.). US Department of Heath and Human Services. Available at: <http://www.cms.gov/medicare-coverage-database/details/nca-decision-memo.aspx?NCAId=256>; accessed 04 September 2013.

Jamtvedt, G., Dahm, K.T., Holm, I., and Flottorp, S. (2008) Measuring physiotherapy performance in patients with osteoarthritis of the knee: a prospective study. *BMC Health Serv Res*, **8**, 145–52.

Jamtvedt, G., Dahm, K.T., Holm, I., Odegaard-Jensen, J., and Flottorp, S. (2010) Choice of treatment modalities was not influenced by pain, severity or co-morbidity in patients with knee osteoarthritis. *Physiother Res Int*, **15**, 16–23.

Janko, M., and Trontelj, J.V. (1980) Transcutaneous electrical nerve stimulation: a microneurographic and perceptual study. *Pain*, **9**, 219–30.

Jelinek, H.F., and McIntyre, R. (2010) Electric pulse frequency and magnitude of perceived sensation during electrocutaneous forearm stimulation. *Arch Phys Med Rehabil*, **91**, 1378–82.

Jeong, Y., Baik, E., Nam, T., and Paik, K. (1995) Effects of iontophoretically applied naloxone, picrotoxin and strychnine on dorsal horn neuron activities treated with high frequency conditioning stimulation in cats. *Yonsei Med J*, **36**, 336–47.

Jin, D.M., Xu, Y., Geng, D.F., and Yan, T.B. (2010) Effect of transcutaneous electrical nerve stimulation on symptomatic diabetic peripheral neuropathy: a meta-analysis of randomized controlled trials. *Diabetes Res Clin Pract*, **89**, 10–15.

Johansson, F., Almay, B.G., and von Knorring, L. (1981) Personality factors related to the outcome of treatment with transcutaneous nerve stimulation. *Psychiatr Clin (Basel)*, **14**, 96–104.

Johansson, F., Almay, B.G., Von Knorring, L., and Terenius, L. (1980) Predictors for the outcome of treatment with high frequency transcutaneous electrical nerve stimulation in patients with chronic pain. *Pain*, **9**, 55–61.

Johnson, M. (1998) Acupuncture-like transcutaneous electrical nerve stimulation (AL-TENS) in the management of pain. *Physical Therapy Reviews*, **3**, 73–93.

Johnson, M. (1999) The mystique of interferential currents. *Physiotherapy*, **85**, 294–7.

Johnson, M. (2001a) Transcutaneous electrical nerve stimulation (TENS) and TENS-like devices. Do they provide pain relief? *Pain Reviews*, **8**, 121–8.

Johnson, M.I. (2008) Transcutaneous Electrical Nerve Stimulation. In Watson, T. (ed.) *Electrotherapy: Evidence based practice*. Churchill Livingstone, Edinburgh, 253–96.

Johnson, M.I, Ashton, C.H., and Thompson, J.W. (1992a) Long term use of transcutaneous electrical nerve stimulation at Newcastle Pain Relief Clinic. *J R Soc Med*, **85**, 267–8.

Johnson, M., and Martinson, M. (2007) Efficacy of electrical nerve stimulation for chronic musculoskeletal pain: a meta-analysis of randomized controlled trials. *Pain*, **130**, 157–65.

Johnson, M., Oxberry, S., and Robb, K. (2008) Stimulation-induced analgesia. In Sykes, N., Bennett, M., Yuan, C.-S. (eds) *Cancer Pain*. Hodder Arnold, London, 235–50.

Johnson, M.I. (1997) Transcutaneous electrical nerve stimulation (TENS) in the management of labour pain: the experience of over ten thousand women. *British Journal of Midwifery*, **5**, 400–05.

Johnson, M.I. (2001b) A critical review of the analgesic effects of TENS-like devices. *Physical Therapy Reviews*, **6**, 153–73.

Johnson, M.I. (2005) Physiology of chronic pain. In Banks, C., Mackrodt, K. (eds) *Chronic Pain Management* Whurr Publishers Ltd, London, 36–74.

Johnson, M.I., Ashton, C.H., Bousfield, D.R., and Thompson, J.W. (1991a) Analgesic effects of different pulse patterns of transcutaneous electrical nerve stimulation on cold-induced pain in normal subjects. *J Psychosom Res*, **35**, 313–21.

Johnson, M.I., Ashton, C.H., and Thompson, J.W. (1991b) The consistency of pulse frequencies and pulse patterns of transcutaneous electrical nerve stimulation (TENS) used by chronic pain patients. *Pain*, **44**, 231–4.

Johnson, M.I., Ashton, C.H., and Thompson, J.W. (1991c) An in-depth study of long-term users of transcutaneous electrical nerve stimulation (TENS). Implications for clinical use of TENS. *Pain*, **44**, 221–9.

Johnson, M.I., Ashton, C.H., and Thompson, J.W. (1992b) Analgesic effects of Acupuncture Like TENS on cold pressor pain in normal subjects. *Eur J Pain*, **13**, 101–8.

Johnson, M.I., Ashton, C.H., and Thompson, J.W. (1992c) Long term use of transcutaneous electrical nerve stimulation at Newcastle Pain Relief Clinic. *J R Soc Med*, **85**, 267–8.

Johnson, M.I., Ashton, C.H., and Thompson, J.W. (1993) A prospective investigation into factors related to patient response to transcutaneous electrical nerve stimulation (TENS): the importance of cortical responsivity. *Eur J Pain*, **14**, 1–9.

Johnson, M.I., and Bagley, J. (2009) Transcutaneous electrical nerve stimulation in perioperative settings. In Cox, F. (ed.) *Perioperative pain management*. Wiley-Blackwell, Chichester, 248–76.

Johnson, M.I., and Bjordal, J.M. (2011) Transcutaneous electrical nerve stimulation for the management of painful conditions: focus on neuropathic pain. *Expert Rev Neurother*, **11**, 735–53.

Johnson, M.I., and Din, A. (1997) Ethnocultural differences in the analgesic effects of placebo transcutaneous electrical nerve stimulation (TENS) on cold-induced pain in healthy subjects. A preliminary study. *Complementary Therapies in Medicine*, **5**, 74–79.

Johnson, M.I., and Walsh, D.M. (2010) Pain: continued uncertainty of TENS' effectiveness for pain relief. *Nat Rev Rheumatol*, **6**, 314–16.

Kaada, B. (1982) Vasodilation induced by transcutaneous nerve stimulation in peripheral ischemia (Raynaud's phenomenon and diabetic polyneuropathy). *Eur Heart J*, **3**, 303–14.

Kalra, A., Urban, M.O., and Sluka, K.A. (2001) Blockade of opioid receptors in rostral ventral medulla prevents antihyperalgesia produced by transcutaneous electrical nerve stimulation (TENS). *J Pharmacol Exp Ther*, **298**, 257–63.

Kantor, G., Alon, G., and Ho, H.S. (1994) The effects of selected stimulus waveforms on pulse and phase characteristics at sensory and motor thresholds. *Phys Ther*, **74**, 951–62.

Kara, M., Ozcakar, L., Gokcay, D., Ozcelik, E., Yorubulut, M., Guneri, S., Kaymak, B., Akinci, A., and Cetin, A. (2010) Quantification of the effects of transcutaneous electrical nerve stimulation with functional magnetic resonance imaging: a double-blind randomized placebo-controlled study. *Arch Phys Med Rehabil*, **91**, 1160–5.

Keller, T., Lawrence, M., Kuhn, A., and Morari, M. (2006) New multi-channel transcutaneous electrical stimulation technology for rehabilitation. *Conf Proc IEEE Eng Med Biol Soc*, **1**, 194–7.

Khadilkar, A., Odebiyi, D.O., Brosseau, L., and Wells, G.A. (2008) Transcutaneous electrical nerve stimulation (TENS) versus placebo for chronic low-back pain. *Cochrane Database Syst Rev*, CD003008.

Khalil, Z., and Merhi, M. (2000) Effects of aging on neurogenic vasodilator responses evoked by transcutaneous electrical nerve stimulation: relevance to wound healing. *J Gerontol A Biol Sci Med Sci*, **55**, B257–63.

Kiernan, M.C., Hales, J.P., Gracies, J.M., Mogyoros, I., and Burke, D. (1997) Paraesthesiae induced by prolonged high frequency stimulation of human cutaneous afferents. *J Physiol*, **501** (Pt 2), 461–71.

Kim, J., Ho, C.H., Wang, X., and Bogie, K. (2010) The use of sensory electrical stimulation for pressure ulcer prevention. *Physiother Theory Pract*, **26**, 528–36.

King, A. (1998) *King's guide to TENS: A user's guide to transcutaneous electrical nerve stimulation*. Kings Medical, ISBN 9780953562305.

King, A. (1999) *King's Pocket Book of Acupuncture Points for TENS and other Methods of Stimulation. A Health Professionals Guide*. Kings Medical, ISBN: 978-9535623-1-2.

King, E.W., Audette, K., Athman, G.A., Nguyen, H.O., Sluka, K.A., and Fairbanks, C.A. (2005) Transcutaneous electrical nerve stimulation activates peripherally located alpha-2A adrenergic receptors. *Pain*, **115**, 364–73.

King, E.W., and Sluka, K.A. (2001) The effect of varying frequency and intensity of transcutaneous electrical nerve stimulation on secondary mechanical hyperalgesia in an animal model of inflammation. *J Pain*, **2**, 128–33.

Koke, A.J., Schouten, J.S., Lamerichs-Geelen, M.J., Lipsch, J.S., Waltje, E.M., van Kleef, M., and Patijn, J. (2004) Pain reducing effect of three types of transcutaneous electrical nerve stimulation in patients with chronic pain: a randomized crossover trial. *Pain*, **108**, 36–42.

Koklu, S., Koklu, G., Ozguclu, E., Kayani, G.U., Akbal, E., and Hascelik, Z. (2010) Clinical trial: interferential electric stimulation in functional dyspepsia patients - a prospective randomized study. *Aliment Pharmacol Ther*, **31**, 961–8.

Kolen, A.F., de Nijs, R.N., Wagemakers, F.M., Meier, A.J., and Johnson, M.I. (2012) Effects of spatially targeted transcutaneous electrical nerve stimulation using an electrode array that measures skin resistance on pain and mobility in patients with osteoarthritis in the knee: a randomized controlled trial. *Pain*, **153**, 373–81.

Krabbenbos, I.P., Brandsma, D., van Swol, C.F., Boezeman, E.H., Tromp, S.C., Nijhuis, H.J., and van Dongen, E.P. (2009) Inhibition of cortical laser-evoked potentials by transcutaneous electrical nerve stimulation. *Neuromodulation*, **12**, 141–5.

Kraus, T., Hosl, K., Kiess, O., Schanze, A., Kornhuber, J., and Forster, C. (2007) BOLD fMRI deactivation of limbic and temporal brain structures and mood enhancing effect by transcutaneous vagus nerve stimulation. *J Neural Transm*, **114**, 1485–93.

Kroeling, P., Gross, A., Goldsmith, C.H., Burnie, S.J., Haines, T., Graham, N., and Brant, A. (2009) Electrotherapy for neck pain. *Cochrane Database Syst Rev*, CD004251.

Kuhn, A., Keller, T., Lawrence, M., and Morari, M. (2010) The influence of electrode size on selectivity and comfort in transcutaneous electrical stimulation of the forearm. *IEEE Trans Neural Syst Rehabil Eng*, **18**, 255–62.

Kuhn, A., Keller, T., Micera, S., and Morari, M. (2009) Array electrode design for transcutaneous electrical stimulation: a simulation study. *Med Eng Phys*, **31**, 945–51.

Lampl, C., Kreczi, T., and Klingler, D. (1998) Transcutaneous electrical nerve stimulation in the treatment of chronic pain: predictive factors and evaluation of the method. *Clin J Pain*, **14**, 134–42.

Lancet (1973) Acupuncture analgesia. *Lancet*, **1**, 1372.

Lander, J., and Fowler-Kerry, S. (1993) TENS for children's procedural pain. *Pain*, **52**, 209–16.

Lang, T., Barker, R., Steinlechner, B., Gustorff, B., Puskas, T., Gore, O., and Kober, A. (2007) TENS relieves acute posttraumatic hip pain during emergency transport. *J Trauma*, **62**, 184–8.

Laufer, Y., and Elboim-Gabyzon, M. (2011) Does sensory transcutaneous electrical stimulation enhance motor recovery following a stroke? A systematic review. *Neurorehabil Neural Repair*, **25**, 799–809.

Lauretti, G.R., Chubaci, E.F., and Mattos, A.L. (2013) Efficacy of the use of two simultaneously TENS devices for fibromyalgia pain. *Rheumatol Int*, **33**, 2117–22.

Law, P.P., and Cheing, G.L. (2004) Optimal stimulation frequency of transcutaneous electrical nerve stimulation on people with knee osteoarthritis. *J Rehabil Med*, **36**, 220–5.

Lazarou, L., Kitsios, A., Lazarou, I., Sikaras, E., and Trampas, A. (2009) Effects of intensity of transcutaneous electrical nerve stimulation (TENS) on pressure pain threshold and blood pressure in healthy humans: a randomized, double-blind, placebo-controlled trial. *Clin J Pain*, **25**, 773–80.

Le Bars, D., Dickenson, A.H., and Besson, J.M. (1979) Diffuse noxious inhibitory controls (DNIC). I. Effects on dorsal horn convergent neurones in the rat. *Pain*, **6**, 283–304.

Leandri, M., Parodi, C.I., Corrieri, N., and Rigardo, S. (1990) Comparison of TENS treatments in hemiplegic shoulder pain. *Scand J Rehabil Med*, **22**, 69–71.

Lee, A., and Fan, L.T. (2009) Stimulation of the wrist acupuncture point P6 for preventing postoperative nausea and vomiting. *Cochrane Database Syst Rev*, CD003281.

Leem, J.W., Park, E.S., and Paik, K.S. (1995) Electrophysiological evidence for the antinociceptive effect of transcutaneous electrical stimulation on mechanically evoked responsiveness of dorsal horn neurons in neuropathic rats. *Neurosci Lett*, **192**, 197–200.

Leonard, G., Cloutier, C., and Marchand, S. (2011) Reduced analgesic effect of acupuncture-like TENS but not conventional TENS in opioid-treated patients. *J Pain*, **12**, 213–21.

Leong, L.C., Yik, Y.I., Catto-Smith, A.G., Robertson, V.J., Hutson, J.M., and Southwell, B.R. (2011) Long-term effects of transabdominal electrical stimulation in treating children with slow-transit constipation. *J Pediatr Surg*, **46**, 2309–12.

Leroi, A.M., Siproudhis, L., Etienney, I., Damon, H., Zerbib, F., Amarenco, G., Vitton, V., Faucheron, J.L., Thomas, C., Mion, F., Roumeguere, P., Gourcerol, G., Bouvier, M., Lallouche, K., Menard, J.F., and Queralto, M. (2012) Transcutaneous electrical tibial nerve stimulation in the treatment of fecal incontinence: a randomized trial (CONSORT 1a). *Am J Gastroenterol*, **107**, 1888–96.

Levin, M.F., and Hui-Chan, C.W. (1993) Conventional and acupuncture-like transcutaneous electrical nerve stimulation excite similar afferent fibers. *Arch Phys Med Rehabil*, **74**, 54–60.

Lewis, S.M., Clelland, J.A., Knowles, C.J., Jackson, J.R., and Dimick, A.R. (1990) Effects of auricular acupuncture-like transcutaneous electric nerve stimulation on pain levels following wound care in patients with burns: a pilot study. *J Burn Care Rehabil*, **11**, 322–9.

Liebano, R.E., Abla, L.E., and Ferreira, L.M. (2006) Effect of high frequency transcutaneous electrical nerve stimulation on viability of random skin flap in rats. *Acta Cir Bras*, **21**, 133–8.

Liebano, R.E., Abla, L.E., and Ferreira, L.M. (2008) Effect of low-frequency transcutaneous electrical nerve stimulation (TENS) on the viability of ischemic skin flaps in the rat: an amplitude study. *Wound Repair Regen*, **16**, 65–9.

Liebano, R.E., Rakel, B., Vance, C.G., Walsh, D.M., and Sluka, K.A. (2011) An investigation of the development of analgesic tolerance to TENS in humans. *Pain*, **211**, 335–42.

Lima, M.C., and Fregni, F. (2008) Motor cortex stimulation for chronic pain: systematic review and meta-analysis of the literature. *Neurology*, **70**, 2329–37.

Linderoth, B., and Foreman, R.D. (2006) Mechanisms of spinal cord stimulation in painful syndromes: role of animal models. *Pain Med*, 7 Suppl 1, S14–26.

Lindsay, D.M., Dearness, J., and McGinley, C.C. (1995) Electrotherapy usage trends in private physiotherapy practice in Alberta. *Physiother Can*, **47**, 30–4.

Loeser, J., Black, R., and Christman, A. (1975) Relief of pain by transcutaneous electrical nerve stimulation. *J Neurosurg*, **42**, 308–14.

Lofgren, M., and Norrbrink, C. (2009) Pain relief in women with fibromyalgia: a cross-over study of superficial warmth stimulation and transcutaneous electrical nerve stimulation. *J Rehabil Med*, **41**, 557–62.

Long, D.M. (1974) External electrical stimulation as a treatment of chronic pain. *Minn Med*, **57**, 195–8.

Lu, M.C., Tsai, C.C., Chen, S.C., Tsai, F.J., Yao, C.H., and Chen, Y.S. (2009) Use of electrical stimulation at different current levels to promote recovery after peripheral nerve injury in rats. *J Trauma*, **67**, 1066–72.

Lund, I., Lundeberg, T., Kowalski, J., and Svensson, E. (2005) Gender differences in electrical pain threshold responses to transcutaneous electrical nerve stimulation (TENS). *Neurosci Lett*, **375**, 75–80.

Ma, Y.T., and Sluka, K.A. (2001) Reduction in inflammation-induced sensitization of dorsal horn neurons by transcutaneous electrical nerve stimulation in anesthetized rats. *Exp Brain Res*, **137**, 94–102.

Macefield, G., and Burke, D. (1991) Long-lasting depression of central synaptic transmission following prolonged high-frequency stimulation of cutaneous afferents: a mechanism for post-vibratory hypaesthesia. *Electroencephalogr Clin Neurophysiol*, **78**, 150–8.

Machado, L.A., Kamper, S.J., Herbert, R.D., Maher, C.G., and McAuley, J.H. (2009) Analgesic effects of treatments for non-specific low back pain: a meta-analysis of placebo-controlled randomized trials. *Rheumatology (Oxford)*, **48**, 520–7.

MacPherson, H., Altman, D.G., Hammerschlag, R., Li, Y., Wu, T., White, A., and Moher, D. (2010) Revised STandards for Reporting Interventions in Clinical Trials of Acupuncture (STRICTA): extending the CONSORT statement. *Acupunct Med*, **28**, 83–93.

Maeda, Y., Lisi, T.L., Vance, C.G., and Sluka, K.A. (2007) Release of GABA and activation of GABA(A) in the spinal cord mediates the effects of TENS in rats. *Brain Res*, **1136**, 43–50.

Mann, C. (1996) Respiratory compromise: a rare complication of transcutaneous electrical nerve stimulation for angina pectoris. *J Accid Emerg Med*, **13**, 68.

Mannheimer, J., and Lampe, G. (1988) Factors that hinder enhance and restore the effectiveness of TENS: physiological and theoretical considerations. In Mannheimer, J., and Lampe, G. (eds) *Clinical Transcutaneous Electrical Nerve Stimulation*. FA Davis Company, Philadelphia, PA, 529–70.

Marchand, S., Bushnell, M.C., and Duncan, G.H. (1991) Modulation of heat pain perception by high frequency transcutaneous electrical nerve stimulation (TENS). *Clin J Pain*, **7**, 122–9.

Marchand, S., Charest, J., Li, J., Chenard, J.R., Lavignolle, B., and Laurencelle, L. (1993) Is TENS purely a placebo effect? A controlled study on chronic low back pain. *Pain*, **54**, 99–106.

Marchand, S., Li, J., and Charest, J. (1995) Effects of caffeine on analgesia from transcutaneous electrical nerve stimulation. *N Engl J Med*, **333**, 325–6.

McDonough, S. (2008) Neuromuscular and muscular electrical stimulation In Watson, T. (ed.) *Electrotherapy: Evdence based Practice*. Churchill Livingstone, Edinburgh, Elsevier, 231–52.

McIntosh, G., and Hall, H. (2011) Low back pain (acute). *Clin Evid (Online)*, online version of *BMJ Clinical Evidence*, (see: <http://www.clinicalevidence.com>), **2011**.

Medicines and Healthcare Products Regulatory Agency (2006) Advice from the CSM Expert working group on analgesic options in treatment of mild to moderate pain. Available online at: <http://www.mhra.gov.uk/home/groups/pl-a/documents/websiteresources/con2023013.pdf>.

Meechan, J.G., Gowans, A.J., and Welbury, R.R. (1998) The use of patient-controlled transcutaneous electronic nerve stimulation (TENS) to decrease the discomfort of regional anaesthesia in dentistry: a randomised controlled clinical trial. *J Dent*, **26**, 417–20.

Meesen, R.L., Cuypers, K., Rothwell, J.C., Swinnen, S.P., and Levin, O. (2011) The effect of long-term TENS on persistent neuroplastic changes in the human cerebral cortex. *Hum Brain Mapp*, **32**, 872–82.

Mello, L.F., Nobrega, L.F., and Lemos, A. (2011) Transcutaneous electrical stimulation for pain relief during labor: a systematic review and meta-analysis. *Rev Bras Fisioter*, **15**, 175–84.

Melzack, R., Jeans, M.E., Stratford, J.G., and Monks, R.C. (1980) Ice massage and transcutaneous electrical stimulation: comparison of treatment for low-back pain. *Pain*, **9**, 209–17.

Melzack, R., and Wall, P.D. (1965) Pain mechanisms: a new theory. *Science*, **150**, 971–9.

Mense, S. (1993) Nociception from skeletal muscle in relation to clinical muscle pain. *Pain*, **54**, 241–89.

Merkel, S.I., Gutstein, H.B., and Malviya, S. (1999) Use of transcutaneous electrical nerve stimulation in a young child with pain from open perineal lesions. *J Pain Symptom Manage*, **18**, 376–81.

Miller, L., Mattison, P., Paul, L., and Wood, L. (2007) The effects of transcutaneous electrical nerve stimulation (TENS) on spasticity in multiple sclerosis. *Mult Scler*, **13**, 527–33.

Miller, M.G., Cheatham, C.C., Holcomb, W.R., Ganschow, R., Michael, T.J., and Rubley, M.D. (2008) Subcutaneous tissue thickness alters the effect of NMES. *J Sport Rehabil*, **17**, 68–75.

Mittal, A., Masuria, B.L., and Bajaj, P. (1998) Transcutaneous electrical nerve stimulation in treatment of post herpetic neuralgia. *Indian J Dermatol Venereol Leprol*, **64**, 45–47.

Mollon, B., da Silva, V., Busse, J.W., Einhorn, T.A., and Bhandari, M. (2008) Electrical stimulation for long-bone fracture-healing: a meta-analysis of randomized controlled trials. *J Bone Joint Surg Am*, **90**, 2322–30.

Moore, R., and Chester, M. (2001) Neuromodulation for chronic refractory angina. *Br Med Bull*, **59**, 269–78.

Moore, R.A., Derry, S., McQuay, H.J., Straube, S., Aldington, D., Wiffen, P., Bell, R.F., Kalso, E., and Rowbotham, M.C. (2010) Clinical effectiveness: an approach to clinical trial design more relevant to clinical practice, acknowledging the importance of individual differences. *Pain*, **149**, 173–6.

Moran, F., Leonard, T., Hawthorne, S., Hughes, C.M., McCrum-Gardner, E., Johnson, M.I., Rakel, B.A., Sluka, K.A., and Walsh, D.M. (2011) Hypoalgesia in response to transcutaneous electrical nerve stimulation (TENS) depends on stimulation intensity. *J Pain*, **12**, 929–35.

Morrish, R.B., Jr. (1997) Suppression and prevention of the gag reflex with a TENS device during dental procedures. *Gen Dent*, **45**, 498–501.

Morton, C.R., Du, H.J., Xiao, H.M., Maisch, B., and Zimmermann, M. (1988) Inhibition of nociceptive responses of lumbar dorsal horn neurones by remote noxious afferent stimulation in the cat. *Pain*, **34**, 75–83.

Mulvey, M.R., Bagnall, A.M., Johnson, M.I., and Marchant, P.R. (2010) Transcutaneous electrical nerve stimulation (TENS) for phantom pain and stump pain following amputation in adults. *Cochrane Database Syst Rev*, **5**, CD007264.

Mulvey, M.R., Fawkner, H.J., Radford, H., and Johnson, M.I. (2009) The use of transcutaneous electrical nerve stimulation (TENS) to aid perceptual embodiment of prosthetic limbs. *Med Hypotheses*, **72**, 140–2.

Mulvey, M.R., Radford, H.E., Fawkner, H.J., Hirst, L., Neumann, V., and Johnson, M.I. (2012) Transcutaneous electrical nerve stimulation for phantom pain and stump pain in adult amputees. *Pain Pract*, **13**, 289–96.

Murakami, T., Takino, R., Ozaki, I., Kimura, T., Iguchi, Y., and Hashimoto, I. (2010) High-frequency transcutaneous electrical nerve stimulation (TENS) differentially modulates sensorimotor cortices: an MEG study. *Clin Neurophysiol*, **121**, 939–44.

Mutlu, B., Paker, N., Bugdayci, D., Tekdos, D., and Kesiktas, N. (2013) Efficacy of supervised exercise combined with transcutaneous electrical nerve stimulation in women with fibromyalgia: a prospective controlled study. *Rheumatol Int*, **33**, 649–55.

Nadler, S.F., Prybicien, M., Malanga, G.A., and Sicher, D. (2003) Complications from therapeutic modalities: results of a national survey of athletic trainers. *Arch Phys Med Rehabil*, **84**, 849–53.

Naimy, N., Lindam, A.T., Bakka, A., Faerden, A.E., Wiik, P., Carlsen, E., and Nesheim, B.I. (2007) Biofeedback vs. electrostimulation in the treatment of postdelivery anal incontinence: a randomized, clinical trial. *Dis Colon Rectum*, **50**, 2040–6.

Nam, T.S., Choi, Y., Yeon, D.S., Leem, J.W., and Paik, K.S. (2001) Differential antinociceptive effect of transcutaneous electrical stimulation on pain behavior sensitive or insensitive to phentolamine in neuropathic rats. *Neurosci Lett*, **301**, 17–20.

Nardone, A., and Schieppati, M. (1989) Influences of transcutaneous electrical stimulation of cutaneous and mixed nerves on subcortical and cortical somatosensory evoked potentials. *Electroencephalogr Clin Neurophysiol*, **74**, 24–35.

National Institute for Health and Clinical Excellence (2007) NICE clinical guideline 55 Intrapartum care: care of healthy women and their babies during childbirth. NICE, London, 1–65.

National Institute for Health and Clinical Excellence (2008) NICE clinical guideline 59 Osteoarthritis: the care and management of osteoarthritis in adults. NICE, London, 1–22.

National Institute for Health and Clinical Excellence (2009a) NICE clinical guideline 79 Rheumatoid arthritis: the management of rheumatoid arthritis in adults. NICE, London, 1–35.

National Institute for Health and Clinical Excellence (2009b) NICE clinical guideline 88 Early management of persistent non-specific low back pain. NICE, London, 1–25.

National Institute for Health and Clinical Excellence (2011) NICE clinical guideline 126. Management of stable angina. NICE, London.

National Institute for Health and Clinical Excellence (2003) NICE clinical guideline 8. Multiple Sclerosis. National clinical guideline for diagnosis and management in primary and secondary care. NICE, London.

Ng, S.S., and Hui-Chan, C.W. (2009) Does the use of TENS increase the effectiveness of exercise for improving walking after stroke? A randomized controlled clinical trial. *Clin Rehabil*, **23**, 1093–1103.

Ngai, S.P., and Jones, A.Y. (2012) Changes in skin impedance and heart rate variability with application of Acu-TENS to BL 13 (Feishu). *J Altern Complement Med*, **19**, 558–63.

Nielzen, S., Sjölund, B.H., and Eriksson, M.B. (1982) Psychiatric factors influencing the treatment of pain with peripheral conditioning stimulation. *Pain*, **13**, 365–71.

Nigam, A.K., Taylor, D.M., and Valeyeva, Z. (2011) Non-invasive interactive neurostimulation (InterX) reduces acute pain in patients following total knee replacement surgery: a randomised, controlled trial. *J Orthop Surg Res*, **6**, 45–56.

Nilsson, H.J., Levinsson, A., and Schouenborg, J. (1997) Cutaneous field stimulation (CFS): a new powerful method to combat itch. *Pain*, **71**, 49–55.

Nilsson, H.J., Psouni, E., and Schouenborg, J. (2003) Long term depression of human nociceptive skin senses induced by thin fibre stimulation. *Eur J Pain*, **7**, 225–33.

Nnoaham, K.E., and Kumbang, J. (2008) Transcutaneous electrical nerve stimulation (TENS) for chronic pain. *Cochrane Database Syst Rev*, CD003222.

Norrbrink, C. (2009) Transcutaneous electrical nerve stimulation for treatment of spinal cord injury neuropathic pain. *J Rehabil Res Dev*, **46**, 85–93.

Norton, C., and Cody, J.D. (2012) Biofeedback and/or sphincter exercises for the treatment of faecal incontinence in adults. *Cochrane Database Syst Rev*, 7, CD002111.

O'Brien, W.J., Rutan, F.M., Sanborn, C., and Omer, G.E. (1984) Effect of transcutaneous electrical nerve stimulation on human blood beta-endorphin levels. *Phys Ther*, **64**, 1367–74.

O'Connell, N.E., Wand, B.M., Marston, L., Spencer, S., and Desouza, L.H. (2011) Non-invasive brain stimulation techniques for chronic pain. A report of a Cochrane systematic review and meta-analysis. *Eur J Phys Rehabil Med*, **47**, 309–26.

Olyaei, G.R., Talebian, S., Hadian, M.R., Bagheri, H., and Momadjed, F. (2004) The effect of transcutaneous electrical nerve stimulation on sympathetic skin response. *Electromyogr Clin Neurophysiol*, **44**, 23–8.

Oncel, M., Sencan, S., Yildiz, H., and Kurt, N. (2002) Transcutaneous electrical nerve stimulation for pain management in patients with uncomplicated minor rib fractures. *Eur J Cardiothorac Surg*, **22**, 13–17.

Oosterhof, J., De Boo, T.M., Oostendorp, R.A., Wilder-Smith, O.H., and Crul, B.J. (2006) Outcome of transcutaneous electrical nerve stimulation in chronic pain: short-term results of a double-blind, randomised, placebo-controlled trial. *J Headache Pain*, **7**, 196–205.

Oosterhof, J., Samwel, H.J., de Boo, T.M., Wilder-Smith, O.H., Oostendorp, R.A., and Crul, B.J. (2008) Predicting outcome of TENS in chronic pain: a prospective, randomized, placebo controlled trial. *Pain*, **136**, 11–20.

Ordog, G.J. (1987) Transcutaneous electrical nerve stimulation versus oral analgesic: a randomized double-blind controlled study in acute traumatic pain. *Am J Emerg Med*, **5**, 6–10.

Ottawa Panel (2004) Ottawa Panel Evidence-Based Clinical Practice Guidelines for Electrotherapy and Thermotherapy Interventions in the Management of Rheumatoid Arthritis in Adults. *Phys Ther*, **84**, 1016–43.

Pallett, E., Rentowl P, Johnson, M.I., and Watson, P. (2013) Implementation fidelity of self-administered transcutaneous electrical nerve stimulation (TENS) in patients with chronic back pain: an observational study. *Clin J Pain*, **29**(2), 146–53.

Palmer, S., and Martin, D. (2008) Interferential Current. In Watson, T. (ed.) *Electrotherapy. Evidence-Based Practice*. Churchill Livingstone Elsevier, Edinburgh, 217–315.

Panel, P. (2001) Philadelphia Panel evidence-based clinical practice guidelines on selected rehabilitation interventions: overview and methodology. *Phys Ther*, **81**, 1629–40.

Pantaleao, M.A., Laurino, M.F., Gallego, N.L., Cabral, C.M., Rakel, B., Vance, C., Sluka, K.A., Walsh, D.M., and Liebano, R.E. (2011) Adjusting pulse amplitude during transcutaneous electrical nerve stimulation (TENS) application produces greater hypoalgesia. *J Pain*, **12**, 581–90.

Patriciu, A., Yoshida, K., Struijk, J.J., DeMonte, T.P., Joy, M.L., and Stodkilde-Jorgensen, H. (2005) Current density imaging and electrically induced skin burns under surface electrodes. *IEEE Trans Biomed Eng*, **52**, 2024–31.

Pertovaara, A., Kemppainen, P., Johansson, G., and Karonen, S.L. (1982) Dental analgesia produced by non-painful low-frequency stimulation is not influenced by stress or reversed by naloxone. *Pain*, **13**, 379–84.

Peterson, M., Elmfeldt, D., and Svardsudd, K. (2005) Treatment practice in chronic epicondylitis: a survey among general practitioners and physiotherapists in Uppsala County, Sweden. *Scand J Prim Health Care*, **23**, 239–41.

Petrofsky, J., Laymon, M., Prowse, M., Gunda, S., and Batt, J. (2009) The transfer of current through skin and muscle during electrical stimulation with sine, square, Russian and interferential waveforms. *J Med Eng Technol*, **33**, 170–81.

Pieber, K., Herceg, M., and Paternostro-Sluga, T. (2010) Electrotherapy for the treatment of painful diabetic peripheral neuropathy: a review. *J Rehabil Med*, **42**, 289–95.

Ping Ho Chung, B., and Kam Kwan Cheng, B. (2010) Immediate effect of transcutaneous electrical nerve stimulation on spasticity in patients with spinal cord injury. *Clin Rehabil*, **24**, 202–10.

Poitras, S., and Brosseau, L. (2008) Evidence-informed management of chronic low back pain with transcutaneous electrical nerve stimulation, interferential current, electrical muscle stimulation, ultrasound, and thermotherapy. *Spine J*, **8**, 226–33.

Poltawski, L., and Watson, T. (2009) Bioelectricity and microcurrent therapy for tissue healing – a narrative review. *Physical Therapy Reviews*,**14**, 104–14.

Pop, T., Austrup, H., Preuss, R., Niedzialek, M., Zaniewska, A., Sobolewski, M., Dobrowolski, T., and Zwolinska, J. (2010) Effect of TENS on pain relief in patients with degenerative disc disease in lumbosacral spine. *Ortop Traumatol Rehabil*, **12**, 289–300.

Pope, G.D., Mockett, S.P., and Wright, J.P. (1995) A survey of electrotherapeutic modalities: ownership and use in the NHS in England. *Physiotherapy*, **81**, 82–91.

Prabhakar, R., and Ramteke, G. (2011) Cervical spinal mobilization versus TENS in the management of cervical radiculopathy: a comparative, experimental, randomized controlled trial. *Indian Journal of Physiotherapy and Occupational Therapy*, **5**, 128–33.

Price, C.I., and Pandyan, A.D. (2000) Electrical stimulation for preventing and treating post-stroke shoulder pain. *Cochrane Database Syst Rev*, CD001698.

Price, C.I., and Pandyan, A.D. (2001) Electrical stimulation for preventing and treating post-stroke shoulder pain: a systematic Cochrane review. *Clin Rehabil*, **15**, 5–19.

Proctor, M.L., Smith, C.A., Farquhar, C.M., and Stones, R.W. (2003) Transcutaneous electrical nerve stimulation and acupuncture for primary dysmenorrhoea (Cochrane Review). *Cochrane Database of Syst Rev*, CD002123.

Radhakrishnan, R., King, E.W., Dickman, J.K., Herold, C.A., Johnston, N.F., Spurgin, M.L., and Sluka, K.A. (2003) Spinal 5-HT(2) and 5-HT(3) receptors mediate low, but not high, frequency TENS-induced antihyperalgesia in rats. *Pain*, **105**, 205–13.

Radhakrishnan, R., and Sluka, K.A. (2003) Spinal muscarinic receptors are activated during low or high frequency TENS-induced antihyperalgesia in rats. *Neuropharmacology*, **45**, 1111–19.

Radhakrishnan, R., and Sluka, K.A. (2005) Deep tissue afferents, but not cutaneous afferents, mediate transcutaneous electrical nerve stimulation-Induced antihyperalgesia. *J Pain*, **6**, 673–80.

Rajpurohit, B., Khatri, S.M., Metgud, D., and Bagewadi, A. (2010) Effectiveness of transcutaneous electrical nerve stimulation and microcurrent electrical nerve stimulation in bruxism associated with masticatory muscle pain—a comparative study. *Indian J Dent Res*, **21**, 104–6.

Rakel, B., Cooper, N., Adams, H.J., Messer, B.R., Frey Law, L.A., Dannen, D.R., Miller, C.A., Polehna, A.C., Ruggle, R.C., Vance, C.G., Walsh, D.M., and Sluka, K.A. (2010) A new transient sham TENS device allows for investigator blinding while delivering a true placebo treatment. *J Pain*, **11**, 230–8.

Rakel, B., and Frantz, R. (2003) Effectiveness of transcutaneous electrical nerve stimulation on postoperative pain with movement. *J Pain*, **4**, 455–64.

Rao, V.R., Wolf, S.L., and Gersh, M.R. (1981) Examination of electrode placements and stimulating parameters in treating chronic pain with conventional transcutaneous electrical nerve stimulation (TENS). *Pain*, **11**, 37–47.

Rasmussen, M., Hayes, D., Vlietstra, R., and Thorsteinsson, G. (1988) Can transcutaneous electrical nerve stimulation be safely used in patients with permanent cardiac pacemakers? *Mayo Clin Proc*, **63**, 443–5.

Ratna, T., and Rekha, P. (2004) Comparative study of transcutaneous electrical nerve stimulation (TENS) and tramadol hydrochloride for pain relief in labour. *J Obstet Gynecol India*, **54**, 346.

Rawashdeh, Y.F., Austin, P., Siggaard, C., Bauer, S.B., Franco, I., de Jong, T.P., and Jorgensen, T.M. (2012) International Children's Continence Society's recommendations for therapeutic intervention in congenital neuropathic bladder and bowel dysfunction in children. *Neurourol Urodyn*, **31**, 615–20.

Reeve, J., Menon, D., and Corabian, P. (1996) Transcutaneous electrical nerve stimulation (TENS): a technology assessment. *Int J Technol Assess Health Care*, **12**, 299–324.

Reeves, J.L., 2nd, Graff-Radford, S.B., and Shipman, D. (2004) The effects of transcutaneous electrical nerve stimulation on experimental pain and sympathetic nervous system response. *Pain Med*, **5**, 150–61.

Resende, M.A., Sabino, G.G., Candido, C.R., Pereira, L.S., and Francischi, J.N. (2004) Local transcutaneous electrical stimulation (TENS) effects in experimental inflammatory edema and pain. *Eur J Pharmacol*, **504**, 217–22.

Reynolds, D.V. (1969) Surgery in the rat during electrical analgesia induced by focal brain stimulation. *Science*, **164**, 444–5.

Richardson, D.E., and Akil, H. (1977) Pain reduction by electrical brain stimulation in man. Part 1: Acute administration in periaqueductal and periventricular sites. *J Neurosurg*, **47**, 178–83.

Robb, K.A., Bennett, M.I., Johnson, M.I., Simpson, K.J., and Oxberry, S.G. (2008) Transcutaneous electric nerve stimulation (TENS) for cancer pain in adults. *Cochrane Database Syst Rev*, CD006276.

Robbins, S.M., Houghton, P.E., Woodbury, M.G., and Brown, J.L. (2006) The therapeutic effect of functional and transcutaneous electric stimulation on improving gait speed in stroke patients: a meta-analysis. *Arch Phys Med Rehabil*, **87**, 853–9.

Robertson, V., Chipchase, L., and Laakso, E. (2001) *Guidelines for the clinical use of electrophysical agents*. Australian Physiotherapy Association, Melbourne.

Robertson, V., Ward, A., Low, J., and Reed, A. (2006) *Electrotherapy Explained: principles and practice*. 4th edn, Butterworth-Heinemann, Oxford.

Robertson, V.J., and Spurritt, D. (1998) Electrophysical agents: implications of their availability and use in undergraduate clinical placements. *Physiotherapy*, **84**, 335–44.

Roche, P.A., Gijsbers, K., Belch, J.J., and Forbes, C.D. (1985) Modification of haemophiliac haemorrhage pain by transcutaneous electrical nerve stimulation. *Pain*, **21**, 43–8.

Rodriguez-Fernandez, A.L., Garrido-Santofimia, V., Gueita-Rodriguez, J., and Fernandez-de-Las-Penas, C. (2011) Effects of burst-type transcutaneous electrical nerve stimulation on cervical range of motion and latent myofascial trigger point pain sensitivity. *Arch Phys Med Rehabil*, **92**, 1353–8.

Rorsman, I., and Johansson, B. (2006) Can electroacupuncture or transcutaneous nerve stimulation influence cognitive and emotional outcome after stroke? *J Rehabil Med*, **38**, 13–19.

Rosted, P. (2001) Repetitive epileptic fits—a possible adverse effect after transcutaneous electrical nerve stimulation (TENS) in a post-stroke patient. *Acupunct Med*, **19**, 46–9.

Rutgers, M., Van-Romunde, L., and Osman, P. (1988) A small randomised comparative trial of acupuncture verses transcutaneous electrical neurostimulation in postherpetic neuralgia. *Pain Clinic*, **2**, 87–9.

Rutjes, A.W., Nuesch, E., Sterchi, R., Kalichman, L., Hendriks, E., Osiri, M., Brosseau, L., Reichenbach, S., and Juni, P. (2009) Transcutaneous electrostimulation for osteoarthritis of the knee. *Cochrane Database Syst Rev*, CD002823.

Sabino, G.S., Santos, C.M., Francischi, J.N., and de Resende, M.A. (2008) Release of endogenous opioids following transcutaneous electric nerve stimulation in an experimental model of acute inflammatory pain. *J Pain*, **9**, 157–63.

Sadowsky, C.L. (2001) Electrical stimulation in spinal cord injury. *NeuroRehabilitation*, **16**, 165–9.

Saggini, R., Carniel, R., Coco, V., Cancelli, F., Ianieri, M., and Maccanti, D. (2004) Gonarthrosis: treatment with horizontal therapy electrotherapy. A mulitcentred study *European Medical Physics*, **40**, 549–9.

Salar, G., Job, I., Mingrino, S., Bosio, A., and Trabucchi, M. (1981) Effect of transcutaneous electrotherapy on CSF beta-endorphin content in patients without pain problems. *Pain*, **10**, 169–72.

Sandkühler, J. (2000) Long-lasting analgesia following TENS and acupuncture: spinal mechanisms beyond gate control. In: Devor, M., Rowbotham, M.C., and Wiesenfeld-Hallin, Z.M. (eds), Vol. 16, 9th World Congress on Pain: Progress in Pain Research and Management. IASP Press, Seattle, WA, 359–69.

Sandkühler, J., Chen, J.G., and Cheng, G. (1997) Low-frequency stimulation of afferent adelta -fibers induces long-term depression at primary afferent synapses with substantia gelatinosa neurons in the rat. *J Neurosci*, **17**, 6483–91.

Sang, C.N., Max, M.B., and Gracely, R.H. (2003) Stability and reliability of detection thresholds for human A-Beta and A-delta sensory afferents determined by cutaneous electrical stimulation. *J Pain Symptom Manage*, **25**, 64–73.

Sato, K.L., Sanada, L.S., Rakel, B.A., and Sluka, K.A. (2012) Increasing intensity of TENS prevents analgesic tolerance in rats. *J Pain*, **13**, 884–90.

Satter, E.K. (2008) Third-degree burns incurred as a result of interferential current therapy. *Am J Dermatopathol*, **30**, 281–3.

Sbruzzi, G., Silveira, S.A., Silva, D.V., Coronel, C.C., and Plentz, R.D. (2012) Transcutaneous electrical nerve stimulation after thoracic surgery: systematic review and meta-analysis of 11 randomized trials. *Rev Bras Cir Cardiovasc*, **27**, 75–87.

Schabrun, S.M., Cannan, A., Mullens, R., Dunphy, M., Pearson, T., Lau, C., and Chipchase, L.S. (2012) The effect of interactive neurostimulation therapy on myofascial trigger points associated with mechanical neck pain: a preliminary randomized, sham-controlled trial. *J Altern Complement Med*, **18**, 946–52.

Schaefer, N., Schafer, H., Maintz, D., Wagner, M., Overhaus, M., Hoelscher, A.H., and Turler, A. (2008) Efficacy of direct electrical current therapy and laser-induced interstitial thermotherapy in local treatment of hepatic colorectal metastases: an experimental model in the rat. *J Surg Res*, **146**, 230–40.

Scherder, E.J., Luijpen, M.W., and van Dijk, K.R. (2003) Activation of the dorsal raphe nucleus and locus coeruleus by transcutaneous electrical nerve stimulation in Alzheimer's disease: a reconsideration of stimulation-parameters derived from animal studies. *Chin J Physiol*, **46**, 143–50.

Scherder, E.J., Van Someren, E.J., Bouma, A., and v d Berg, M. (2000) Effects of transcutaneous electrical nerve stimulation (TENS) on cognition and behaviour in aging. *Behav Brain Res*, **111**, 223–5.

Scherder, E.J., Van Someren, E.J., and Swaab, D.F. (1999) Transcutaneous electrical nerve stimulation (TENS) improves the rest-activity rhythm in midstage Alzheimer's disease. *Behav Brain Res*, **101**, 105–7.

Schreiner, L., dos Santos, T.G., Knorst, M.R., and da Silva Filho, I.G. (2010) Randomized trial of transcutaneous tibial nerve stimulation to treat urge urinary incontinence in older women. *Int Urogynecol J*, **21**, 1065–70.

Schroder, A., Wist, E.R., and Homberg, V. (2008) TENS and optokinetic stimulation in neglect therapy after cerebrovascular accident: a randomized controlled study. *Eur J Neurol*, **15**, 922–7.

Schuhfried, O., Crevenna, R., Fialka-Moser, V., and Paternostro-Sluga, T. (2012) Non-invasive neuromuscular electrical stimulation in patients with central nervous system lesions: an educational review. *J Rehabil Med*, **44**, 99–105.

Searle, R.D., Bennett, M.I., Johnson, M.I., Callin, S., and Radford, H. (2008) Letter to editor: transcutaneous electrical nerve stimulation (TENS) for cancer bone pain. *Palliat Med*, **22**, 878–9.

Shealy, C.N., Mortimer, J.T., and Reswick, J.B. (1967) Electrical inhibition of pain by stimulation of the dorsal columns: preliminary clinical report. *Anesth Analg*, **46**, 489–91.

Simpson, B.A. (ed.) (2003) *Electrical stimulation and the relief of pain*. Elsevier, Amsterdam.

Singla, S., Prabhakar, V., and Singla, R.K. (2011) Role of transcutaneous electric nerve stimulation in the management of trigeminal neuralgia. *J Neurosci Rural Pract*, **2**, 150–2.

Sjölund, B., and Eriksson, M. (1976) Electro-acupunture and endogenous morphines. *Lancet*, **2**, 1085.

Sjölund, B., Terenius, L., and Eriksson, M. (1977) Increased cerebrospinal fluid levels of endorphins after electro-acupuncture. *Acta Physiol Scand*, **100**, 382–4.

Sjölund, B.H. (1985) Peripheral nerve stimulation suppression of C-fiber-evoked flexion reflex in rats. Part 1: Parameters of continuous stimulation. *J Neurosurg*, **63**, 612–16.

Sjölund, B.H. (1988) Peripheral nerve stimulation suppression of C-fiber-evoked flexion reflex in rats. Part 2: Parameters of low-rate train stimulation of skin and muscle afferent nerves. *J Neurosurg*, **68**, 279–83.

Sjölund, B.H., and Eriksson, M.B. (1979) The influence of naloxone on analgesia produced by peripheral conditioning stimulation. *Brain Res*, **173**, 295–301.

Sluka, K.A., Bailey, K., Bogush, J., Olson, R., and Ricketts, A. (1998) Treatment with either high or low frequency TENS reduces the secondary hyperalgesia observed after injection of kaolin and carrageenan into the knee joint. *Pain*, **77**, 97–102.

Sluka, K.A., Bjordal, J.M., Marchand, S., and Rakel, B.A. (2013) What makes transcutaneous electrical nerve stimulation work? Making sense of the mixed results in the clinical literature. *Phys Ther*, **93**(10), 1426–7.

Sluka, K.A., and Chandran, P. (2002) Enhanced reduction in hyperalgesia by combined administration of clonidine and TENS. *Pain*, **100**, 183–90.

Sluka, K.A., Deacon, M., Stibal, A., Strissel, S., and Terpstra, A. (1999) Spinal blockade of opioid receptors prevents the analgesia produced by TENS in arthritic rats. *J Pharmacol Exp Ther*, **289**, 840–6.

Sluka, K.A., Judge, M.A., McColley, M.M., Reveiz, P.M., and Taylor, B.M. (2000) Low frequency TENS is less effective than high frequency TENS at reducing inflammation-induced hyperalgesia in morphine-tolerant rats. *Eur J Pain*, **4**, 185–93.

Sluka, K.A., Lisi, T.L., and Westlund, K.N. (2006) Increased release of serotonin in the spinal cord during low, but not high, frequency transcutaneous electric nerve stimulation in rats with joint inflammation. *Arch Phys Med Rehabil*, **87**, 1137–40.

Sluka, K.A., Vance, C.G., and Lisi, T.L. (2005) High-frequency, but not low-frequency, transcutaneous electrical nerve stimulation reduces aspartate and glutamate release in the spinal cord dorsal horn. *J Neurochem*, **95**, 1794–801.

Smith, T.J., Coyne, P.J., Parker, G.L., Dodson, P., and Ramakrishnan, V. (2010) Pilot trial of a patient-specific cutaneous electrostimulation device (MC5-A Calmare®) for chemotherapy-induced peripheral neuropathy. *J Pain Symptom Manage*, **40**, 883–91.

Snyder, A.R., Perotti, A.L., Lam, K.C., and Bay, R.C. (2010) The influence of high-voltage electrical stimulation on edema formation after acute injury: a systematic review. *J Sport Rehabil*, **19**, 436–51.

Somers, D.L., and Clemente, F.R. (1998) High-frequency transcutaneous electrical nerve stimulation alters thermal but not mechanical allodynia following chronic constriction injury of the rat sciatic nerve. *Arch Phys Med Rehabil*, **79**, 1370–6.

Somers, D.L., and Clemente, F.R. (2006a) Transcutaneous electrical nerve stimulation for the management of neuropathic pain: the effects of frequency and electrode position on prevention of allodynia in a rat model of complex regional pain syndrome type II. *Phys Ther*, **86**, 698–709.

Somers, D.L., and Clemente, F.R. (2006b) Transcutaneous electrical nerve stimulation for the management of neuropathic pain: the effects of frequency and electrode position on prevention of allodynia in a rat model of complex regional pain syndrome type II. *Phys Ther*, **86**, 698–709.

Somers, D.L., and Clemente, F.R. (2009) Contralateral high or a combination of high- and low-frequency transcutaneous electrical nerve stimulation reduces mechanical allodynia and alters dorsal horn neurotransmitter content in neuropathic rats. *J Pain*, **10**, 221–9.

Sommer, P., Kluschina, O., Schley, M., Namer, B., Schmelz, M., and Rukwied, R. (2011) Electrically induced quantitative sudomotor axon reflex test in human volunteers. *Auton Neurosci*, **159**, 111–16.

Soomro, N.A., Khadra, M.H., Robson, W., and Neal, D.E. (2001) A crossover randomized trial of transcutaneous electrical nerve stimulation and oxybutynin in patients with detrusor instability. *J Urol*, **166**, 146–9.

Staahl, C., and Drewes, A.M. (2004) Experimental human pain models: a review of standardised methods for preclinical testing of analgesics. *Basic Clin Pharmacol Toxicol*, **95**, 97–111.

Steier, J., Seymour, J., Rafferty, G.F., Jolley, C.J., Solomon, E., Luo, Y., Man, W.D., Polkey, M.I., and Moxham, J. (2011) Continuous transcutaneous submental electrical stimulation in obstructive sleep apnea: a feasibility study. *Chest*, **140**, 998–1007.

Sun, R.Q., Wang, H.C., Wan, Y., Jing, Z., Luo, F., Han, J.S., and Wang, Y. (2004) Suppression of neuropathic pain by peripheral electrical stimulation in rats: mu-opioid receptor and NMDA receptor implicated. *Exp Neurol*, **187**, 23–9.

Sussmilch-Leitch, S.P., Collins, N.J., Bialocerkowski, A.E., Warden, S.J., and Crossley, K.M. (2012) Physical therapies for Achilles tendinopathy: systematic review and meta-analysis. *J Foot Ankle Res*, **5**, 15–31.

Swett, J.E., and Law, J.D. (1983) Analgesia with Peripheral-Nerve Stimulation—Absence of a Peripheral Mechanism. *Pain*, **15**, 55–70.

Szeto, A.Y. (1985) Relationship between pulse rate and pulse width for a constant-intensity level of electrocutaneous stimulation. *Ann Biomed Eng*, **13**, 373–83.

Szuminsky, N.J., Albers, A.C., Unger, P., and Eddy, J.G. (1994) Effect of narrow, pulsed high voltages on bacterial viability. *Phys Ther*, **74**, 660–7.

Tashani, O., and Johnson, M. (2009) Transcutaneous electrical nerve stimulation (TENS) a possible aid for pain relief in developing countries? *Libyan J Med*, **4**, 62–5.

Taylor, R.J., and Taylor, R.S. (2005) Spinal cord stimulation for failed back surgery syndrome: a decision-analytic model and cost-effectiveness analysis. *Int J Technol Assess Health Care*, **21**, 351–8.

Tekeoglu, Y., Adak, B., and Goksoy, T. (1998) Effect of transcutaneous electrical nerve stimulation (TENS) on Barthel Activities of Daily Living (ADL) index score following stroke. *Clin Rehabil*, **12**, 277–80.

Thomas, I.L., Tyle, V., Webster, J., and Neilson, A. (1988) An evaluation of transcutaneous electrical nerve stimulation for pain relief in labour. *Aust N Z J Obstet Gynaecol*, **28**, 182–9.

Thompson, J., and Filshie, J. (1998) Transcutaneous electrical nerve stimulation (TENS) and acupuncture. In Doyle, D., Hanks, G., and MacDonald, N. (eds) *Oxford Textbook of Palliative Medicine*. Oxford University Press, Oxford, 421–37.

Thompson, J.W., Bower, S., and Tyrer, S.P. (2008) A double blind randomised controlled clinical trial on the effect of transcutaneous spinal electroanalgesia (TSE) on low back pain. *Eur J Pain*, **12**, 371–7.

Thompson, J.W., and Cummings, M. (2008) Investigating the safety of electroacupuncture with a Picoscope. *Acupunct Med*, **26**, 133–9.

Thorsen, S.W., and Lumsden, S.G. (1997) Trigeminal neuralgia: sudden and long-term remission with transcutaneous electrical nerve stimulation. *J Manipulative Physiol Ther*, **20**, 415–19.

Timofeeva, M.A., Ar'kov, V.V., Andreev, R.A., Trushkin, E.V., and Tonevitsky, A.G. (2011) Changes in parameters of laser-induced potentials after transcutaneous electroneurostimulation. *Bull Exp Biol Med*, **150**, 479–80.

Tinegate, H., and McLelland, J. (2002) Transcutaneous electrical nerve stimulation may improve pruritus associated with haematological disorders. *Clin Lab Haematol*, **24**, 389–90.

Tong, K.C., Lo, S.K., and Cheing, G.L. (2007) Alternating frequencies of transcutaneous electric nerve stimulation: does it produce greater analgesic effects on mechanical and thermal pain thresholds? *Arch Phys Med Rehabil*, **88**, 1344–9.

Torquati, K., Franciotti, R., Della Penna, S., Babiloni, C., Rossini, P.M., Romani, G.L., and Pizzella, V. (2007) Conditioning transcutaneous electrical nerve stimulation induces delayed gating effects on cortical response: a magnetoencephalographic study. *Neuroimage*, **35**, 1578–85.

Torquati, K., Pizzella, V., Della Penna, S., Franciotti, R., Babiloni, C., Romani, G.L., and Rossini, P.M. (2003) "Gating" effects of simultaneous peripheral electrical stimulations on human secondary somatosensory cortex: a whole-head MEG study. *Neuroimage*, **20**, 1704–13.

Tsujimoto, T., Takano, M., Ishikawa, M., Tsuruzono, T., Matsumura, Y., Kitano, H., Yoneda, S., Yoshiji, H., Yamao, J., and Fukui, H. (2004) Onset of ischemic colitis following use of electrical muscle stimulation (EMS) exercise equipment. *Intern Med*, **43**, 693–5.

Tugay, N., Akbayrak, T., Demirturk, F., Karakaya, I.C., Kocaacar, O., Tugay, U., Karakaya, M.G., and Demirturk, F. (2007) Effectiveness of transcutaneous electrical nerve stimulation and interferential current in primary dysmenorrhea. *Pain Med*, **8**, 295–300.

Urasaki, E., Wada, S., Yasukouchi, H., and Yokota, A. (1998) Effect of transcutaneous electrical nerve stimulation (TENS) on central nervous system amplification of somatosensory input. *J Neurol*, **245**, 143–8.

van der Heide, E.M., Buitenweg, J.R., Marani, E., and Rutten, W.L. (2009) Single pulse and pulse train modulation of cutaneous electrical stimulation: a comparison of methods. *J Clin Neurophysiol*, **26**, 54–60.

van Dijk, K.R., Scherder, E.J., Scheltens, P., and Sergeant, J.A. (2002) Effects of transcutaneous electrical nerve stimulation (TENS) on non-pain related cognitive and behavioural functioning. *Rev Neurosci*, **13**, 257–70.

van Middelkoop, M., Rubinstein, S.M., Kuijpers, T., Verhagen, A.P., Ostelo, R., Koes, B.W., and van Tulder, M.W. (2011) A systematic review on the effectiveness of physical and rehabilitation interventions for chronic non-specific low back pain. *Eur Spine J*, **20**, 19–39.

Vance, C.G., Radhakrishnan, R., Skyba, D.A., and Sluka, K.A. (2007) Transcutaneous electrical nerve stimulation at both high and low frequencies reduces primary hyperalgesia in rats with joint inflammation in a time-dependent manner. *Phys Ther*, **87**, 44–51.

Vance, C.G., Rakel, B.A., Blodgett, N.P., DeSantana, J.M., Amendola, A., Zimmerman, M.B., Walsh, D.M., and Sluka, K.A. (2012) Effects of transcutaneous electrical nerve stimulation on pain, pain sensitivity, and function in people with knee osteoarthritis: a randomized controlled trial. *Phys Ther*, **92**, 898–910.

Veiga, M.L., Lordelo, P., Farias, T., and Barroso, U., Jr. (2013) Evaluation of constipation after parasacral transcutaneous electrical nerve stimulation in children with lower urinary tract dysfunction—A pilot study. *J Pediatr Urol*, **9**, 622–6.

Vivo, M., Puigdemasa, A., Casals, L., Asensio, E., Udina, E., and Navarro, X. (2008) Immediate electrical stimulation enhances regeneration and reinnervation and modulates spinal plastic changes after sciatic nerve injury and repair. *Exp Neurol*, **211**, 180–93.

Wall, P.D., and Sweet, W.H. (1967) Temporary abolition of pain in man. *Science*, **155**, 108–9.

Waller, A., and Bercovitch, M. (2000) Treatment of lymphoedema with TENS. *Lymphoedema*. Radcliffe Medical Press, Oxford, 27–184.

Walsh, D.M. (1996) Transcutaneous electrical nerve stimulation and acupuncture points. *Complementary Therapies in Medicine*, **4**, 133–7.

Walsh, D.M. (1997) *TENS: Clinical Applications and Related Theory*. Churchill Livingstone, Edinburgh.

Walsh, D.M., Howe, T.E., Johnson, M.I., and Sluka, K.A. (2009) Transcutaneous electrical nerve stimulation for acute pain. *Cochrane Database Syst Rev*, CD006142.

Walsh, D.M., Lowe, A.S., McCormack, K., Willer, J.C., Baxter, G.D., and Allen, J.M. (1998) Transcutaneous electrical nerve stimulation: effect on peripheral nerve conduction, mechanical pain threshold, and tactile threshold in humans. *Arch Phys Med Rehabil*, **79**, 1051–8.

Walsh, N.E., and Hurley, M.V. (2009) Evidence based guidelines and current practice for physiotherapy management of knee osteoarthritis. *Musculoskeletal Care*, **7**, 45–56.

Wang, S.F., Lee, J.P., and Hwa, H.L. (2009) Effect of transcutaneous electrical nerve stimulation on primary dysmenorrhea. *Neuromodulation*, **12**, 302–9.

Warke, K., Al-Smadi, J., Baxter, D., Walsh, D.M., and Lowe-Strong, A.S. (2006) Efficacy of transcutaneous electrical nerve stimulation (tens) for chronic low-back pain in a multiple sclerosis population: a randomized, placebo-controlled clinical trial. *Clin J Pain*, **22**, 812–9.

Watson, T. (2000) The role of electrotherapy in contemporary physiotherapy practice. *Man Ther*, **5**, 132–41.

Watson, T. (2008) Electrical Stimulation for Enhanced Wound Healing. In Watson, T. (ed.) *Electrotherapy: Evdence based Practice*. Churchill Livingstone Elsevier, Edinburgh, 329–46.

Weng, C., Shu, S., and Chen, C. (2005) The evaluation of two modulated frequency modes of acupuncture-like TENS on the treatment of tennis elbow pain. *Biomed Eng Appl Basis Comm*, **17**, 236–42.

White, A., Cummings, M., Barlas, P., Cardini, F., Filshie, J., Foster, N.E., Lundeberg, T., Stener-Victorin, E., and Witt, C. (2008a) Defining an adequate dose of acupuncture using a neurophysiological approach—a narrative review of the literature. *Acupunct Med*, **26**, 111–20.

White, A., Cummings, M., and Filshie, J. (2008b) *An Introduction to Western Medical Acupuncture*. Churchill Livingstone Elsevier, Edinburgh.

Wikstrom, S.O., Svedman, P., Svensson, H., and Tanweer, A.S. (1999) Effect of transcutaneous nerve stimulation on microcirculation in intact skin and blister wounds in healthy volunteers. *Scand J Plast Reconstr Surg Hand Surg*, **33**, 195–201.

Woolf, C.J., Mitchell, D., and Barrett, G.D. (1980) Antinociceptive effect of peripheral segmental electrical stimulation in the rat. *Pain*, **8**, 237–52.

Wu, L.L., Su, C.H., and Liu, C.F. (2012) Effects of noninvasive electroacupuncture at Hegu (LI4) and Sanyinjiao (SP6) acupoints on dysmenorrhea: a randomized controlled trial. *J Altern Complement Med*, **18**, 137–42.

Xiao, W.B., and Liu, Y.L. (2004) Rectal hypersensitivity reduced by acupoint TENS in patients with diarrhea-predominant irritable bowel syndrome: a pilot study. *Dig Dis Sci*, **49**, 312–19.

Yan, T., and Hui-Chan, C.W. (2009) Transcutaneous electrical stimulation on acupuncture points improves muscle function in subjects after acute stroke: a randomized controlled trial. *J Rehabil Med*, **41**, 312–16.

Yoshimoto, S., Babygirija, R., Dobner, A., Ludwig, K., and Takahashi, T. (2012) Anti-stress effects of transcutaneous electrical nerve stimulation (TENS) on colonic motility in rats. *Dig Dis Sci*, **57**, 1213–21.

Zaghi, S., Acar, M., Hultgren, B., Boggio, P.S., and Fregni, F. (2010) Noninvasive brain stimulation with low-intensity electrical currents: putative mechanisms of action for direct and alternating current stimulation. *Neuroscientist*, **16**, 285–307.

Zaghi, S., Thiele, B., Pimentel, D., Pimentel, T., and Fregni, F. (2011) Assessment and treatment of pain with non-invasive cortical stimulation. *Restor Neurol Neurosci*, **29**, 439–51.

Zambito, A., Bianchini, D., Gatti, D., Rossini, M., Adami, S., and Viapiana, O. (2007) Interferential and horizontal therapies in chronic low back pain due to multiple vertebral fractures: a randomized, double blind, clinical study. *Osteoporos Int*, **18**, 1541–5.

Index